# Essentials of Cardiology

ADAM D. TIMMIS
MA, MD, MRCP
*Consultant Cardiologist*
*London Chest and*
*Newham General Hospitals*

ANTHONY W. NATHAN
MD, FRCP
*Consultant Cardiologist*
*St Bartholomew's Hospital*
*London*

SECOND EDITION

OXFORD

BLACKWELL SCIENTIFIC PUBLICATIONS

LONDON EDINBURGH BOSTON

MELBOURNE PARIS BERLIN VIENNA

© 1988, 1993 by
Blackwell Scientific Publications
Editorial Offices:
Osney Mead, Oxford OX2 0EL
25 John Street, London WC1N 2BL
23 Ainslie Place, Edinburgh EH3 6AJ
238 Main Street, Cambridge
    Massachusetts 02142, USA
54 University Street, Carlton
    Victoria 3053, Australia

Other Editorial Offices:
Librairie Arnette SA
2, rue Casimir−Delavigne
75006 Paris
France

Blackwell Wissenschafts−Verlag
Meinekestrasse 4
D-1000 Berlin 15
Germany

Blackwell MZV
Feldgasse 13
A-1238 Wien
Austria

First published 1988
Reprinted 1989
Four Dragons edition 1989
Second edition 1993
Four Dragons edition 1993

Set by Excel Typesetters Company,
Hong Kong
Printed and bound in Great Britain
at the University Press, Cambridge

DISTRIBUTORS

  Marston Book Services Ltd
  PO Box 87
  Oxford OX2 0DT
  (*Orders*: Tel: 0865 791155
             Fax: 0865 791927
             Telex: 837515)

USA
  Blackwell Scientific Publications, Inc.
  238 Main Street
  Cambridge, MA 02142
  (*Orders*: Tel: 800 759-6102
                  617 876-7000)

Canada
  Times Mirror Professional Publishing Ltd
  130 Flaska Drive
  Markham, Ontario L6G 1B8
  (*Orders*: Tel: 800 268−4178
                  416 470−6739)

Australia
  Blackwell Scientific Publications
  Pty Ltd
  54 University Street
  Carlton, Victoria 3053
  (*Orders*: Tel: 03 347-5552)

A catalogue record for this title
is available from the British Library

ISBN 0-632-03367-3
     0-632-03482-3 (Four Dragons)


Library of Congress
Cataloging-in-Publication Data

Timmis, Adam D.
    Essentials of cardiology /
  Adam D. Timmis, Anthony W. Nathan. —
  2nd edn.
        p.         cm.
    Includes bibliographical references and
index.
    ISBN 0-632-03367-3
    1. Cardiology.   2. Heart − Diseases.
I. Nathan, Anthony W.   II. Title.
    [DNLM: 1. Heart Diseases − diagnosis.
2. Heart Diseases − therapy.
WG 100 T584e]
RC667.T56   1993
616.1′2 − dc20

# Essentials of Cardiology

# Contents

v

# Preface

Clinical cardiology has seen remarkable technological and therapeutic developments in the 5 years since the first edition of *Essentials of Cardiology*. Nowhere have these developments been more marked than in cardiac electrophysiology which has now emerged as a major subspecialty in its own right. For this reason the decision has been taken to expand the authorship of the book to include Anthony Nathan who is an expert in this complex and challenging field. A new section on arrhythmia detection has been included in Chapter 2 of the book while the chapters on conduction tissue disease and cardiac arrhythmias have been completely rewritten. The reader will now find a detailed account of the current recommendations for pacemaker therapy in conduction tissue disease, with emphasis given to the diminishing role of ventricular inhibited units as the use of atrial and dual chamber units increases. Important changes in the management of life-threatening tachyarrhythmias are also described with the balance shifting away from antiarrhythmic drugs towards nonpharmacological methods that include sophisticated catheter ablation techniques and implantable cardioverter defibrillators.

These recent advances in cardiac electrophysiology themselves provide sufficient justification for a new edition of *Essentials of Cardiology*. However, during the same period many other areas of clinical cardiology have seen important developments that have required inclusion within the text. Thus, the chapter on coronary artery disease now documents the dramatic changes that have occurred in the management of acute myocardial infarction, the prognosis of which has been substantially improved by thrombolytic and aspirin therapy, with intravenous beta blockers contributing in selected patients. The chapter also includes new information about the role of the atheromatous plaque in the pathogenesis of acute coronary syndromes and describes the expanding role of balloon angioplasty in the treatment of patients with disabling angina. Indeed, every one of the 17 chapters in this book has been updated and several new illustrations and tables have been added. In addition, each chapter now starts with a short summary that provides an overview of the subject, and ends with a reading list drawn mainly from recent review articles in the cardiovascular literature.

*Essentials of Cardiology* has undergone substantial revision but still aims to provide a concise, highly illustrated account of current cardiological practice. We hope that readers of this book will come to share some of our enthusiasm for this fascinating subject which remains one of the most exciting fields in clinical medicine.

Adam D. Timmis and Anthony W. Nathan

# List of Abbreviations

| | |
|---|---|
| ACE | angiotensin-converting enzyme |
| AF | atrial fibrillation |
| AIDS | acquired immunodeficiency syndrome |
| AMI | acute myocardial infarction |
| APB | atrial premature beat |
| AR | aortic regurgitation |
| AS | aortic stenosis |
| ASD | atrial septal defect |
| AV | atrioventricular |
| AVJRT | atrioventricular junctional re-entrant tachycardia |
| CK | creatine kinase |
| CSM | carotid sinus massage |
| CT | computed tomography |
| CVA | cerebrovascular accident |
| CXR | chest X-ray |
| 2D | two-dimensional |
| DC | direct current |
| DNA | deoxyribonucleic acid |
| DVT | deep venous thrombosis |
| ECG | electrocardiogram |
| EPS | electrophysiological study |
| ESR | erythrocyte sedimentation rate |
| GI | gastrointestinal |
| GOT | glutamic oxaloacetic transaminase |
| GU | genitourinary |
| ICD | implantable cardioverter defibrillator |
| IV | intravenous |
| IVC | inferior vena cava |
| JVP | jugular venous pulse |
| LDH | lactic dehydrogenase |
| LGL | Lown–Ganong–Levine |
| LV | left ventricle or left ventricular |
| LVF | left ventricular failure |
| MI | myocardial infarction |
| MR | mitral regurgitation |
| MRI | magnetic resonance imaging |
| MS | mitral stenosis |
| NYHA | New York Heart Association |

| | |
|---|---|
| P1 | pulmonary component of first heart sound |
| PA | pulmonary artery |
| PAT | paroxysmal atrial tachycardia |
| PDA | patent ductus arteriosus |
| PE | pulmonary embolism |
| PS | pulmonary stenosis |
| RA | right atrium |
| RHF | right heart failure |
| RV | right ventricle or right ventricular |
| RVF | right ventricular failure |
| S1 | first heart sound |
| SA | sinoatrial |
| SAM | systolic anterior motion |
| SVT | supraventricular tachycardia |
| SVC | superior vena cava |
| TB | tuberculosis |
| TR | tricuspid regurgitation |
| TS | tricuspid stenosis |
| VA | ventriculoatrial |
| VF | ventricular fibrillation |
| VPB | ventricular premature beat |
| VSD | ventricular septal defect |
| VT | ventricular tachycardia |
| WPW | Wolff–Parkinson–White |

# 1 Symptoms and Signs of Heart-disease

## Summary

A careful history and examination are potentially diagnostic of most of the common cardiac disorders. Chest pain caused by myocardial ischaemia is called angina and is identified by its location, character and relation to provocative stimuli, particularly exertion. Dyspnoea and fatigue are important symptoms of heart failure and, like angina, are associated with exertion, though dyspnoea may also be provoked by lying flat, in which case it is called orthopnoea. Palpitation may be symptomatic of cardiac arrhythmia, particularly when its onset and termination is abrupt: description of the rate, rhythm (regular or irregular), duration and relation to provocative stimuli is required for accurate diagnosis. Cardiac syncope is always the result of abrupt cerebral hypoperfusion and, by definition, must be brief if death is to be avoided. Causes range from the trivial (vasovagal or postural attacks) to the serious (Stokes–Adams attacks, aortic stenosis).

During the cardiac examination, the patient should recline at a 45° angle while note is made of body habitus and general appearance. The radial pulse is examined for rate and rhythm but the carotid pulse provides more useful information about volume and waveform, a slow upstroke indicating aortic stenosis and a rapid upstroke aortic regurgitation. Blood-pressure is measured by sphygmomanometry, phase V (disappearance of Korotkoff sounds) providing the best measure of diastolic pressure. The jugular venous pulse (JVP) reflects right atrial pressure and is elevated in right heart failure. It has a flickering character due to 'a' and 'v' waves, abnormalities of which provide additional diagnostic information. On examination of the chest, the position of the apex beat and the character of the left and right ventricular impulses should be noted. Auscultation of the heart requires identification of the first sound (S1) and both aortic and pulmonary components of the second sound (S2), which should split physiologically during inspiration. Abnormalities of S2 are an important sign of heart-disease. Low-frequency rapid-filling sounds early (S3) and late (S4) in diastole may be physiological in the young and elderly, respectively, but in other contexts are abnormal, often reflecting advanced ventricular dysfunction. Valve opening is usually silent but causes an early diastolic 'opening snap' in mitral stenosis and may also cause an early systolic 'ejection click' in aortic stenosis when the valve is bicuspid. Turbulent flow through diseased heart valves produces characteristic murmurs, the loudness, quality, location and timing of which should all be noted.

## Symptoms

The extent to which a patient is limited by symptoms of heart-disease provides the basis for the New York Heart Association (NYHA) functional classification:

*Class 1*   asymptomatic (no functional limitation).

*Class 2*   symptomatic on extra exertion.

*Class 3*   symptomatic on mild exertion.

*Class 4*   symptomatic at rest or on minimal exertion (severe functional limitation).

This classification provides a simple means of describing functional capacity but it does not always reflect accurately the severity of disease in individual patients. Nevertheless, in large groups, the classification has been shown to provide a useful indication of disease severity and prognosis.

### *Chest pain*

The common cardiovascular causes of chest pain are myocardial ischaemia, myocardial infarction, pericarditis, aortic dissection and pulmonary embolism.

*Myocardial ischaemia* results from an imbalance between myocardial oxygen supply and demand, which produces pain called angina. Angina is usually a symptom of coronary artery disease (which impedes oxygen supply) but may also occur when left ventricular hypertrophy or rapid tachyarrhythmias cause excessive oxygen demand. Sensory impulses from the myocardium enter the upper cervical spine at the same level as impulses from the anterior chest wall, arm, throat and jaw. Angina is usually experienced in the anterior chest wall as a retrosternal constricting discomfort but it may radiate into any other of these areas. A number of anginal syndromes are recognized (see p. 105) but the most common is chronic stable angina, in which the pain is provoked by stimuli that increase myocardial oxygen demand, particularly exertion and emotion. Symptoms are relieved within 2–10 min by rest. The location and character of the pain, its relation to provocative stimuli and its duration are essential criteria for the clinical diagnosis of chronic stable angina.

*Myocardial infarction* produces pain that is similar in location and character to angina. However, the pain is usually more severe, occurring at rest without provocation, and may last for several hours.

In *pericarditis*, chest pain is central or left-sided and is characteristically sharp. It is aggravated by deep inspiration, coughing or changes in posture and often lasts for several days.

*Aortic dissection* produces intense, tearing pain in either the front or back of the chest. The onset of symptoms is abrupt, unlike the crescendo quality of ischaemic cardiac pain.

Massive *pulmonary embolism* may cause central chest pain difficult to distinguish from myocardial ischaemia. Small pulmonary embolism, however, is often asymptomatic unless it causes a pulmonary infarct, when pleuritic pain occurs over the affected area.

Rare cardiovascular causes of chest pain include mitral valve disease associated with massive left atrial dilatation. This causes discomfort in the back, which is sometimes associated with dysphagia due to oesophageal compression. Aortic aneurysms can also cause pain in the chest due to local compression.

## Dyspnoea

Dyspnoea is an abnormal awareness of breathing, occurring at rest or at an unexpectedly low level of exertion. It is a prominent symptom in a wide variety of cardiac disorders, including coronary, myocardial, valvular and pericardial disease. Nevertheless, left heart failure is the major cardiac cause of dyspnoea.

### Acute left heart failure

The left atrium is in continuity with the pulmonary capillaries through the pulmonary venous bed. There are no valves in the pulmonary veins and the elevated left atrial pressure that characterizes acute left heart failure produces corresponding elevation of the pulmonary capillary pressure. This increases fluid transudation into the pulmonary interstitium and, as pressure rises, interstitial oedema progresses to alveolar oedema. The oedematous lung is stiff and the extra effort required for ventilation produces the sensation of dyspnoea. In alveolar oedema, impaired gas exchange leads to hypoxaemia, which exacerbates dyspnoea by its effect on the respiratory centre. Reduction of left atrial pressure with diuretics and opiates leads to prompt relief of dyspnoea.

### Chronic left heart failure

Chronic left heart failure, caused by left ventricular or mitral disease, is also associated with elevation of the left atrial pressure, which rises still further on lying flat (due to gravitational effects), causing orthopnoea (Fig. 1.1a). Thus patients with left heart failure prefer to sleep with extra pillows. In advanced cases, frank pulmonary oedema in the supine

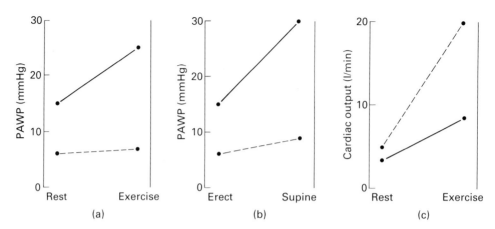

**Fig. 1.1** Orthopnoea (a), exertional dyspnoea (b) and fatigue (c) in left heart failure. Responses of normal individuals (broken line) are compared with those of patients with heart failure (continuous line). Note that, in patients with heart failure, lying supine and exercise both cause a sharp increase in the pulmonary artery wedge pressure (an indirect measure of left atrial pressure), in contrast to normal patients, in whom the wedge pressure is lower and shows little tendency to change. Despite the sharp rise in wedge pressure with exercise, however, the cardiac output response is markedly attenuated in heart failure compared with normal individuals.

position causes paroxysmal nocturnal dyspnoea. This usually occurs during sleep and wakens the patient with distressing shortness of breath and fear of imminent death. These symptoms are corrected by sitting or standing upright, when gravitational pooling of blood lowers left atrial pressure. Exertional dyspnoea (Fig. 1.1b) is the most troublesome symptom in left heart failure. The mechanism is complex because, although left atrial pressure rises abnormally in response to exercise, it correlates poorly with the severity of dyspnoea. Moreover, drugs that lower left atrial pressure do not always improve exercise tolerance. Thus, other factors must contribute to exertional dyspnoea in left heart failure. These may include respiratory muscle fatigue, increases in physiological dead space in the lungs and metabolic signals such as exertional acidosis.

## *Fatigue* (Fig. 1.1c)

Exertional fatigue is an important symptom of both left and right heart failure. It is caused by inadequate oxygen delivery to exercising skeletal muscle and reflects the combined effects of arteriolar vasoconstriction and impaired cardiac output. Drugs which improve the output response to exercise may correct fatigue if regional arteriolar vasodilatation allows the increased output to be distributed to skeletal muscle.

## Palpitation

Palpitation is awareness of the heartbeat. It is common during vigorous exertion or heightened emotion but under other circumstances it is usually symptomatic of a cardiac arrhythmia. Occasional awareness of either the pause or the forceful beat that follows an extrasystole is a common complaint but rarely reflects important heart-disease. Patients with brady-arrhythmias may be aware of the slow heartbeat but tachyarrhythmias are a more common cause of symptoms. The abrupt onset and termination of paroxysmal tachyarrhythmias are particularly noticeable. Irregular palpitation indicates atrial fibrillation or ectopic beats but regular palpitation may be caused by atrial or ventricular arrhythmias. A history of arrhythmia termination by vagal manoeuvres (Valsalva, rubbing the neck or eyes) suggests a re-entry tachycardia, either within the atrioventricular (AV) node or involving an accessory pathway.

## Dizziness and syncope

Cardiac disorders produce dizziness and syncope by abrupt reductions in blood-pressure, associated with disturbance of cerebral perfusion. Prolonged attacks (longer than 4 min) are inevitably fatal because of the brain's obligatory oxygen requirement. Thus, almost by definition, recovery from cardiac dizziness and syncope occurs within a minute or two, unlike most other common causes of unconsciousness (e.g. stroke, epilepsy, overdose), in which full recovery may be delayed for several hours.

*Postural hypotension* becomes more troublesome with advancing age. It is due to inadequate baroreceptor-mediated reflex vasoconstriction on standing up from the lying or sitting position. This produces a pronounced fall in blood-pressure and cerebral perfusion, which may cause the patient to fall to the ground, whereupon the condition corrects itself. Vasodilator drugs must be avoided and patients should be encouraged to change posture gradually. There is no specific treatment.

*Vasovagal attacks* usually occur in response to emotional or painful stimuli. Autonomic overactivity, manifested by yawning, nausea or sweating, causes vasodilatation in skeletal muscle and inappropriate slowing of the pulse; these combine to reduce blood-pressure and cerebral perfusion. Recovery is rapid if the patient lies down.

*Carotid sinus syncope* affects the elderly. It arises when an exaggerated vagal discharge occurs in response to stimulation of the carotid sinus. Reflex vasodilatation and excessive slowing of the pulse lower the blood-pressure and lead to dizziness and syncope. Simple stimuli such as a tight shirt collar or shaving the neck may trigger attacks and should be avoided by the patient. Pacemaker therapy is not always effective because, although it prevents slow heart rates, it has less effect on reductions in blood-pressure caused by reflex vasodilatation.

*Stokes–Adams attacks* are caused by self-limiting episodes of asystole or ventricular tachyarrhythmias, during which there is no effective cardiac output. Blood-pressure becomes unrecordable and the patient loses consciousness. Recovery is rapid following restoration of normal rhythm when flushing occurs, as circulation through the cutaneous bed is restored. Attacks caused by intermittent asystole are readily prevented by pacemaker therapy. Paroxysmal ventricular tachyarrhythmias are more difficult to treat (see p. 244).

*Valvular obstruction*, either fixed or intermittent, is an important cardiac cause of syncope. In aortic stenosis, syncope typically occurs during exertion, due to fixed valvular obstruction, which prevents a normal increase in cardiac output into the dilated skeletal muscle vascular bed. Reductions in blood-pressure and cerebral perfusion lead to syncope. Paroxysmal ventricular arrhythmias (Stokes–Adams attacks) also cause syncope in aortic stenosis. Intermittent valvular obstruction is usually caused by left atrial myxoma or ball thrombus (Fig. 1.2). These are mobile tumours which fall into the mitral valve orifice during diastole, thereby obstructing ventricular filling. The abrupt decline in cardiac output and cerebral perfusion causes syncope and if obstruction is unrelieved death may ensue.

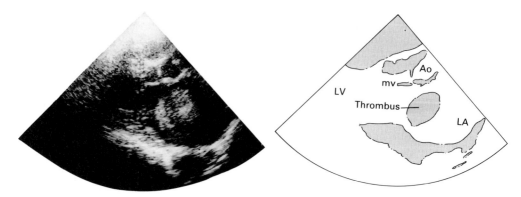

**Fig. 1.2**  Left atrial ball thrombus. This two-dimensional echocardiogram (parasternal long-axis view) shows massive dilatation of the left atrium in a patient with severe mitral valve disease. A large echogenic thrombus is clearly visible within the left atrium, partially obstructing the mitral valve.

## Other symptoms

Other symptoms of heart-disease include *cough* and *haemoptysis* in left heart failure due to congestion of the bronchial tree. *Fever* and *flu-like* symptoms accompany infective endocarditis. A variety of other systemic disorders involve the cardiovascular system (Chapter 16).

## Signs

### General examination

The general examination should first concentrate on the appearance of the patient. Severe obesity may be associated with diabetes, hyperlipidaemia or hypertension, while malnutrition and cachexia occur in advanced heart failure. Other signs of heart failure include tachypnoea, oedema, cyanosis and scleral jaundice. The distinctive features of specific congenital syndromes should be recognized because they are often associated with cardiovascular disorders (see Table 15.2). *Splinter haemorrhages* in the nail-beds are a common but non-specific manifestation of infective endocarditis. Other 'classical' manifestations of this condition (clubbing, Osler's nodes, Janeway lesions) are now rarely seen.

A white ring around the iris is common in the elderly (*arcus senilis*), but in younger patients it may indicate hypercholesterolaemia. *Xanthelasmata* — yellowish, fatty deposits in the eyelids — are also a non-specific sign of hypercholesterolaemia. However, *tendon xanthomas* are considerably more specific and are commonly associated with premature coronary artery disease. *Argyll Robertson pupils* (irregular, unequal and reacting to accommodation but not to light) are diagnostic of syphilis, which was an important cause of coronary and aortic disease in the past. Fundoscopy may reveal signs of hypertensive or diabetic vascular disease, both of which are commonly associated with coronary artery disease.

*Inspiratory crackles* at the lung base occur commonly in left heart failure. *Hepatic* and *splenic enlargement* reflect visceral engorgement in right heart failure. In advanced heart failure, signs of *ascites* may also be present. Abdominal *aortic aneurysms* can usually be located by deep palpation and may be the cause of bruits heard during auscultation of the abdomen. Bruits over the renal area are a sign of renal artery stenosis (an important and potentially reversible cause of hypertension), while carotid and femoral bruits provide additional evidence of vascular disease.

### Oedema

Oedema which pits in response to digital pressure is an important sign of congestive heart failure. The salt and water retention which characterizes heart failure expands plasma volume and increases capillary hydrostatic pressure. As pressure rises, the equilibrium between hydrostatic forces driving fluid out of the capillary and osmotic forces reabsorbing it cannot be maintained and oedema fluid accumulates in the interstitial space. The effect of gravity on capillary hydrostatic pressure ensures that dependent parts of the body are worst affected. Thus, oedema is most prominent in the ankles in the ambulant patient and over the sacrum in the bedridden patient. Worsening salt and water overload leads to oedema of the legs, genitalia and trunk, with engorgement of the abdominal viscera. Hepatic engorgement produces abdominal discomfort and nausea; jaundice may develop if hepatic dysfunction is severe. In advanced cases ascites occurs, particularly when disordered protein synthesis in the liver lowers plasma osmotic pressure. Effusion into the pleural and pericardial spaces may also occur.

## Cyanosis

Cyanosis is a blue discoloration of the skin and mucous membranes caused by an increased concentration of reduced haemoglobin (greater than 5 g/100 ml) in the superficial blood-vessels.

### Peripheral cyanosis

Peripheral cyanosis affects the skin and the lips but spares the mucous membranes of the palate. It is caused by cutaneous vasoconstriction, which slows flow and increases oxygen extraction in the skin. Peripheral cyanosis is physiological during exposure to cold but is also an important manifestation of heart failure, when sympathetically mediated cutaneous vasoconstriction occurs in response to reduced cardiac output. In severe mitral stenosis, cyanosis is often prominent over the cheeks, producing the characteristic mitral facies.

### Central cyanosis

Central cyanosis is caused by reduced arterial oxygen saturation and affects the skin and the mucous membranes of the mouth. Important cardiac causes of central cyanosis are acute pulmonary oedema and congenital heart-disease. In acute pulmonary oedema, oxygenation of the blood is inadequate due to alveolar flooding. In congenital heart-disease, central cyanosis is usually the result of right-to-left ('reversed') shunting of blood through a septal defect or a patent ductus arteriosus. Desaturated venous blood bypasses the lungs and enters the arterial circulation. Cyanosis caused by reversed shunting through a patent ductus arteriosus may be more prominent in the lower part of the body (differential cyanosis) because desaturated venous blood enters the aorta below the origins of the carotid and subclavian arteries. In adults, cyanotic congenital heart-disease is usually associated with digital clubbing.

## Skin temperature

Skin temperature provides a useful indication of cutaneous flow. In high-output states, such as pregnancy, the skin is vasodilated and warm, while in low-output states, such as heart failure or haemorrhage, reflex vasoconstriction causes cooling of the skin. Measurements of skin temperature are widely used in intensive care units for monitoring changes in cardiac output in response to treatment.

## Clubbing of the fingers and toes

Congenital cyanotic heart-disease is almost invariably associated with the development of clubbing during infancy; it is not present at birth. Clubbing may also be seen in pulmonary heart-disease, but it is now a rare manifestation of infective endocarditis.

## Arterial pulse and blood-pressure

The arterial pulse is generated by the systolic contractions of the left ventricle. At the onset of ejection, the aortic valve is forced open and arterial pressure rises rapidly to a peak. The early decline in arterial pressure is checked by the dicrotic notch, which marks aortic valve closure. There follows a more gradual decline in pressure as blood runs off into the peripheral circulation. Peak systolic pressure rises progressively as distance from the heart increases, because reflected pressure waves from the branch arteries summate with the main wave (Fig. 1.3). Pressure in the legs may be 20 mmHg higher than in the thoracic aorta. A small decline in peak systolic pressure occurs during inspiration, due to the increased vascular capacity of the inflated lung, which reduces pulmonary venous return to the left atrium. Full examination of the pulse requires documentation of rate, rhythm and character. Finally, the symmetry of the peripheral pulses should be assessed and the blood-pressure measured.

### Rate and rhythm

Both are traditionally assessed by palpation of the right radial artery. Pulse rate, expressed in beats per minute, is measured by counting over a timed period of at least 15 sec. If the rhythm is irregular, the rate should be measured by auscultation at the cardiac apex, because beats

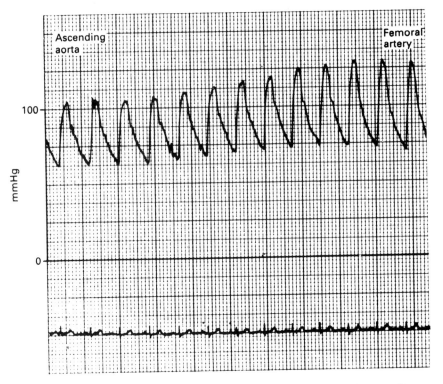

**Fig. 1.3**   Arterial pressure recording during catheter withdrawal from the ascending thoracic aorta to the femoral artery. Note the progressive rise in pressure as distance from the heart increases.

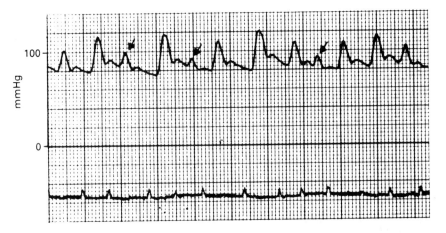

**Fig. 1.4**   Arterial pressure recording in atrial fibrillation. The ECG shows the irregularly irregular rhythm of atrial fibrillation. There is beat-to-beat variation of arterial pressure. The pulse pressure is lowest in those beats which follow very short diastolic intervals (arrowed).

that follow very short diastolic intervals may not generate sufficient pressure to be palpable at the radial artery. In rapid atrial fibrillation the apex–radial pulse deficit may be greater than 20 beats/min (Fig. 1.4).

The rhythm is described as regular or irregular. Normal sinus rhythm is regular but may show phasic variation in rate during respiration (sinus arrhythmia), particularly in young patients. Frequent ectopic beats cause an irregular rhythm which may be difficult to distinguish from atrial fibrillation unless they occur predictably in bigeminal or trigeminal sequence. The irregularly irregular rhythm that characterizes atrial fibrillation is shown in Fig. 1.4.

### Character

The character of the pulse, defined by its volume and waveform, should be evaluated at the (right) carotid artery. This is closest to the heart and

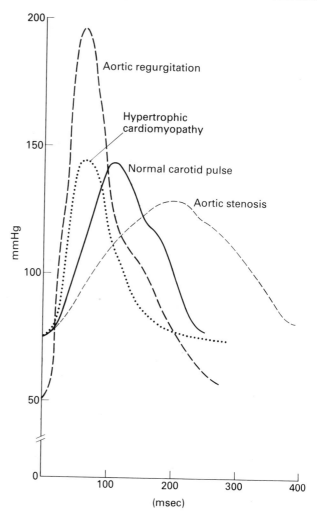

**Fig. 1.5**  The normal carotid arterial pulse recording compared with recordings in hypertrophic cardiomyopathy, aortic regurgitation and aortic stenosis. Note the very rapid upstroke of the pulse in hypertrophic cardiomyopathy and aortic regurgitation compared with the slow upstroke in aortic stenosis. The pulse pressure in aortic regurgitation is widened because of the exaggerated systolic peak and the diastolic collapse.

is least subject to damping and distortion during passage through the arterial tree. A small, *low-volume* pulse reflects reduced stroke volume and occurs in advanced heart failure. Conversely, a *large-volume* pulse reflects increased stroke volume, which characterizes aortic regurgitation and conditions associated with a hyperkinetic circulation (such as anaemia, pregnancy, fever or thyrotoxicosis).

Of greater diagnostic importance is the *waveform* of the pulse (Fig. 1.5). A *slow upstroke* pulse with a delayed peak characterizes aortic stenosis and reflects left ventricular outflow obstruction. In aortic regurgitation, backflow through the valve volume-loads the left ventricle in diastole, stimulating vigorous systolic ejection (Starling's law), with a *rapid upstroke* pulse and an exaggerated systolic peak; backflow also causes abrupt collapse of the pulse in early diastole, with an exaggerated diastolic nadir. Thus, the pulse pressure (systolic minus diastolic pressure) is widened and prominent pulsations in the neck (Corrigan's pulse) are clearly visible. A *bisferiens* pulse, in which two systolic peaks can be felt, is characteristic but not diagnostic of mixed aortic stenosis and regurgitation. In hypertrophic cardiomyopathy, left ventricular contraction is vigorous and ejection is near complete by mid-systole. The pulse has a jerky quality, with a rapid upstroke and a very early peak.

An alternating pulse always indicates severe left ventricular failure. The alternating high and low systolic peaks are particularly prominent in

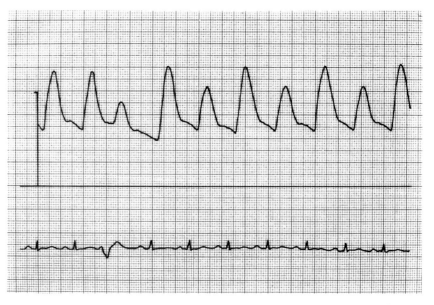

**Fig. 1.6** Alternating pulse — arterial pressure recording in severe left ventricular failure. After the second beat a ventricular premature beat triggers an episode of alternating pulse.

the beats which follow an extrasystole and can usually be detected by palpating the carotid pulse (Fig. 1.6). The mechanism of the alternating pulse is unknown.

Paradoxical pulse is characterized by an exaggeration of the normal inspiratory decline in systolic pressure. A decline greater than 10 mmHg (measured by sphygmomanometry) is usually pathological (Fig. 1.7). It is always present in cardiac tamponade because the normal inspiratory increase in right ventricular output is prevented. This exacerbates the inspiratory reduction in pulmonary venous return to the left atrium. Paradoxical pulse also occurs, albeit less frequently, in constrictive pericarditis and obstructive pulmonary disease.

## Symmetry

The presence and symmetry of the following pulses should always be confirmed: radial, brachial, carotid, femoral, popliteal, posterior tibial and dorsalis pedis. A pulse that is absent or reduced in volume indicates an obstructive lesion more proximally in the arterial tree, which is usually due to atherosclerosis or thromboembolism. Auscultation over the abdomen, or the carotid or femoral pulses, may reveal arterial bruits due to turbulent flow within the diseased vessels. Coarctation of the aorta is an important cause of symmetrical reduction of the femoral pulses, which are 'delayed' compared with the radial pulses (radiofemoral delay).

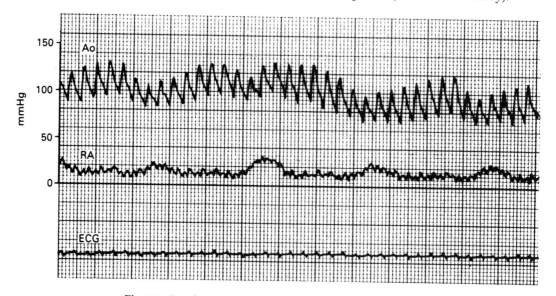

**Fig. 1.7** Paradoxical pulse and Kussmaul's sign. Pericardial effusion (evidenced by the small voltage deflexions on the ECG) has caused tamponade. Respiratory fluctuations in the aortic (Ao) and right atrial (RA) pressure signals are seen. During inspiration aortic pressure falls markedly (paradoxical pulse) and right atrial pressure rises (Kussmaul's sign).

## Measurement of blood-pressure

Blood-pressure is measured indirectly, using a sphygmomanometer. Supine and erect measurements should be recorded to provide an assessment of baroreceptor function. A cuff attached to a mercury or aneroid manometer is placed around the arm above the elbow. The width of the cuff should be at least 40% the circumference of the arm, in order to avoid overestimation of blood-pressure, and in obese patients a large 'thigh cuff' may be required. The cuff is inflated until the brachial pulse disappears and then gradually deflated during auscultation over the brachial artery, which should be held at the same level as the heart. Five phases of Korotkoff sounds can be distinguished during deflation of the cuff:

*Phase I*   the first appearance of an audible Korotkoff sound, marking systolic blood-pressure.

*Phase II/III*   increasingly loud turbulence as blood flows through the constricted artery.

*Phase IV*   abrupt muffling of the Korotkoff sounds.

*Phase V*   disappearance of the Korotkoff sounds. This is usually within 10 mmHg of phase IV.

In pregnancy, aortic regurgitation or patients with large arteriovenous fistulae, phase V may be difficult to identify and phase IV should be used as the measure of diastolic pressure. In all other situations, phase V should be used, not only because it corresponds more closely with directly measured diastolic pressure but also because its identification is less subjective.

## Jugular venous pulse (JVP)

Fluctuations in right atrial pressure during the cardiac cycle generate a pulse which is transmitted backwards into the internal jugular vein. Although the JVP is rarely palpable it may be visualized using a tangential light source while the patient reclines at a 45° angle. A more horizontal position may be required to visualize the pulse if right atrial pressure is low; or manual pressure applied to the upper abdomen may be used to produce a transient increase in venous return to the heart, which elevates the JVP. The (vertical) level of the pulse above the sternal angle provides a measure of right atrial pressure, while analysis of the waveform provides more specific diagnostic information.

## Level of JVP

The upper limit of normal is 4 cm vertically above the sternal angle, corresponding to a right atrial pressure of 6 mmHg. Elevation indicates increase of right atrial pressure, unless the superior vena cava is obstructed, producing engorgement of the neck veins.

During inspiration, pressure within the chest falls and there is a corresponding fall in the level of the JVP, despite an increase in venous return to the heart. In constrictive pericarditis, however, and less commonly in tamponade, the increased venous return during inspiration cannot be accommodated within the constricted right ventricle. This produces a paradoxical inspiratory rise in the level of the JVP — Kussmaul's sign (Fig. 1.7).

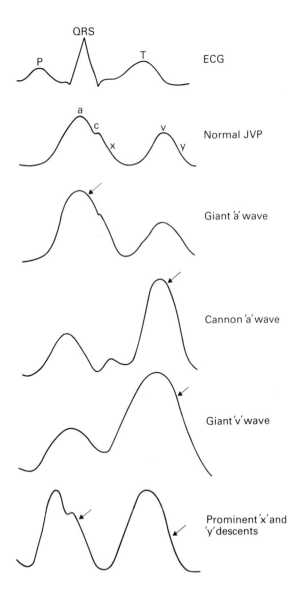

**Fig. 1.8**  The jugular venous pulse. Electrical events always precede mechanical events. Thus, the P wave of the ECG (representing atrial depolarization) and the QRS complex (representing ventricular depolarization) precede the 'a' wave and the 'v' wave of the JVP, respectively.

## *Waveform of JVP* (Fig. 1.8)

The JVP has a flickering character due to 'a' and 'v' waves separated by 'x' and 'y' descents. The 'a' wave, produced by atrial systole, precedes tricuspid valve closure, and is followed by the 'x' descent, marking the descent of the tricuspid valve ring. The 'x' descent is interrupted by the diminutive 'c' wave, marking tricuspid closure. Atrial pressure then rises again ('v' wave) as the chamber fills passively during ventricular systole. The decline in atrial pressure as the tricuspid valve opens to allow ventricular filling produces the 'y' descent. These events are difficult to distinguish on inspection, although they are clear on pressure recordings. The 'a' wave, however, is usually the most prominent deflexion and precedes ventricular systole, which can be identified by simultaneous palpation of the carotid pulse on the opposite side of the neck.

### Giant 'a' wave

Forceful atrial contraction against a stenosed tricuspid valve or a non-compliant hypertrophied right ventricle produces an unusually prominent (giant) 'a' wave.

### Cannon 'a' wave (see Fig. 10.6)

Atrial systole against a closed tricuspid valve also produces prominent 'a' waves, called cannon waves, which occur irregularly when atrial and ventricular rhythms are dissociated in complete heart block or ventricular tachycardia. They mark the random coincidence of atrial and ventricular systole. In junctional tachycardias, atrial and ventricular systole are simultaneous; cannon 'a' waves are therefore regular. Note that, because cannon 'a' waves occur during ventricular systole, their timing is coincident with the normal 'v' wave.

### Giant 'v' wave (see Fig. 9.11)

This is an important sign of tricuspid regurgitation. The regurgitant jet produces pulsatile systolic waves in the jugular veins, which coincide with the period normally associated with passive atrial filling. They are therefore called giant 'v' waves, even though they are generated by an entirely different mechanism from the normal 'v' wave.

### Prominent 'x' and 'y' descents (see Fig. 7.7)

Prominence of either the 'x' or the 'y' descent produces an unusually dynamic jugular venous pulse, although clinical distinction between these two negative waves is difficult. Tamponade produces a prominent 'x' descent because the vigorous right ventricular contraction causes exaggerated descent of the tricuspid valve ring. In constrictive pericarditis, ventricular contraction often shows variable impairment and the 'x' descent may not be so marked. The 'y' descent, however, is always prominent because ventricular filling is unusually rapid following the tricuspid valve opening, due to the elevated right atrial pressure.

## Examination of the heart

### Inspection of the chest

Common chest-wall deformities include *pectus excavatum* (depressed sternum) and *straight back syndrome* (loss of dorsal curvature of thoracic spine), either of which may compress the heart and displace the apex beat laterally, giving a spurious impression of cardiac enlargement. Cardiac compression may also cause turbulence in the ventricular outflow tracts and produce 'innocent' ejection murmurs without affecting cardiac function. *Pectus carinatum* (pigeon chest) is sometimes associated with Marfan's syndrome but does not itself affect the heart. Large ventricular or aortic aneurysms may produce visible pulsations on the chest wall. Obstructions of the superior or inferior vena cava produce prominent venous collaterals on the anterior chest wall, with caudal or cranial flow, respectively.

### Palpation of the chest

The *apex beat* is the lowest and most lateral point on the chest wall at which the cardiac impulse is palpable while the patient sits upright. Location of the beat inferior or lateral to the intersection of the mid-clavicular line and the fifth intercostal space usually indicates cardiac enlargement.

The quality of the apex beat (as opposed to its location) is best appreciated with the patient lying on the left side. A *thrusting* impulse occurs in patients with left ventricular enlargement (dilatation or hypertrophy), particularly if stroke volume is increased, e.g. aortic regurgitation. A *double* apical impulse may occur in patients with third or fourth heart sounds (see below). Indeed, these low-frequency added heart sounds are often more easy to feel than to hear.

Ventricular aneurysms and non-aneurysmal dyskinetic segments, following myocardial infarction, can be palpated as a more diffuse impulse medial to the apex beat. Right ventricular enlargement produces a systolic thrust in the left parasternal area.

The turbulent flow responsible for heart murmurs may produce palpable vibrations, called *thrills*, on the chest wall. The location of thrills and their timing in the cardiac cycle are the same as the location and timing of the murmur with which they are associated. Thrills are most commonly associated with aortic stenosis, but the murmurs of aortic regurgitation, mitral regurgitation, ventricular septal defect and patent ductus arteriosus may also be palpable if turbulence is sufficiently vigorous.

## Percussion of the heart

Percussion plays no useful role in the cardiac examination. Although the area of cardiac dullness provides a crude measure of heart size, the location of the apex beat and the chest X-ray provide more accurate information.

## Auscultation of the heart

A stethoscope with a diaphagm and bell must be used for appreciation of high-pitched and low-pitched auscultatory events, respectively. The apex, lower left, upper left and upper right sternal edge should be auscultated in turn. These correspond to the mitral, tricuspid, pulmonary and aortic areas, respectively, and loosely identify the sites at which murmurs from the four heart valves are best heard.

The *diaphragm* must be used at each of these sites but the *bell* is only used at the apex and lower left sternal edge, where the important low-frequency sounds and murmurs occur. During auscultation the patient should recline at 45°; the sitting forward and lateral decubitis positions accentuate sounds and murmurs from the base (aortic and pulmonary areas) and apex of the heart, respectively.

To ensure identification of all auscultatory events in the cardiac cycle, a systematic approach should be adopted, listening to the first and second heart sounds and the systolic and diastolic intervals in sequence. Simultaneous palpation of the carotid pulse distinguishes systole from diastole when there is doubt about timing.

### Heart sounds

**First sound (S1)**

This coincides with mitral and tricuspid valve closure at the onset of ventricular systole. The valve leaflets themselves do not produce S1, the precise cause of which is unknown. Electromechanical events on the right side of the heart are slightly delayed with respect to the left side, and narrow splitting of S1 into mitral followed by tricuspid components can occasionally be appreciated. Mitral closure makes the major contribution to S1. The normal mitral valve leaflets fall together following atrial systole, such that at the onset of ventricular systole the valve is already partially closed. In *mitral stenosis*, however, diastolic filling of the ventricle through the restricted mitral orifice is prolonged and the valve leaflets remain widely separated at the onset of ventricular systole. Valve closure therefore generates unusually vigorous vibrations and S1 is accentuated. In very advanced mitral stenosis, the valve is rigid and immobile and S1 becomes soft again.

### Second sound (S2)

This coincides with aortic and pulmonary valve closure and marks the end of ventricular ejection (Fig. 1.9). S2 may be heard as a single sound

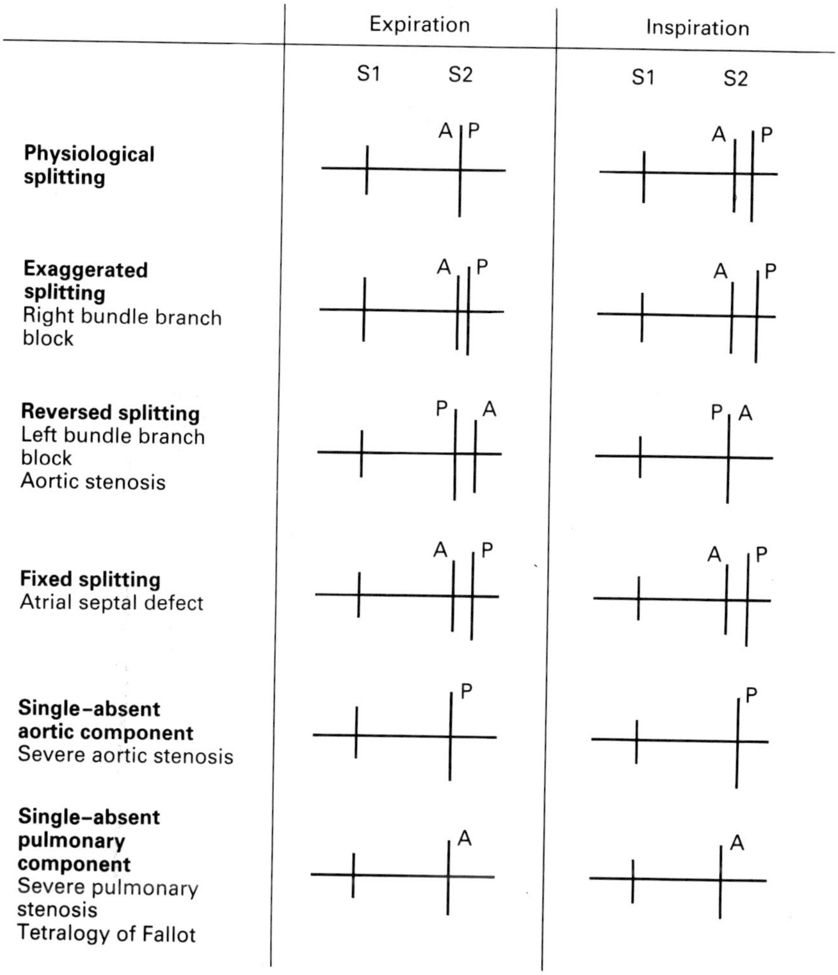

Fig. 1.9   Splitting of the second heart sound.

during expiration, but during inspiration the increased venous return to the right side of the heart delays pulmonary valve closure, to produce physiological splitting into aortic followed by pulmonary components. *Right bundle branch block* delays right ventricular activation and exaggerates the normal splitting of S2. Conditions associated with delayed aortic valve closure (*left bundle branch block, aortic stenosis*) produce reversed splitting of S2; pulmonary followed by aortic components are heard separately during expiration, but during inspiration the physiological delay in the pulmonary component produces a single sound. In *atrial septal defect*, fixed splitting of S2 occurs throughout the respiratory cycle. The left-to-right shunt increases right ventricular stroke volume and delays pulmonary valve closure, resulting in a split S2; during inspiration, increased venous return to the right atrium reduces the shunt such that the split remains fixed. S2 is single throughout the respiratory cycle when either the aortic or pulmonary component is absent. This occurs in severe *aortic* or *pulmonary stenosis*, and also in *tetralogy of Fallot* (absent pulmonary component). The aortic and pulmonary components of S2 are loud in *systemic* and *pulmonary hypertension*, respectively.

### Third and fourth heart sounds (S3, S4)

These low-frequency diastolic sounds are associated with rapid ventricular filling, which occurs early in diastole (S3), following atrioventricular valve opening, and again later in diastole (S4), due to atrial contraction. When present, they give a characteristic gallop to the cardiac rhythm — best heard at the apex with the bell of the stethoscope.

In children and young adults, the left ventricle is relatively thin and relaxes rapidly, permitting rapid filling in early diastole. S3 is therefore physiological in this age-group, but tends to disappear beyond the age of 40, as increase in ventricular mass reduces the velocity of relaxation. S3 may also be present in high-output states caused by anaemia, fever, pregnancy or thyrotoxicosis. After the age of 40, S3 is nearly always pathological, usually indicating left ventricular failure or, less commonly, mitral regurgitation or constrictive pericarditis (see Fig. 4.6).

S4 is usually pathological but may be physiological in the very elderly. It occurs when vigorous atrial contraction late in diastole is required to augment filling of a hypertrophied non-compliant left ventricle — for example in hypertension, aortic stenosis or hypertrophic cardiomyopathy.

### Systolic clicks and opening snaps

In the normal heart, valve opening is silent (unlike valve closure) and cannot be detected during auscultation. Under certain circumstances, however, aortic or pulmonary valve opening produces an *ejection click* in early diastole, while mitral valve opening produces an *opening snap* in early diastole (tricuspid opening is only rarely audible). An *aortic ejection click* is heard in aortic stenosis if the valve leaflets are mobile. The click precedes the ejection murmur and is particularly prominent in patients with a congenitally bicuspid valve (see Fig. 9.7). In advanced calcific disease, the aortic leaflets are rigid and do not generate an ejection click. A *pulmonary ejection click* occurs in conditions associated with dilatation of the main pulmonary artery, including pulmonary hypertension and valvular pulmonary stenosis. A click later in systole (*mid-systolic click*) usually signifies mitral valve prolapse. It may be followed by a murmur if mitral regurgitation is present (see Fig. 9.5).

The *mitral opening snap* is best heard at the cardiac apex and is pathognomonic of mitral stenosis. It is related to forceful opening of the valve due to elevated left atrial pressure (see Fig. 9.4). As mitral stenosis worsens, left atrial pressure rises and leaflet rigidity increases; these cause the opening snap to occur progressively earlier in diastole and to become progressively quieter, respectively. The timing of the opening snap is unaffected by respiration, helping to distinguish it from the pulmonary component of the second heart sound.

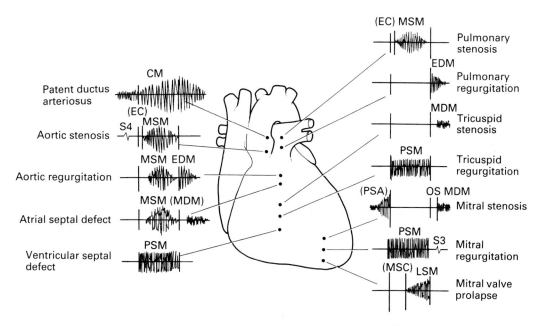

**Fig. 1.10**  Heart murmurs: CM — continuous murmur; MSM — mid-systolic murmur; PSM — pansystolic murmur; LSM — late systolic murmur; EDM — early diastolic murmur; MDM — mid-diastolic murmur; PSA — presystolic accentuation of murmur; EC — ejection click; MSC — mid-systolic click; OS — opening snap; S3 — third heart sound; S4 — fourth heart sound. Parentheses indicate those auscultatory findings which are not constant.

**Table 1.1**   Grading system for describing the loudness of heart murmurs

| | |
|---|---|
| 1 | The faintest detectable murmur |
| 2 | Faint murmur, readily detectable |
| 3 | Moderately loud murmur |
| 4 | Loud murmur |
| 5 | Very loud murmur |
| 6 | Extra-loud murmur, detectable with stethoscope raised off the chest wall |

**Heart murmurs**

Heart murmurs detected during auscultation are vibrations caused by turbulent flow within the heart (Fig. 1.10). Murmurs are defined by four characteristics: loudness, quality, location and timing.

The *loudness* of a murmur is graded from 1 to 6 (Table 1.1) and is determined principally by the degree of turbulence, which in turn relates to volume and velocity of flow rather than to the severity of the cardiac lesion. Indeed, although turbulent flow often reflects valvular disease or an intracardiac shunt, it may also occur when the volume or velocity of flow through a normal valve is exaggerated. Thus, the hyperdynamic circulation in anaemia or pregnancy may cause turbulence in the ventricular outflow tracts and produce 'innocent' murmurs that are difficult to distinguish from those associated with aortic or pulmonary stenosis.

A variety of adjectives have been used to describe the *quality* of heart murmurs (blowing, musical, honking, rumbling) but their interpretation is very subjective. The quality relates to its frequency (or pitch) and is therefore best described as low-, medium- or high-pitched. The mid-diastolic murmurs of mitral and tricuspid stenosis are low-pitched, the systolic murmurs of aortic and pulmonary stenosis and mitral and tricuspid regurgitation are medium-pitched and the early diastolic murmurs of aortic and pulmonary regurgitation are high-pitched. The *location* of a murmur on the chest wall is determined by its origin, while its *radiation* is determined by the direction of the blood flow. The location of the aortic, pulmonary, tricuspid and mitral areas has already been described (p. 18) and murmurs from the respective valves are usually best heard in these areas. Localization is not always specific and aortic systolic murmurs, for example, are often clearly audible all over the left precordium. Significant radiation of murmurs occurs only when flow velocity is rapid. The high-velocity systolic flow in *mitral regurgitation* and *aortic stenosis* is directed towards the left axilla and the neck, respectively. Thus, murmurs related to these lesions radiate to the same area. The high-velocity diastolic flow in *aortic regurgitation* is directed towards the left sternal edge, where the murmur is often more clearly audible than at the aortic area.

It is inadequate to describe the *timing* of a murmur as systolic or diastolic without more specific reference to the length of the murmur and the phase of systole or diastole during which it is heard: *systolic* murmurs are either mid-systolic, pansystolic or late systolic; *diastolic* murmurs are either early diastolic, mid-diastolic or presystolic in timing. Continuous murmurs are audible in both phases of the cardiac cycle.

A *mid-systolic* (*ejection*) murmur is caused by turbulence in the left or right ventricular outflow tracts during ejection. It starts following opening of the aortic or pulmonary valve, reaches a crescendo in mid-systole and disappears before the second heart sound. The murmur is loudest in the aortic area (with radiation to the neck) when it arises from the left ventricular outflow tract, and in the pulmonary area when it arises from the right ventricular outflow tract. It is best heard with the diaphragm of the stethoscope while the patient sits forward. Important causes of *aortic ejection murmurs* are aortic stenosis and hypertrophic cardiomyopathy. Aortic regurgitation also produces an ejection murmur due to increased stroke volume and velocity of ejection. *Pulmonary ejection murmurs* may be caused by pulmonary stenosis or infundibular stenosis (Fallot's tetralogy). In atrial septal defect the pulmonary ejection murmur results from right ventricular volume-loading and does not indicate organic valvular disease. '*Innocent*' *murmurs* unrelated to heart-disease are always mid-systolic in timing, usually reflecting a hyperkinetic circulation in conditions such as anaemia, pregnancy, thyrotoxicosis or fever. They are rarely louder than grade 3, often vary with posture and may disappear on exertion, and are not associated with other signs of organic heart-disease.

*Pansystolic murmurs* are audible throughout systole from the first to the second heart sounds. They are caused by regurgitation through incompetent atrioventricular valves and by ventricular septal defects. The pansystolic murmur of *mitral regurgitation* is loudest at the cardiac apex and radiates into the left axilla. It is best heard with the diaphragm of the stethoscope with the patient lying on the left side. The murmurs of *tricuspid regurgitation* and *ventricular septal defect* are loudest at the lower left sternal edge. Inspiration accentuates the murmur of tricuspid regurgitation because the increased venous return to the right side of the heart increases the regurgitant volume. *Mitral valve prolapse* may also produce a pansystolic murmur but, more commonly, prolapse occurs in mid-systole, producing a click followed by a late-systolic murmur (see Fig. 9.5).

*Early diastolic* murmurs are high-pitched and start immediately after the second heart sound, fading away in mid-diastole. They are caused by regurgitation through incompetent aortic and pulmonary valves and are best heard using the diaphragm of the stethoscope while the patient leans forward. The early diastolic murmur of *aortic regurgitation* radiates from the aortic area to the left sternal edge, where it is usually easier to hear. *Pulmonary regurgitation* is loudest at the pulmonary area.

*Mid-diastolic murmurs* are caused by turbulent flow through the atrioventricular valves. They start following valve opening, relatively late after the second sound, and continue for a variable period during mid-diastole. *Mitral stenosis* is the principal cause of a mid-diastolic murmur, which is best heard at the cardiac apex, using the bell of the stethoscope while the patient lies on the left side. Increased flow across a non-stenotic mitral valve occurs in *ventricular septal defect* and *mitral regurgitation* and may produce a mid-diastolic murmur. In severe *aortic regurgitation*, preclosure of the anterior leaflet of the mitral valve by the regurgitant jet may produce mitral turbulence, associated with a mid-diastolic murmur (Austin Flint murmur). A mid-diastolic murmur at the lower left sternal edge, accentuated by inspiration, is caused by *tricuspid stenosis* and also by conditions which increase tricuspid flow, e.g. atrial septal defect, tricuspid regurgitation.

In *mitral* or *tricuspid stenosis*, atrial systole produces a presystolic murmur immediately before the first heart sound. The murmur is perceived as an accentuation of the mid-diastolic murmur associated with these conditions. Because presystolic murmurs are generated by atrial systole they do not occur in patients with atrial fibrillation.

*Continuous murmurs* are heard during systole and diastole, and are uninterrupted by valve closure. The commonest cardiac cause is *patent ductus arteriosus*, in which flow from the high-pressure aorta to the low-pressure pulmonary artery continues throughout the cardiac cycle, producing a murmur over the base of the heart, which, though continuously audible, is loudest at end systole and diminishes during diastole. Ruptured sinus of Valsalva aneurysm also produces a continuous murmur (see Fig. 13.2).

In patients with a hyperkinetic circulation, flow in the jugular veins is sometimes audible as a continuous hum over the base of the heart, abolished by the patient lying supine.

## Pericardial friction rub

In *pericarditis*, the movement of the visceral layer of the pericardium against the parietal layer produces a high-pitched, scratching noise called a friction rub. This may be audible during any part of the cardiac cycle and over any part of the left precordium, depending on the extent of pericardial involvement. It is best heard using the diaphragm of the stethoscope while the patient sits forward.

## Further reading

Anonymous. Clinical signs in heart failure. *Lancet* 1989, **ii**, 309–10.

Constant J. *Bedside Cardiology*, 3rd edn. Boston, Little, Brown and Co., 1985.

Craige E. Should auscultation be rehabilitated? *N. Engl. J. Med.* 1988, **318**, 1611–13.

Henkind S.J., Benis A.M. and Teichholz L.E. The paradox of pulsus paradoxus. *Am. Heart J.* 1987, **114**, 198–203.

Leatham A. Auscultation and phonocardiography: a personal view of the past 40 years. *Br. Heart J.* 1987, **57**, 397–403.

Timmis A.D. The third heart sound. *Br. Med. J.* 1987, **294**, 326–7.

# 2 The Electrocardiogram and Arrhythmia Detection

## Summary

The electrocardiogram (ECG) records the electrical activity of the heart at the skin surface and consists of three bipolar leads (I, II, III) and nine unipolar leads (aVR, aVL, aVF, V1–V6). The orientation of each lead with respect to the heart is different and consequently the positive and negative depolarization changes recorded by each lead are also different. However, in normal sinus rhythm, the sequence of changes is always the same, each sinus impulse initiating atrial depolarization (P wave) followed by ventricular depolarization (QRS complex) and ventricular repolarization (T wave). In analysing the ECG, the rate, rhythm and frontal plane QRS axis should first be noted. Examination of P wave and QRS morphology provides evidence not only of myocardial disease involving the atria and ventricles but also of conducting tissue disease as it affects the PR interval, the duration of the QRS complex and the P wave–QRS association. ST segment analysis is important for diagnosis of acute ischaemia, myocardial infarction and pericarditis.

The ECG is the most useful tool for arrhythmia detection, and if a 12-lead recording can be obtained during symptoms it is usually diagnostic. For patients with intermittent arrhythmias, a recording may be obtained by ambulatory ECG monitoring, either in hospital, using a central monitoring station, or as an out-patient, using a small portable recording device. When the history suggests arrhythmias in association with specific activities, the ECG recorded during provocative testing may be helpful, using stress testing for exercise-induced symptoms or tilt testing for postural symptoms. In some cases, electrophysiological study (EPS) is required, in which one or more electrode catheters are positioned within the cardiac chambers to record the intracardiac electrogram and to deliver electrical impulses for stimulating and terminating arrhythmias. More recently, EPS has also been used for delivering therapy in patients requiring catheter ablation of conducting tissue and arrhythmogenic foci.

## The electrocardiogram (ECG)

The ECG is a record of the electrical activity of the heart recorded at the skin surface. A good quality 12-lead ECG is essential for the proper evaluation of the cardiac patient.

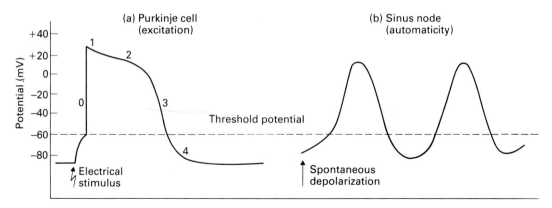

**Fig. 2.1** Action potential recordings from (a) a Purkinje cell and (b) a pacemaker cell of the sinus node. Depolarization of the Purkinje cell occurs in response to excitation but in the sinus node depolarization is spontaneous.

## Generation of electrical activity

The interior of the resting cardiac cell is electrically negative relative to the exterior, due to active extrusion of sodium ions, which maintain a transmembrane voltage difference of approximately −90 mV. Reduction of the voltage difference to a threshold of −60 mV triggers a self-perpetuating action potential.

In the Purkinje cell (Fig. 2.1a), this occurs in response to electrical stimulation, which reduces the voltage difference to threshold by increasing membrane permeability to sodium ions. The action potential has five parts:

**0** Rapid depolarization caused by rapid influx of sodium ions.

**1** Early repolarization caused by efflux of sodium ions.

**2** Plateau during which depolarization is temporarily arrested by slow influx of calcium ions.

**3** Rapid repolarization due to completion of cation efflux.

**4** Diastole during which the resting transmembrane voltage difference remains at −90 mV until the cell is once again stimulated.

In the sinus and atrioventricular (AV) nodes (Fig. 2.1b), depolarization to threshold occurs spontaneously and is not dependent upon electrical stimulation. All the specialized conduction tissues are capable of spontaneous depolarization (*automaticity*) but, because the sinus node has the fastest intrinsic rate, it provides the pacemaker for the normal heart. The action potential of the sinus node pacemaker cells is principally dependent on the influx of calcium ions, and exhibits a different contour from that of the His–Purkinje cells.

In the normal heart, the impulse generated by the sinus node spreads first through the atria, producing atrial systole, and then through the AV

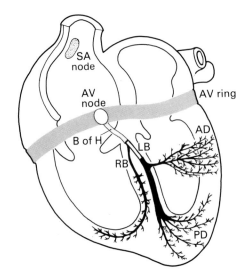

**Fig. 2.2** Normal conducting pathways: SA — sinoatrial; AV — atrioventricular; B of H — bundle of His; LB — left bundle; RB — right bundle. Note that the left bundle branch divides into anterior and posterior divisions (AD and PD). The electrically inert atrioventricular ring tissue is indicated by the shaded band.

node and His–Purkinje tissue, producing ventricular systole (Fig. 2.2). The AV node and bundle of His provide the only pathway connecting atria and ventricles; the remainder of the AV ring tissue is electrically inert. Moreover, impulse conduction through the AV node is slow and cannot proceed above a certain rate. These anatomical and physiological properties of AV conduction ensure that:

1   Ventricular filling is complete before the onset of systole.
2   The ventricles will not respond to excessively rapid atrial rates.

Within the ventricles, the impulse is conducted rapidly through the bundle of His into the upper part of the interventricular septum and thence through the left and right bundle branches to the free walls of the ventricles. The wave of depolarization that spreads through the heart during each cardiac cycle has vector properties defined by its direction and magnitude. At any instant depolarization occurs in multiple directions as the activation wave is propagated. Thus, the instantaneous direction of the wave recorded at the skin surface is the resultant of multiple 'minivectors' throughout the heart. Since the sinus node is in the high right atrium, the predominant direction of the activation wave is downwards and to the left. This produces the P wave on the ECG. Ventricular depolarization is initiated in the upper part of the septum, following passage of the impulse through the AV node into the bundle of His. The predominant direction of the activation wave is downwards and slightly leftwards due to the greater thickness of the wall of the left ventricle. This produces the QRS complex on the ECG.

An activation wave approaching the recording electrode produces, by convention, a *positive* deflexion on the ECG, whilst a wave moving in the opposite direction produces a *negative* deflexion. Importantly, if the

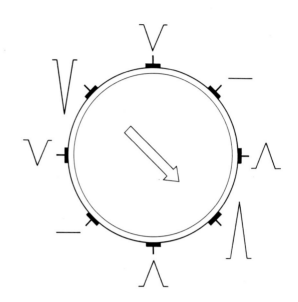

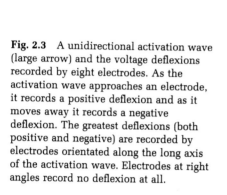

**Fig. 2.3**   A unidirectional activation wave (large arrow) and the voltage deflexions recorded by eight electrodes. As the activation wave approaches an electrode, it records a positive deflexion and as it moves away it records a negative deflexion. The greatest deflexions (both positive and negative) are recorded by electrodes orientated along the long axis of the activation wave. Electrodes at right angles record no deflexion at all.

direction of the wave is at right angles to the recording electrode it produces no deflexion at all. Thus, every gradation of deflexion (positive and negative) can be produced by the same activation wave, depending on the precise orientation of the recording electrode (Fig. 2.3). During the normal depolarization process, the (resultant) direction of the activation wave is continuously changing as it spreads throughout the heart. The ECG deflexions change accordingly during each cardiac cycle, being positive at one moment and negative at another.

The magnitude of the activation wave is a function of muscle mass and therefore the ECG deflexion produced by depolarization of the atrium (the P wave) is smaller than that produced by depolarization of the more muscular ventricles (QRS complex). Consequently, patients with *ventricular hypertrophy* tend to have exaggerated QRS voltage deflexions on the ECG. As previously stated, the magnitude of the activation wave perceived by a recording electrode is also influenced by its direction, the deflexions, regardless of muscle mass, becoming progressively smaller as the orientation of the recording electrode to the activation wave approaches right angles.

## Inscription of the QRS complex

The shape of the QRS complex is determined by the ventricular depolarization vector and the orientation of the recording electrode with respect to the heart. The ventricular depolarization vector can, for convenience, be resolved into two components (Fig. 2.4): the first, septal depolarization, spreads from left to right while the second, ventricular free wall depolarization, spreads from endocardium to epicardium.

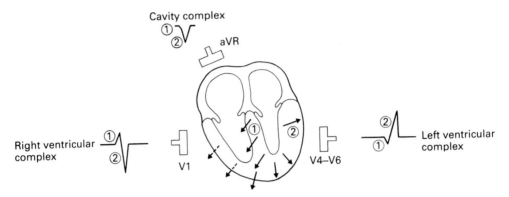

**Fig. 2.4** Inscription of the QRS complex. The first (1) and second (2) ventricular depolarization vectors as perceived by recording electrodes orientated towards the right ventricle (V1) and the left ventricle (V4–V6). Note that lead aVR is orientated towards the ventricular cavities and therefore records an entirely negative deflexion.

Because the left ventricular depolarization vector dominates that of the thin-walled right ventricle, the net direction of the second vector component is from right to left. Therefore, leads orientated to the *left ventricle* record a small negative deflexion (Q wave) as the septal depolarization vector moves away, followed by a large positive deflexion (R wave) as the ventricular depolarization vector moves towards the recording electrode. The sequence of deflexions in leads orientated towards the *right ventricle* is in the opposite direction, to give an RS complex (Fig. 2.4).

## *Mean frontal QRS axis*

This is the mean direction of the ventricular depolarization vector in those leads (1 to aVF) which lie in the frontal plane of the heart. Although the direction of the depolarization vector is continuously changing, its mean direction can be determined by identifying the limb lead in which the net QRS deflexion (positive and negative) is least pronounced, i.e. the lead where positive and negative deflexions are most equal. The mean frontal QRS axis is at right angles to this lead and is quantified using a hexaxial reference system (Fig. 2.5).

The principal importance of the mean frontal QRS axis relates to its wide range of normality, from $-30°$ to $90°$. This explains the wide variation of limb lead QRS patterns that are consistent with a normal ECG. Correct interpretation of the ECG, therefore, must take account of the mean frontal QRS axis. An abnormal axis often indicates heart-disease but does not itself identify the nature of the disorder. Nevertheless, *left axis deviation* is usually associated with conduction block in the anterior

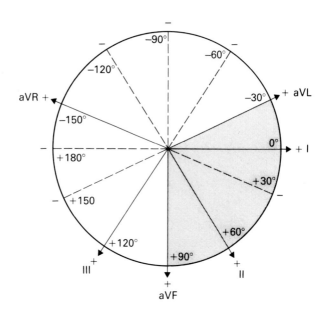

**Fig. 2.5** Hexaxial reference system. When the mean frontal QRS axis is directed towards lead 1, it is arbitrarily defined as 0°; the dominant positive deflexion is in lead I and the equiphasic deflexion is in aVF. Axis shifts are ascribed a negative sign if directed leftwards (towards aVL) and a positive sign if directed rightwards (towards aVF). Axes between −30° and +90° are normal (shaded area). Axes less than −30° (left axis deviation) or greater than +90° (right axis deviation) are abnormal.

fascicle of the left bundle branch (left anterior hemiblock, see p. 135) while *right axis deviation* may indicate right ventricular strain or a block in the posterior fascicle of the left bundle branch (left posterior hemiblock).

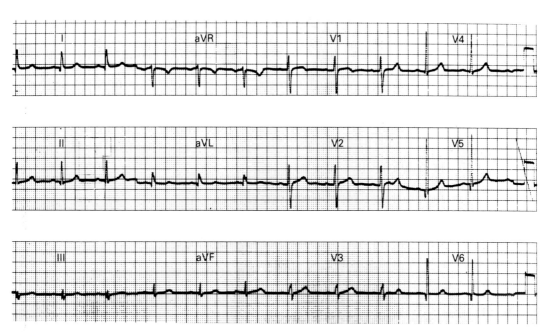

**Fig. 2.6** Standard 12-lead ECG. Normal recording. Note that lead III is equiphasic and at right angles to aVR, which is dominantly negative. Thus, the mean frontal QRS axis is +30°.

### The normal ECG

Figure 2.6 shows a standard 12-lead ECG. The recording is normal. Note the following features:

**1**  There are six limb leads. Leads I to III are the bipolar limb leads. Leads aVR to aVF are the augmented unipolar limb leads.

**2**  There are six unipolar chest leads, V1 to V6.

**3**  The orientation of each lead to the wave of depolarization is different. Consequently the perceived direction and magnitude of the wave show considerable variation, as reflected by the difference in the shapes of the complexes.

**4**  Despite this variation the sequence of deflexions is identical in each lead. The small P wave (atrial depolarization) is followed by the larger QRS complex (ventricular depolarization) and the T wave (ventricular repolarization).

**5**  The paper speed is 25 mm/sec so that each small square (1 mm) represents 0.04 sec and each large square (5 mm) represents 0.20 sec.

**6**  The square wave is a calibration signal: 1 cm vertical deflexion = 1 mV.

### The limb leads

The standard bipolar leads (I to III) each measure the potential difference between two limbs:

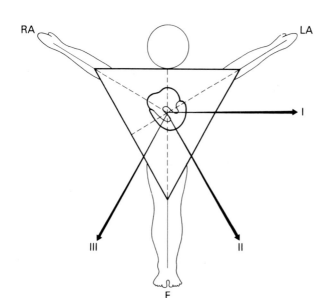

**Fig. 2.7**  Einthoven's triangle. Lead I measures the potential difference between the left and right arms. Since the right arm carries the negative electrode, the resultant direction of the lead I vector is obtained by bisecting the angle between the left arm and a point directly opposite the right arm. The resultant directions of leads II and III are obtained in a similar way. RA — right arm; LA — left arm; F — foot.

Lead I     left arm – right arm.
Lead II    left leg – right arm.
Lead III   left leg – right arm.

An earth electrode is attached to the right leg to minimize electrical interference.

The heart may be considered as the centre of an equilateral triangle (Einthoven's triangle) formed by the two arms and the left leg (Fig. 2.7). By simple subtraction of vectors, the orientation of each standard lead with reference to the heart may be calculated.

The augmented unipolar limb leads (aVR to aVF) each consist of an exploring electrode connected to a limb: an indifferent electrode is connected to the other two limbs through high electrical resistance. The potential of the indifferent electrode is thus reduced to a very low level. This has two important effects:

**1**   The voltage deflexion on the ECG is augmented.

**2**   The orientation of the augmented lead with reference to the heart is very close to that of the limb to which the exploring electrode is attached. Thus, in Fig. 2.7 the orientation of the limbs (RA, LA, F) is essentially the same as the orientation of aVR, aVL and aVF with reference to the heart.

## The chest leads

Each of the unipolar leads V1 to V6 consists of an exploring electrode on the chest wall (Fig. 2.8) and an indifferent electrode connected to the three limbs through high electrical resistance. The very low (effectively zero) potential of the indifferent electrode ensures that the orientation of

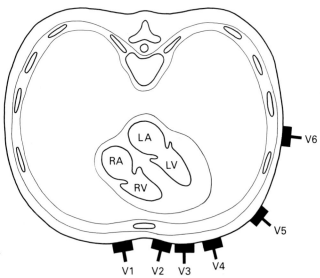

**Fig. 2.8**   The chest leads. This horizontal section through the chest shows the orientation of the chest leads with respect to the chambers of the heart. V1 is orientated towards the right ventricle, V2 and V3 face the interventricular septum, and V4–V6 extend around the free wall of the left ventricle.

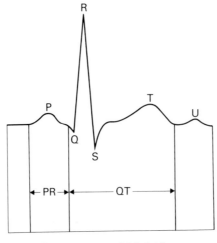

P wave:       0.06–0.10 sec
PR interval:  0.12–0.20 sec
QRS complex: 0.08–0.12 sec
QT interval:  0.35–0.45 sec

**Fig. 2.9**  The normal ECG complex.

each chest lead with respect to the heart is defined almost exactly by the position of the exploring electrode on the chest wall.

## Analysis of the ECG

Figure 2.9 illustrates the normal ECG complex.

### Heart rate

The ECG is usually recorded at a paper speed of 25 mm/sec such that each large square (5 mm) represents 0.20 sec. Heart rate is conveniently calculated by counting the number of large squares between consecutive R waves and dividing this into 300.

### Rhythm

In normal sinus rhythm, P waves precede each QRS complex. The rhythm is regular or shows phasic variations in rate with respiration (sinus arrhythmia). Absence of P waves and an irregular rhythm indicate atrial fibrillation. Other arrhythmias are discussed in Chapters 10 and 11.

### Electrical axis

Evaluation of the mean frontal plane QRS axis is described on p. 30.

## P-wave morphology

The P wave is a small deflexion caused by atrial depolarization. Upper limits of normal for height and duration are 3.0 mm and 0.1 sec respectively. The deflexion is negative in aVR and often biphasic in III and V1; in all other leads the P wave is positive.

Atrial depolarization is initiated by the sinus node in the high right atrium and proceeds downwards and to the left. *Right atrial enlargement* in pulmonary hypertension accentuates the early depolarization vector, producing a tall, peaked P wave (P pulmonale). *Left atrial enlargement* in left heart failure accentuates the late depolarization vector, producing a broad notched P wave (P mitrale, Fig. 2.10). If an ectopic atrial focus assumes pacemaker function, atrial depolarization proceeds by abnormal pathways, resulting in altered P-wave morphology. This is particularly obvious for foci in the low right atrium around the coronary sinus, when atrial depolarization occurs from below upwards, resulting in an inverted P wave (coronary sinus rhythm).

Failure of atrial depolarization results in absence of the P wave. This occurs in sinus arrest with junctional or ventricular escape. In atrial fibrillation or atrial flutter, P waves are replaced by fibrillation or flutter waves, respectively.

## PR interval

The PR interval is measured from the onset of the P wave to the first deflexion of the QRS complex, and represents the time taken for the sinus node impulse to reach the ventricular myocardium. The normal duration is 0.12–0.20 sec. *Prolongation* of the PR interval occurs when conduction

**Standard lead II**

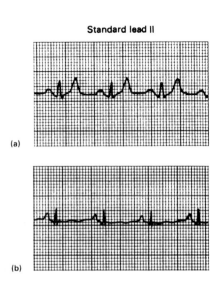

(a)

(b)

**Fig. 2.10**   P wave abnormalities. (a) P mitrale. (b) P pulmonale.

through the AV node is delayed by disease or drugs (first-degree AV block). If AV conduction fails, either intermittently (second-degree AV block) or completely (third-degree AV block), the normal 1:1 relation between the P wave and the QRS complex is lost.

A *short PR interval* (<0.12 sec) occurs when a rapidly conducting accessory pathway bypasses the AV node, permitting early ventricular activation, e.g. Wolff–Parkinson–White or Lown–Ganong–Levine syndromes. Shortening of the PR intervals also occurs in low atrial or coronary sinus escape rhythms, because of the proximity of the escape focus to the AV node.

## QRS morphology

The QRS complex (caused by ventricular depolarization) is the most prominent deflection in the ECG. Its duration should not exceed 0.12 sec. Prolongation indicates slow ventricular depolarization, caused sometimes by pre-excitation (Wolff–Parkinson–White syndrome) or hypokalaemia but most commonly by bundle branch block (Fig. 2.11). In *right bundle branch block* depolarization of the right ventricle is delayed, resulting in a late positive deflection in leads facing the right ventricle (V1) and a late negative deflection in leads facing the left ventricle (I, V6). In *left bundle branch block* the entire sequence of ventricular depolarization is disorganized and the QRS complex is broad and bizarre. Septal depolarization no longer occurs from left to right and the small septal Q waves in leads V4 to V6 are therefore lost.

*Exaggerated QRS deflexions* indicate ventricular hypertrophy (Fig. 2.12). Voltage criteria for *left ventricular hypertrophy* are fulfilled when

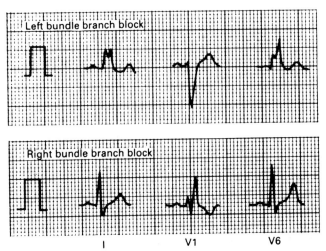

**Fig. 2.11** Bundle branch block with widening of the QRS complex.

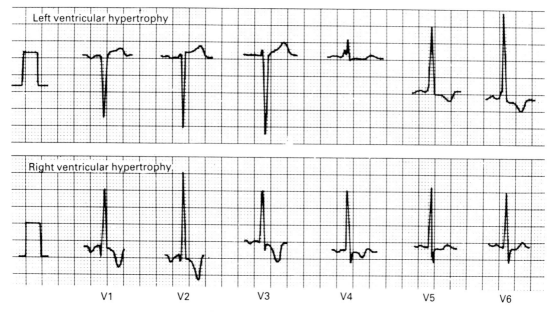

**Fig. 2.12** Left and right ventricular hypertrophy causing exaggerated voltage deflexions in leads V1–V6, often associated with T-wave inversion in leads V5–V6 and V1–V3, respectively ('strain' pattern).

the sum of the S and R wave deflexions in leads V1 and V6, respectively, exceeds 35 mm (3.5 mV). However, these criteria may be normal in narrow-chested individuals. Other ECG manifestations of left ventricular hypertrophy include T-wave inversion in left ventricular leads (strain pattern). *Right ventricular hypertrophy* causes tall R waves in right ventricular leads (V1 and V2), often associated with T-wave inversion.

*Diminished QRS deflexions* occur when pericardial effusion, hyperinflated lungs (emphysema) or severe obesity partially insulate the heart from the skin surface. Myxoedema may also be associated with diminished QRS deflexions.

*Pathological Q waves* (duration >0.04 sec), associated with variable loss of height of the ensuing R wave, usually indicate myocardial infarction. Note, however, that in leads orientated towards the cavity of the left ventricle (aVR and sometimes V1) a deep Q wave is normal and simply reflects the endocardial to epicardial depolarization vector directed away from the lead on the opposite side of the ventricle (see Fig. 2.4).

## ST segment

This is the isoelectric segment between the end of the QRS complex and the start of the T wave. Deviation of the ST segment above or below the isoelectric line may indicate heart-disease (Fig. 2.13). However, minor

ST elevation

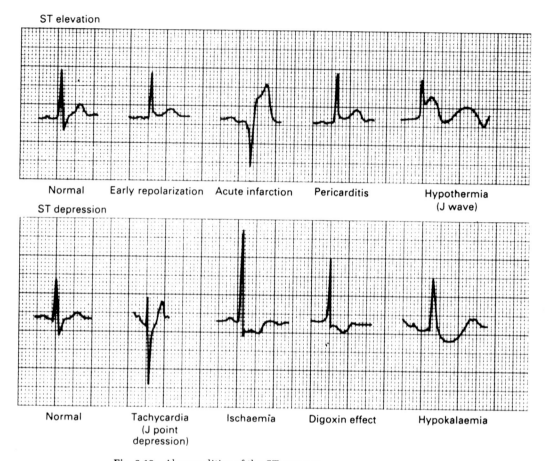

| Normal | Early repolarization | Acute infarction | Pericarditis | Hypothermia (J wave) |

ST depression

| Normal | Tachycardia (J point depression) | Ischaemia | Digoxin effect | Hypokalaemia |

**Fig. 2.13**   Abnormalities of the ST segment.

degrees of ST elevation (early repolarization) occur as a normal variant, particularly in patients of African origin. *Pathological ST elevation is* caused by acute myocardial infarction, variant angina and pericarditis. In acute infarction and variant angina, the ST elevation is typically convex upwards (coved), affecting leads orientated towards the threatened myocardium. In pericarditis, the changes are more widespread and the ST elevation is concave upwards. Elevation of the early part of the ST segment occurs in severe hypothermia and is caused by a J wave at the junction of the QRS complex and the ST segment.

*Depression of the junction* between the QRS complex and the ST segment (J point) with an upwards sloping ST segment is physiological during exertion, unlike the horizontal (planar) ST depression that indicates myocardial ischaemia. In acute myocardial infarction, however, ST depression affecting leads opposite the infarct zone occurs as a reciprocal phenomenon and does not necessarily indicate remote ischaemia. Other important causes of ST depression include digitalis therapy and hypokalaemia, both of which cause sagging of the ST segment which may be difficult to distinguish from ischaemia.

## T wave

The T wave represents ventricular repolarization, and its orientation (positive or negative) is usually the same as the QRS complex. Thus T-wave *inversion* is normal in leads aVR and V1. Widespread T-wave inversion is common in cardiomyopathy and occurs as a non-specific response to viral infection, hypothermia and hyperventilation. More important causes of T-wave inversion include left ventricular hypertrophy and myocardial ischaemia and infarction; in small non-Q-wave infarcts this may be the only abnormality.

Exaggerated *peaking* of the T wave is seen as a hyperacute phenomenon in the early hours of acute myocardial infarction and also occurs in hyperkalaemia.

## QT interval

This is measured from the onset of the QRS complex to the end of the T wave and represents the duration of *electrical* systole (*mechanical* systole starts between the QRS complex and the T wave). The QT interval (0.35–0.45 sec) is very rate-sensitive, shortening as heart rate increases. *Abnormal prolongation* of the QT interval predisposes to ventricular arrhythmias and may be congenital or occur in response to hypokalaemia, rheumatic fever or drugs (e.g. quinidine, amiodarone, tricyclic antidepressants). *Shortening* of the QT interval is caused by hyperkalaemia and digitalis therapy.

## U wave

The cause of the U wave is unknown. It is a small, often invisible, deflexion following the T wave and orientated in the same direction. Although U-wave abnormalities are rarely of diagnostic importance, inversion may occur in ischaemic disease, while peaking is seen in hyperkalaemia.

## Arrhythmia detection

The effective management of cardiac arrhythmias depends upon accurate diagnosis. Although the history and examination are sometimes useful, special investigations are required in most cases in order to obtain electrocardiographic documentation of the arrhythmia.

## *Electrocardiogram*

The ECG is the basic tool for arrhythmia diagnosis. A single lead or monitor strip is sometimes adequate but accurate diagnosis often requires a full 12-lead ECG. If a patient has an arrhythmia at the time of presentation, all efforts should be made to get a 12-lead recording, even if the patient is hypotensive. Appropriate future management may depend on the ECG obtained at that time. Occasionally, special ECG leads are required, particularly when atrial activity is not clearly visible. The electrocardiographic diagnosis of arrhythmias will be discussed in Chapter 11.

## *Ambulatory ECG monitoring*

Many patients present with symptoms suggesting an intermittent arrhythmia or conduction disturbance. Although an ECG obtained during symptoms may be diagnostic, this is often not practical and some form of ambulatory monitoring must be performed.

### *In-hospital ECG monitoring*

Patients who have severe arrhythmias, thought to be life-threatening, should be managed in hospital with continuous ECG monitoring. Unless the patient is being individually nursed, a central monitoring system is required, ideally with a computerized alarm triggered by abrupt alterations in rate or QRS morphology. Patients may be connected directly to the system or monitored at a distance, using radiotelemetry. Either way, continuous surveillance by trained staff is essential.

### *Continuous ambulatory ECG monitoring (24-hour or Holter monitors)*

This utilizes a small recording device (either magnetic tape or solid state) called a 24-hour or Holter monitor, which records at least two ECG channels. It is worn during normal activities while the patient keeps a diary of symptoms; activities known to trigger symptoms should be encouraged during the monitoring period. Tape analysis is computer-assisted and rhythm abnormalities are usually displayed at standard paper speed. Alternatively, a full disclosure of the entire ECG can be displayed at very slow speed (Fig. 2.14). If an arrhythmia is documented, it is usually diagnostic, particularly when it coincides with symptoms entered into the diary.

An advantage of continuous ambulatory monitoring is that symptomatic and asymptomatic arrhythmias may be recorded, and also the start

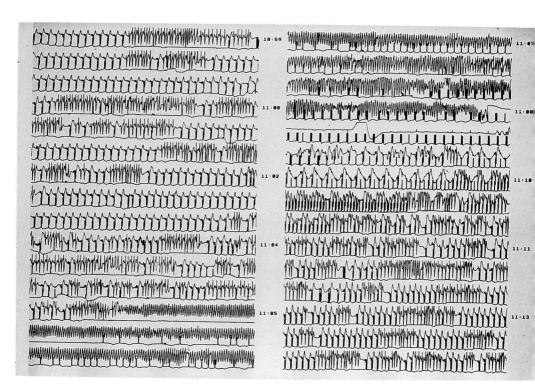

**Fig. 2.14**  Ambulatory (Holter) ECG monitoring: full disclosure from 24-hour recording, played at very slow speed, with recurrent paroxysms of ventricular tachycardia.

and end of attacks (Fig. 2.14). Events leading up to a sustained arrhythmia can be examined in detail. Unfortunately, however, in patients with paroxysmal arrhythmias who do not experience attacks each day, the chances of recording an abnormality by this technique may be small.

### Event recorders

These are useful for patients with infrequent symptoms and often have a facility for telephonic transmission of rhythm recordings, which may then be examined by the cardiologist. The recorder is patient-activated and applied to the chest wall in the event of symptoms in order to obtain the ECG, which is then stored for later analysis. Some units are capable of storing only one arrhythmic episode while others can store several. More sophisticated devices are available which are continuously connected to the patient, recording events that fulfil certain trigger criteria (automatic mode) and also events that provoke symptoms (manual mode). These devices have a loop facility so that, when triggered manually by the patient during symptoms, a record of the ECG in the seconds leading up to the episode is recorded. The most sophisticated of these devices will also alert the patient if a dangerously abnormal rhythm occurs.

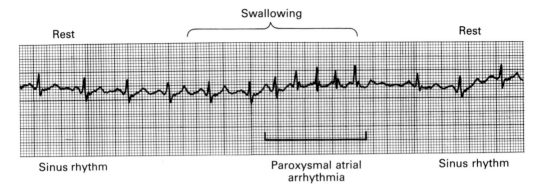

**Fig. 2.15**   Atrial tachycardia induced by swallowing.

### Provocative testing

This is helpful when the history suggests cardiac rhythm disturbance in association with specific activities, for example exercise or swallowing (Fig. 2.15). In certain patients, an ECG obtained during the activity will be diagnostic if the arrhythmia is recorded.

*The exercise ECG* is frequently used for provocation of arrhythmias caused by ischaemia or increased sympathetic activity. However, it must be emphasized that, although ventricular tachycardia, in particular, is usually associated with coronary artery disease, it is not usually triggered by an acute ischaemic episode and for this reason exercise testing is often unhelpful as a provocative test.

*Tilt testing* is another provocative test, particularly useful in the diagnosis of malignant vasovagal syndrome, an autonomic disorder causing brady-cardias and syncope. The patient is placed on a tilt table at 60°, with adequate restraints, and the blood-pressure and ECG are monitored for up to 40 min. Most patients with malignant vasovagal syndrome become suddenly bradycardic and/or hypotensive and lose consciousness unless the table is tilted back to the horizontal.

**Table 2.1**   Indications for EPS

| |
|---|
| 1   Assessing risk (e.g. Wolff–Parkinson–White syndrome, ventricular arrhythmias) |
| 2   Elucidating difficult ECGs |
| 3   Investigating palpitations or syncope when non-invasive techniques have failed |
| 4   Assessing therapy (especially after drugs, ablation, surgery or special devices) |
| 5   Delivering therapy (catheter ablation) |

*Carotid sinus massage* (after excluding carotid bruits) during simultaneous ECG recording is useful for provoking symptomatic bradycardia in the carotid sinus syndrome. The test is positive if it provokes a bradycardia (pauses longer than 3 sec) and reproduces symptoms, usually dizziness or syncope.

### Electrophysiological study (EPS)

Indications for EPS are shown in Table 2.1. It is usually used to investigate tachyarrhythmias, less commonly bradyarrhythmias. Depending on the type of study being performed, one or more multipolar electrode catheters are positioned in the right atrium, right ventricle, across the tricuspid valve (to record the His bundle deflexion), into the coronary sinus (to record left atrial and ventricular activity), into the left ventricle and occasionally into the left atrium (Fig. 2.16). The catheters are used to record the intracardiac electrogram and to deliver electrical impulses for stimulating and terminating arrhythmias. Although the original application of EPS was for arrhythmia diagnosis and monitoring therapy, more recently it has been used for delivering therapy in patients requiring catheter ablation of conducting tissue and arrhythmogenic foci. The EPS

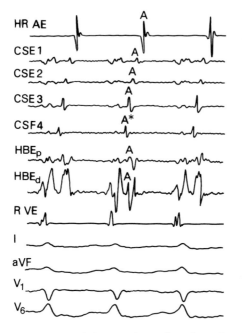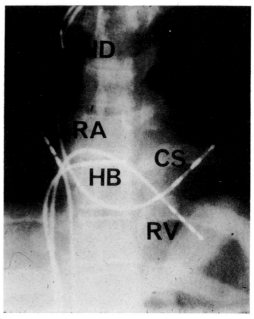

**Fig. 2.16** Electrophysiological study. Surface ECG and intracardiac recordings (left panel) obtained from electrodes positioned strategically within the heart (right panel) in a patient with Wolff–Parkinson–White syndrome. Note that the paper speed is accelerated (100 mm/sec) in order to permit accurate timing of the abnormal atrial activation (A) that characterizes the syndrome. HRAE = high right atrial electrode, CSE = coronary sinus electrodes, HBE = His bundle electrodes, RVE = right ventricular electrode, A* = earliest atrial activation.

is a powerful tool and, though invasive, is usually safe. However, because it may involve deliberate induction of ventricular tachycardia or fibrillation, considerable expertise is required and resuscitation equipment must always be available.

## Special techniques for identifying patients at risk of arrhythmias

In patients recovering from acute myocardial infarction, special techniques may be employed to identify those at greatest risk of developing lethal arrhythmias early after discharge from hospital, so that specific treatment can be given to protect them from sudden death. Electrophysiological studies (see above) to test susceptibility to arrhythmia induction by ventricular stimulation are often used for this purpose. Recently, however, a number of non-invasive methods have been developed to identify patients at risk of arrhythmias.

### *The signal-averaged ECG*

This technique permits identification of low-voltage signals by means of high-gain amplification of the ECG. By recording a large number of cycles, which are superimposed and filtered, electrical noise is averaged out while the low-voltage signal remains amplified. The technique was originally used to record His bundle potentials non-invasively but now finds greater application in the identification of ventricular late potentials (Fig. 2.17). These are low-amplitude deflexions at the end of QRS complex, which indicate a heightened risk of ventricular tachyarrhythmias. Their presence has been used for prognostic assessment after myocardial infarction.

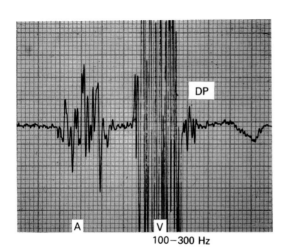

**Fig. 2.17** Signal-averaged ECG showing atrial (A) and ventricular (V) potentials. Delayed potentials (DP) late after ventricular activation are clearly visible.

## *Heart rate variability*

The heart rate varies during the respiratory cycle, autonomic influences causing it to increase during inspiration and decrease during expiration. This may be quantified by 24-hour ECG recording while the patient breathes normally. Loss of heart rate variability is seen in autonomic neuropathy and may also occur early after acute myocardial infarction, when it is a poor prognostic sign.

## Further reading

Ayres S.M. The electrocardiogram in acute coronary syndromes. *J. Am. Coll. Cardiol.* 1990, **16**, 1026–8.

Jaffe A.S., Atkins J.M., Mentzer R.M. *et al.* Recommended guidelines for in-hospital cardiac monitoring of adults for detection of arrhythmias. *J. Am. Coll. Cardiol.* 1991, **18**, 1431–4.

Knoebel S.B., Crawford M.N., Dunn M.I., *et al.* Guidelines for ambulatory electrocardiography. *J. Am. Coll. Cardiol.* 1989, **13**, 249–58.

Krikler D.M. Electrocardiography then and now: where next? *Br. Heart J.* 1987, **57**, 113–17.

Schamroth L. *An Introduction to Electrocardiography*, 7th edn. Oxford, Blackwell Scientific Publications, 1990.

Ward D.E. Can the technicalities of electrophysiological testing for ventricular tachycardia be simplified? *Br. Heart J.* 1987, **58**, 437–40.

Zipes D.P. Sympathetic stimulation and arrhythmias. *N. Engl. J. Med.* 1991, **325**, 656–7.

# 3 Cardiac Imaging and Catheterization

## Summary

*The chest X-ray* permits assessment of heart size, which should not exceed 50% the transverse diameter of the chest. Enlargement is usually caused by dilatation (as opposed to hypertrophy) of one or more cardiac chambers, although only the left atrium can be accurately identified on the posteroanterior (PA) film. The lateral chest X-ray permits assessment of left and right ventricular size, and diseased intracardiac structures may be visible if they are calcified. Lung field abnormalities in cardiovascular disease are caused by alterations of pulmonary flow or increased left atrial pressure. Increased pulmonary flow (e.g. atrial septal defect) causes prominent vascular markings, while reduced flow causes oligaemia, which may be regional (e.g. pulmonary embolism) or global (e.g. Eisenmenger's syndrome). Increased left atrial pressure in left heart failure produces corresponding increments in pulmonary venous and pulmonary capillary pressures. Prominence of the upper lobe veins is an early sign but, as pressure rises, interstitial and alveolar oedema develops, evidenced by Kerley B lines and perihilar air-space consolidation, respectively.

*The echocardiogram* utilizes ultrasound to provide unidimensional (M-mode) and two-dimensional (2D) images of the heart, of particular value for diagnosis of myocardial, pericardial, valvular and congenital defects. The more recent availability of Doppler ultrasound to identify direction and velocity of flow within the heart has extended the role of echocardiography, which can now be used for grading the severity of stenotic and regurgitant valve lesions and for localizing intracardiac shunts through septal defects.

*Radionuclide imaging* with a gamma camera provides an alternative diagnostic method, the application of which depends on the isotope used and its uptake within the cardiopulmonary system. Scintigraphic analysis of ventricular function and myocardial perfusion is widely used in the investigation of patients with heart failure and coronary artery disease, while ventilation–perfusion imaging of the lungs is one of the most reliable methods for diagnosing pulmonary embolism.

Computed tomography and, more recently, *magnetic resonance imaging* represent a quantum leap forwards in terms of image quality (and cost), but the roles of these evolving technologies in clinical cardiology remain largely undetermined.

*Cardiac catheterization* is an invasive method for delivery of radiographic contrast material into the area of interest. This permits angiographic assessment of ventricular function, valvular competence and pulmonary perfusion and is the only reliable technique for imaging the coronary arteries. Cardiac catheterization is also used for intracardiac pressure measurement and for haemodynamic evaluation of valvular stenosis, intracardiac shunts and cardiac output. In addition to its important diagnostic role, catheter technology is now being used increasingly for the interventional management of cardiovascular disease, where procedures such as valvuloplasty and angioplasty are extending the therapeutic role of the cardiologist into areas that were once exclusively surgical.

## Non-invasive imaging

### *The chest X-ray*

Good quality posteroanterior (PA) and lateral chest X-rays contribute importantly to the cardiac assessment.

### *Cardiac silhouette*

Because the radiodensity of cardiac tissue is similar to that of blood, intracardiac structures can rarely be identified unless they are calcified (Fig. 3.1). However, the cardiac silhouette contrasts strongly with the adjacent radiolucent lung fields, permitting accurate appreciation of the heart size. The heart is long and thin in endomorphic individuals but is more bulky in mesomorphic individuals. Nevertheless, the maximum transverse measurement should not exceed 50% that of the chest. Cardiac enlargement is caused either by pericardial effusion or by dilatation of the cardiac chambers and great vessels. Myocardial hypertrophy without chamber dilatation rarely causes radiographic cardiac enlargement.

#### Pericardial effusion

This separates the parietal pericardium from the wall of the heart. The cardiac silhouette enlarges and the contour becomes smooth and globular.

#### Atrial dilatation

Right atrial dilatation is usually due to right ventricular failure and tricuspid regurgitation but occurs as an isolated finding in tricuspid stenosis and Ebstein's anomaly. It produces cardiac enlargement without specific radiographic signs.

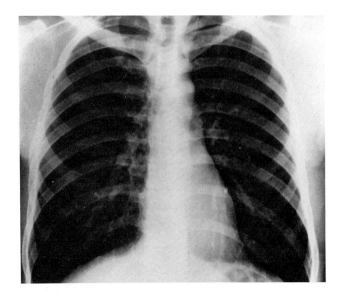

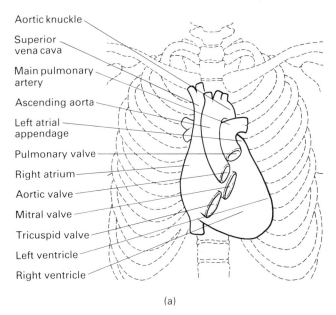

Aortic knuckle

Superior
vena cava

Main pulmonary
artery

Ascending aorta

Left atrial
appendage

Pulmonary valve

Right atrium

Aortic valve

Mitral valve

Tricuspid valve

Left ventricle

Right ventricle

(a)

**Fig. 3.1** (a) Normal chest X-ray —
posteroanterior projection. (b — facing
page) Normal chest X-ray — left lateral
projection.

The left atrium is the only cardiac chamber than can be accurately
identified on the PA chest X-ray. Dilatation occurs in left ventricular
failure and mitral valve disease. This causes (Fig. 3.2):
1   Flattening and later bulging of the left heart border below the main
pulmonary artery due to leftwards displacement of the atrial appendage.
2   Elevation of the left main bronchus with widening of the carina.
3   Appearance of the medial border of the left atrium behind the right
side of the heart (double density sign).

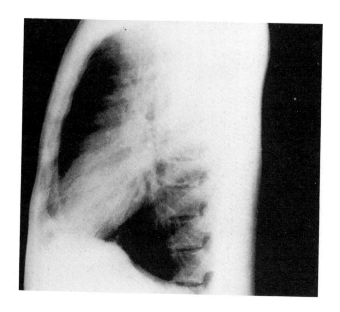

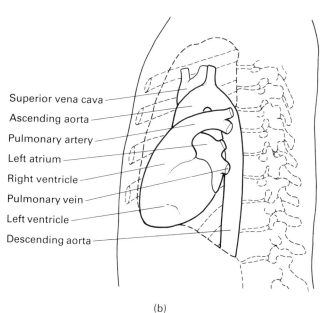

Superior vena cava
Ascending aorta
Pulmonary artery
Left atrium
Right ventricle
Pulmonary vein
Left ventricle
Descending aorta

(b)

### Ventricular dilatation

This commonly accompanies heart failure, particularly when this is caused by myocardial disease or regurgitant valvular disease. Although the PA chest X-ray does not reliably distinguish left from right ventricular dilatation, the lateral view may be more helpful. Thus, dilatation of the posteriorly located left ventricle encroaches on the retrocardiac space,

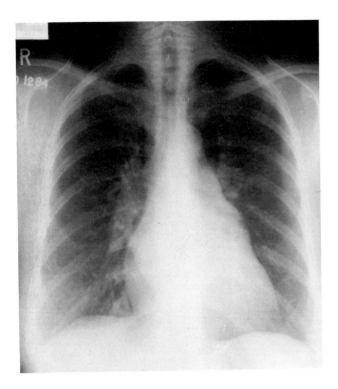

**Fig. 3.2**  Left atrial enlargement in a patient with mitral valve disease. Note the bulging of the left heart border below the main pulmonary artery with elevation of the left main bronchus and the 'double density' at the right heart border.

while dilatation of the anteriorly located right ventricle encroaches on the retrosternal space (see Fig. 9.3).

### Vascular dilatation

Dilatation and lengthening of the thoracic aorta are common in the elderly and produce an unfolded appearance. Aortic dilatation caused by aneurysm or dissection may be focal, but more commonly produces widening of the entire upper mediastinum. Localized dilatation of the proximal aorta occurs in aortic valve disease and produces a prominence in the right upper mediastinum. Dilatation of the main pulmonary artery occurs in pulmonary hypertension and pulmonary stenosis and produces a prominence below the aortic knuckle (Fig. 3.3).

### Intracardiac calcification

Disease of any of the cardiac tissues may result in calcification. Pericardial calcification is characteristic of tuberculous disease but is less common in other causes of constrictive pericarditis (Fig. 3.4). Myocardial calcification may occur in the walls of a ventricular aneurysm and sometimes in the left atrial wall in advanced mitral disease (see Fig. 9.3).

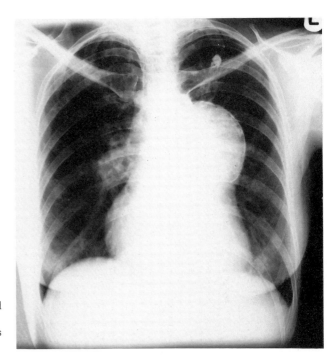

**Fig. 3.3** Pulmonary arterial calcification. The main pulmonary artery is very dilated due to long-standing pulmonary hypertension. Calcification of the artery is clearly visible.

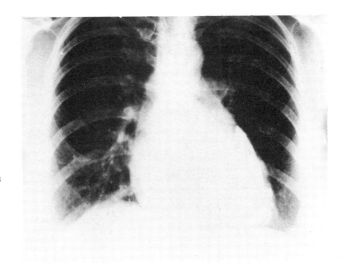

**Fig. 3.4** Pericardial calcification. In this patient with constrictive pericarditis the pericardial calcification is clearly visible on the posteroanterior chest X-ray. In most cases, however, pericardial calcification is better appreciated on the lateral chest X-ray.

Valvular calcification occurs most commonly in aortic and mitral disease and may involve the leaflets, causing stenosis, the ring tissue, when valve function is often unaffected, or both. Identification of the calcified valve usually requires a lateral chest X-ray, in which the aortic valve lies anterior and the mitral valve posterior to the long axis of the heart. Vascular calcification may affect the coronary arteries in atheromatous disease, the wall of the ascending aorta in syphilitic aortitis or the main pulmonary artery in pulmonary hypertension (Fig. 3.3). Most commonly, however, vascular calcification is seen in the aortic arch and represents a benign degenerative process in the elderly.

## Lung fields

In cardiovascular disease, the common lung-field abnormalities are caused either by alterations in pulmonary flow or by increased left atrial pressure.

### Pulmonary flow

*Increased pulmonary flow*, sufficient to cause radiographic abnormalities, is usually caused by a left-to-right intracardiac shunt, e.g. atrial septal defect, ventricular septal defect. Prominence of the vascular markings gives the lung fields a plethoric appearance (see Fig. 15.4).

*Reduced pulmonary flow* may be regional or global. *Regional oligaemia* occurs in emphysema and pulmonary embolism: vascular markings in the affected area are diminished and contrast with the normal vascularity elsewhere in the lung. *Global reduction* occurs in obliterative pulmonary vascular disease (e.g. primary pulmonary hypertension, Eisenmenger's syndrome) and is most marked in the peripheral lung field — peripheral pruning. The main pulmonary artery is always dilated due to long-standing pulmonary hypertension (see Fig. 15.3).

### Increased left atrial pressure

Increased left atrial pressure occurs in mitral valve disease and left ventricular failure and produces a corresponding rise in pulmonary venous and pulmonary capillary pressures. Prominence of the pulmonary veins — most marked in the upper lobes — is an early radiographic sign. As left atrial and pulmonary capillary pressures rise above 18 mmHg, transudation into the lung produces interstitial pulmonary oedema (see Fig. 4.5), characterized by prominence of the interlobular septa, particularly at the lung bases (Kerley B lines). Further rises in pressure lead to alveolar pulmonary oedema, with air-space consolidation in a perihilar ('bat's-wing') distribution (Fig. 3.5).

## Bony abnormalities

Bony abnormalities are unusual in cardiovascular disease, apart from coarctation of the aorta and thoracic outlet syndromes. In coarctation, dilated bronchial collateral vessels erode the inferior aspect of the ribs to

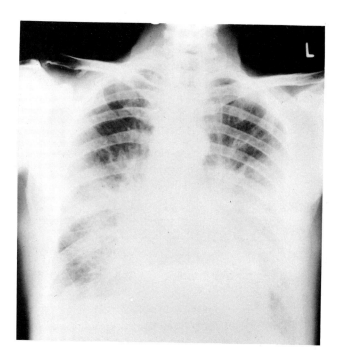

**Fig. 3.5** Alveolar pulmonary oedema. The perihilar 'bat's-wing' distribution of the pulmonary oedema is clearly visible. Small bilateral pleural effusions are also present.

produce notches, although they are rarely present before adolescence (see Fig. 15.15).

Cervical ribs may compress the neurovascular bundle in the thoracic outlet, and special thoracic outlet views are necessary for radiographic diagnosis.

## Echocardiography

Echocardiography is one of the most versatile non-invasive imaging techniques in clinical cardiology. Because it does not utilize ionizing radiation, it is free of known risk and can be used safely throughout pregnancy.

### Principles

A transducer containing a piezoelectric element converts electrical energy into an ultrasound beam, which can be directed towards the heart. The beam is reflected when it strikes an interface between tissues of different density. The reflected ultrasound, or *echo*, is converted back to electrical energy by the piezoelectric element, which permits construction of an image using two basic units of information:

**1** The *intensity* of the echoes, which defines the density difference at tissue interfaces within the heart.

**2** The *time* taken for echoes to arrive back at the transducer, which defines distance from the chest wall.

Density differences within the heart are greatest between the blood-filled chambers and the myocardial and valvular tissues, all of which are clearly visible on the echocardiogram. Because the depth of the myocardial and valvular tissues with respect to the chest wall changes constantly throughout the cardiac cycle, the time taken for echo reflection changes accordingly. Thus, real-time imaging throughout the cardiac cycle provides a dynamic record of cardiac function.

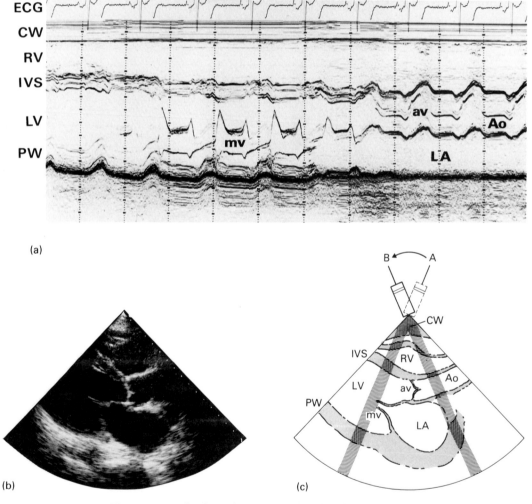

**Fig. 3.6** Normal echocardiogram. (a) The M-mode recording is a sweep from the left ventricular cavity to the ascending aorta and was obtained by angling the transducer through an arc from A to B (c). (b) The two-dimensional recording obtained from the left parasternal area is a long-axis view of the left ventricle as illustrated in (c). CW — chest wall; RV — right ventricle; IVS — interventricular septum; LV — left ventricle; LA — left atrium; PW — posterior wall; mv — mitral valve; av — aortic valve; Ao — aorta.

## M-mode echocardiogram (Fig. 3.6)

This provides a unidimensional 'ice-pick' view through the heart. Continuous recording on light-sensitive paper provides an additional time dimension, thereby permitting appreciation of the dynamic component of the cardiac image. Anteriorly located (right-sided) structures are displayed towards the top of the record and posteriorly located (left-sided) structures are displayed below.

## Two-dimensional echocardiogram (Fig. 3.6)

This provides more detailed information about morphology than the M-mode recording. By projecting a fan of echoes in an arc of up to 80°, a two-dimensional 'slice' through the heart can be obtained, the precise view depending on the location and angulation of the transducer on the chest wall. The most widely used views are shown in Figs 3.6 and 3.7.

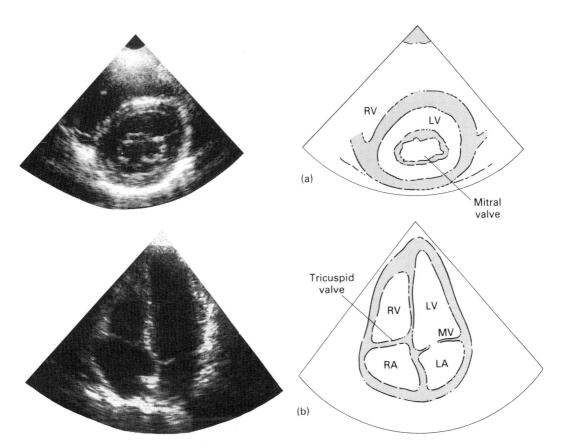

**Fig. 3.7** Normal two-dimensional echocardiogram. (a) A short-axis view through the left ventricle at mitral valve level, obtained from the left parasternal area. (b) A four-chamber view of the heart obtained from the cardiac apex.

Recently available is the *transoesophageal echocardiogram*, in which the transducer is mounted on a probe and positioned in the oesophagus, directly behind the heart. This provides better-quality images because there are no intervening ribs and the probe is closely applied to the posterior aspect of the heart. It is particularly useful for imaging the left atrium, aorta and prosthetic heart valves.

## Clinical applications

### Congenital heart-disease

Echocardiography, particularly the two-dimensional technique, has revolutionized the diagnosis of congenital heart-disease. The relationships of the cardiac chambers and their connections with the great vessels are readily determined. Valvular abnormalities and septal defects can also be recognized. Recent technology has permitted *in utero* fetal imaging for the antenatal diagnosis of cardiac defects.

### Myocardial disease

Echocardiography permits accurate assessment of cardiac dilatation, hypertrophy and contractile function. Congestive cardiomyopathy produces ventricular dilatation with *global* contractile impairment. This must be distinguished from the *regional* contractile impairment which follows myocardial infarction in patients with coronary artery disease. Hypertrophic cardiomyopathy is characterized by thickening (hypertrophy) of the left ventricular myocardium, usually with disproportionate involvement of the interventricular septum (asymmetric septal hypertrophy). In aortic and hypertensive heart-disease, on the other hand, left ventricular hypertrophy is usually symmetrical.

### Valvular disease

Echocardiography is of particular value for identifying both structural and dynamic valvular abnormalities and any associated chamber dilatation or hypertrophy. The severity of valvular involvement in congenital, rheumatic, degenerative and infective disease may thus be defined; the technique is diagnostic of bicuspid aortic valve and mitral valve prolapse, and readily identifies valve thickening and calcification in rheumatic and calcific disease. Vegetations in infective endocarditis can usually be visualized if they are large enough (above 3 mm).

## Pericardial disease

Although the echocardiogram is of little value in constrictive pericarditis, it is the most sensitive technique available for the diagnosis of pericardial effusion. The effusion appears as an echo-free space distributed around the ventricles but usually avoiding the potential space behind the left atrium.

## Other clinical applications

Intracardiac tumours, particularly myxomas and thrombi, are readily visualized by echocardiography, and the transoesophageal instrument has found important application for identifying thrombus in the left atrial appendage. The transoesophageal technique is also helpful for diagnosing aortic disease such as aneurysm and dissection because it provides better views of the aortic arch than are possible with conventional 2D echocardiography.

# Doppler echocardiography

Doppler echocardiography permits evaluation of the direction and velocity of blood flow within the heart and great vessels. The clinical application of this technique has continued to expand, and it is now used widely for measuring the severity of valvular stenosis and for identifying valvular regurgitation and intracardiac shunts through septal defects.

## Principles

According to the Doppler principle, when an ultrasound beam is directed towards the bloodstream the frequency of the ultrasound reflected from the blood cells is altered. The frequency shift or Doppler effect is related to the direction and velocity of flow. If continuous-wave Doppler is used, blood flow at any point along the path of the ultrasound beam is detected, such that a 'clean' Doppler signal from the area of interest may be difficult to obtain. Pulsed Doppler, however, has a range-gating facility which permits frequency sampling from any specific point within the heart, preselected on the echocardiogram. This lends greater precision to the technique. Nevertheless, pulsed Doppler is less able than continuous-wave Doppler to quantitate very high-velocity jets, such as those that occur in aortic stenosis.

The recent introduction of *colour-flow mapping* has been a major technological advance. Instead of the unidirectional ultrasound beam used in continuous-wave and pulsed Doppler imaging, the beam is rotated through an arc. Frequency sampling throughout the arc permits construction of a colour-coded map, red indicating flow towards and blue away from the transducer. Colour-flow data can be superimposed on the standard 2D echocardiogram to identify precisely the patterns of flow within the four chambers of the heart. This simplifies the interpretation of Doppler imaging and provides more useful qualitative data, although it is less useful for quantitative assessment of valve gradients, which requires the precision of the conventional Doppler technique.

## Clinical applications (Fig. 3.8)

In paediatric cardiology, the combination of 2D echocardiography and colour-flow Doppler mapping has made possible the non-invasive diagnosis of the large majority of congenital defects, often without the need for cardiac catheterization. These techniques have also revolutionized the diagnosis of valvular disease in all age-groups. In valvular regurgitation, the retrograde flow that occurs after valve closure is readily detected by Doppler echocardiography, although only an approximate estimate of its severity is possible. In valvular stenosis, peak velocity (as opposed to

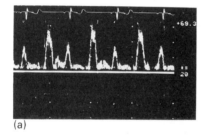
(a)

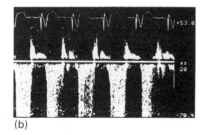
(b)

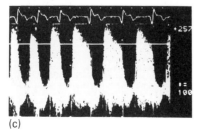
(c)

**Fig. 3.8** Doppler studies of mitral flow. Flow velocity (cm/sec) is represented by the vertical dots according to the scale shown on the right side of each recording. (a) Normal mitral flow shows a biphasic pattern peaking in early diastole immediately after the valve opens and again late in diastole as the left atrium contracts. (b) In mitral regurgitation the normal diastolic flow pattern is preserved, but during systole a high-velocity regurgitant jet is recorded. (c) Mitral stenosis produces a high-velocity jet during diastole. Atrial fibrillation eliminates atrial contraction and ensures complete loss of the normal biphasic flow pattern.

volume) of flow across the valve is directly related to the degree of stenosis. Thus, measurement of Doppler flow velocity (ideally by continuous wave) permits quantification of stenosis by the application of a simple formula.

## Cardiovascular radionuclide imaging

### Principles

All radionuclide techniques require the internal administration of a radioisotope; then the distribution of radioactivity in the area of interest is imaged with a gamma camera. Ideally, the isotope should be distributed homogeneously in that part of the cardiovascular system under investigation: thus, isotopes that remain in the intravascular space during imaging are used for radionuclide angiography. In myocardial perfusion scintigraphy, however, isotopes taken up by the myocardium are required.

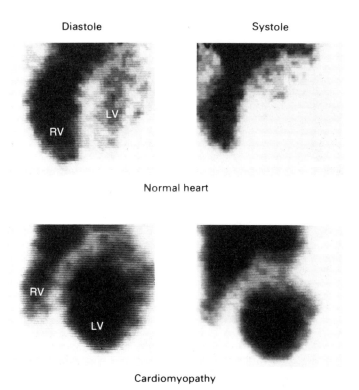

**Fig. 3.9** Radionuclide angiography. The right and left ventricles separated by the interventricular septum are clearly visible. Note that in the normal heart the left ventricular cavity is small and during systole contracts vigorously. In cardiomyopathy the left ventricle is considerably dilated and there is global impairment of contractile function.

Because of their potential toxicity, isotopes with a short half-life are usually used.

## Clinical applications

### Radionuclide angiography

This method is used for assessment of ventricular function. Red cells labelled with technetium-99m are allowed to equilibrate in the blood pool and the heart is then imaged under the gamma camera (Fig. 3.9). The waxing and waning of radioactivity within the ventricular chambers during diastole and systole, respectively, permit construction of a dynamic ventriculogram. Left ventricular contractile function can be evaluated quantitatively, by calculation of ejection fraction, or qualitatively, by observation of wall movement. Global left ventricular impairment is characteristic of cardiomyopathy, while regional defects are seen fol-

Exercise          Rest

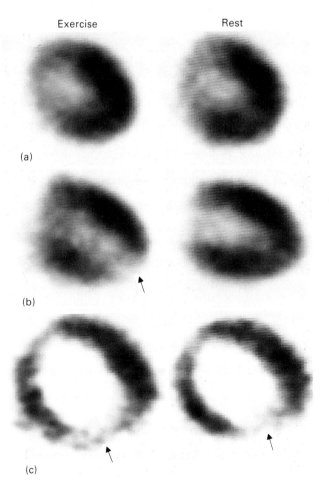

(a)

(b)

(c)

Fig. 3.10 Myocardial perfusion scintigraphy. (a) In the normal LV scintigram there is homogeneous distribution of radioisotope both at peak exercise and at rest (4 hours later). (b) Exercise-induced myocardial ischaemia has produced a reversible perfusion defect (arrowed) towards the apex of the left ventricle, which normalizes during rest. (c) In the patient with myocardial infarction, on the other hand, the perfusion defect of the inferoapical area (arrowed) seen at peak exercise is irreversible and persists during the resting study.

lowing myocardial infarction. Myocardial ischaemia, provoked by exercise or peripheral cold stimulation (cold pressor test), produces reversible regional wall motion abnormalities which are strongly suggestive of coronary artery disease.

### Myocardial perfusion scintigraphy

This method is used for diagnosis of coronary artery disease (Fig. 3.10). The investigation requires a standardized exercise stress test with continuous ECG monitoring in order to provoke myocardial ischaemia in susceptible subjects. Thallium-201 (2–3.5 mCi) is injected intravenously at peak exercise and the heart is imaged under a gamma camera. The isotope is a potassium analogue and distributes homogeneously in normally perfused myocardium, ischaemic or infarcted areas appearing as scintigraphic defects. Repeat imaging after 2–4 hours permits reassessment of scintigraphic defects, those that disappear (reversible defects) indicating areas of exercise-induced ischaemia, those that persist (fixed defects) indicating infarcted myocardium.

### Hot-spot scintigraphy

This method permits diagnosis of acute myocardial infarction but in practice is rarely used (Fig. 3.11). Technetium-99m pyrophosphate is taken up by recently infarcted myocardium, producing a localized 'hot spot' of radioactivity on the scintigram. Diagnostic sensitivity is greatest during the first week following infarction.

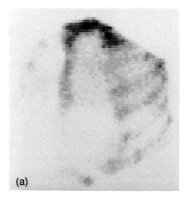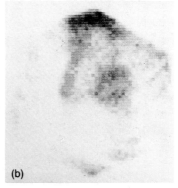

**Fig. 3.11** Hot-spot scintigraphy. Technetium-99m pyrophosphate is taken up by normal bone and in the normal study (a) the ribs are clearly visible. Following myocardial infarction (b) the isotope has localized in the infarcted area of the left ventricle, producing a large 'hot spot', which is clearly visible on the scintigram.

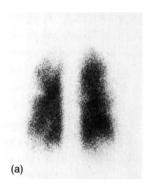 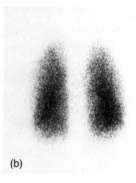

(a)                          (b)

**Fig. 3.12**  Pulmonary ventilation perfusion scintigraphy. In this patient with pulmonary emboli, there are multiple defects visible on the perfusion scan (a). The ventilation scan (b) is entirely normal. Ventilation–perfusion mismatch is highly specific for pulmonary embolism.

### Pulmonary scintigraphy

This method is used for the diagnosis of pulmonary embolism (Fig. 3.12). Technetium-99m-labelled microspheres, injected intravenously, become trapped within the pulmonary capillaries. The normal pulmonary perfusion scintigram shows homogeneous distribution of radioactivity throughout both lung fields. Pulmonary embolism causes regional impairment of pulmonary flow, which results in a perfusion defect of the scintigram; however, the appearance is non-specific and occurs in many other pulmonary disorders, particularly chronic obstructive pulmonary disease. Specificity is enhanced by simultaneous ventilation scintigraphy. Inhaled xenon-133 is distributed homogeneously throughout the normal lung and, in pulmonary embolism (unlike other pulmonary disorders), distribution remains homogeneous. Thus, a scintigraphic perfusion defect not matched by a ventilation defect is highly specific for pulmonary embolism.

## Computed tomography

### Principles

Computed tomography (CT) measures the attenuation of X-rays after they traverse body tissues (Fig. 3.13). Attenuation is greatest for tissues such as bone, which are relatively radio-opaque, and least for tissues such as lung or fat, which are relatively radiotranslucent. From X-ray attenuation measurements, taken as a sensor rotates around the chest, cross-sectional images are constructed. Image resolution is excellent and contrast injection into a peripheral vein provides adequate opacification of the blood pool for identification of intracardiac structures. Until recently, however, the clinical application of CT in cardiology has been limited by image-acquisition times of up to 5 sec, during which the constant motion of the heart leads to image degradation. The new generation of ultrafast CT

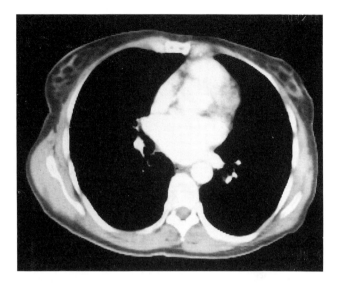

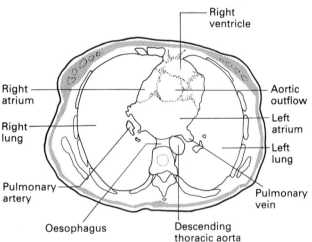

**Fig. 3.13** Computed tomography. A normal thoracic tomogram at left atrial level is shown. The vascular spaces have been enhanced by the injection of contrast medium into the bloodstream.

scanners (with image-acquisition times of less than 1 sec) are now available, and are expected to have a more useful clinical role, with the capacity to provide very high-resolution cardiac images in both static and video mode, and also measurements of blood flow by the application of indicator dilution principles.

## Clinical applications

CT (with contrast enhancement) is widely used for the non-invasive diagnosis of aortic dissection, when two contrast columns separated by an intimal flap can be clearly seen. It is also used for accurate assessment of pericardial thickness in constrictive disease and diagnosis of cardiac tumours. Additional applications of ultrafast CT include the evaluation of graft patency following coronary bypass surgery, analysis of ventricular wall motion, and blood flow quantification in congenital heart-disease, permitting dynamic assessment of shunts and other defects.

## *Magnetic resonance imaging*

### *Principles*

Magnetic resonance imaging (MRI) utilizes the fact that certain nuclei with an intrinsic spin generate magnetic fields and behave like tiny bar magnets. Placed in a magnetic field, these nuclei align and adopt a resonant frequency that is unique to that nucleus and the strength of the magnetic field. If the nuclei are exposed to pulsed radiowaves of that frequency, they resonate and release energy, which allows the location of the nucleus to be determined.

For imaging purposes, the patient lies in a strong magnetic field, which is artificially graded. The hydrogen protons of fat and water are imaged and, on exposure to pulsed radiowaves, they resonate at different frequencies in different parts of the imaging zone. Analysis of the emitted frequencies permits construction of tomographic and three-dimensional images of the heart. If data acquisition is gated to a specific part of the cardiac cycle, motion artefact is eliminated and excellent image resolution can be obtained.

### *Clinical applications*

Potential applications include coronary artery imaging, without the need for contrast material, identification of histological and metabolic disorders of the myocardium, and assessment of myocardial perfusion, using paramagnetic contrast agents. The realization of this exciting potential will ensure an important role for MRI in clinical cardiology.

## **Cardiac catheterization**

Catheters introduced into an artery or vein may be directed into the left or right sides of the heart, respectively. Vascular access is usually percutaneous, using the femoral vessels, or by surgical cut-down, using the antecubital vessels. Originally developed for diagnostic purposes, catheter techniques are now being used increasingly for the interventional management of cardiovascular disease.

### *Diagnostic catheterization*

Catheters introduced into the heart or great vessels are used both for the delivery of radiographic contrast medium (angiography) and for measurement of pressure within the chambers of the heart and cardiac output. The use of catheter techniques in the diagnosis of arrhythmias is discussed in Chapter 11.

## Cardiac angiography

Four diagnostic investigations account for the majority of angiographic procedures:
1  Aortic root angiography.
2  Left ventricular angiography.
3  Coronary arteriography.
4  Pulmonary arteriography.

For coronary arteriography, relatively small volumes of contrast (5–8 ml) injected manually are used but, for other angiographic procedures, much larger amounts (up to 50 ml), introduced by power injection, are required. The images are usually recorded on high-speed cine film, to provide a dynamic record of ventricular wall movement, blood flow and intravascular anatomy. Digital subtraction techniques permit reductions

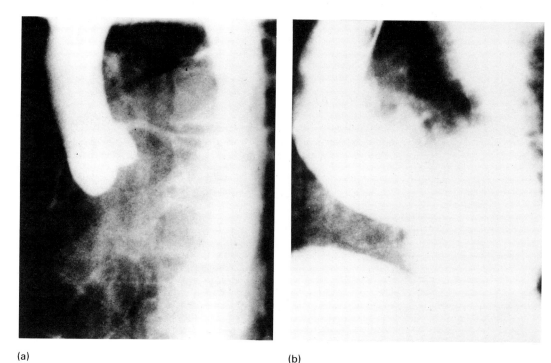

(a) (b)

**Fig. 3.14** Aortic root angiography. Contrast medium has been injected into the ascending aorta. (a) A normal study. (b) Aortic regurgitation causes dilatation of the ascending aorta and opacification of the left ventricle due to diastolic backflow through the diseased aortic valve.

in contrast volume but have, at present, only a limited role in cardio-vascular angiographic diagnosis (see below).

### Aortic root angiography

Contrast injection into the aortic root demonstrates the vascular anatomy in suspected aneurysm or dissection, and also permits evaluation of aortic

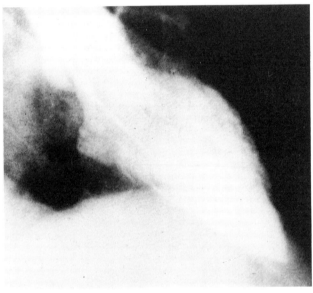

(a)

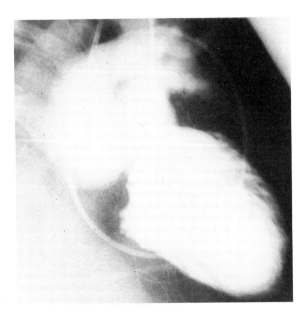

(b)

**Fig. 3.15** Left ventricular angiography. Contrast medium has been injected into the left ventricle. (a) A normal study. (b) Mitral regurgitation causes left ventricular dilatation and opacification of the left atrium due to systolic backflow through the diseased valve.

valve function (Fig. 3.14). The normal aortic valve prevents diastolic backflow of contrast, but in aortic regurgitation variable opacification of the left ventricle occurs, depending on the severity of the valve lesion.

### Left ventricular angiography

Contrast injection into the left ventricle defines ventricular anatomy and wall motion, and also permits evaluation of mitral valve function (Fig. 3.15). Dilatation of the ventricle and contractile dysfunction occur in left ventricular failure. Exaggerated contractile function with systolic obliteration of the cavity occurs in hypertrophic cardiomyopathy. Filling defects within the ventricular lumen may indicate thrombus or neoplasm. The normal mitral valve prevents systolic backflow of contrast into the left atrium, but in mitral regurgitation variable atrial opacification occurs, depending on the severity of the valve lesion.

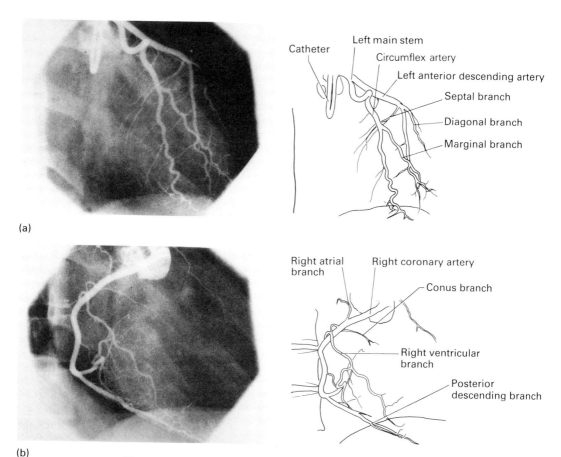

(a)

(b)

**Fig. 3.16**   Contrast medium has been injected into the left (a) and right (b) coronary arteries. These are normal coronary arteriograms.

### Coronary arteriography

This is the only reliable technique for diagnostic imaging of the coronary arteries. It requires selective injection of contrast into the left and right coronary arteries (Fig. 3.16) and multiple views in different projections are necessary for a complete study. Intraluminal filling defects or occlusions indicate coronary artery disease, which is nearly always caused by atherosclerosis.

### Pulmonary arteriography

Injection of contrast medium into the main pulmonary artery opacifies the arterial branches throughout both lung fields. The normal flow distribution is homogeneous. Vascular occlusions with regional perfusion defects usually indicate pulmonary thromboembolism (particularly when intraluminal filling defects are present) but may also occur in advanced emphysema.

### Digital subtraction angiography

This employs computerized subtraction of the background image so that only the contrast medium in the heart and great vessels stands out. Its most enthusiastic proponents hoped this would permit high-resolution imaging with injection of contrast into a peripheral vein without the need for cardiac catheterization. However, this has proved unrealistic because, although contrast resolution is increased, contrast delivery to the area of interest is severely diminished and spatial resolution is poor. At present, therefore, the intravenous digital subtraction technique is useful only for imaging large and relatively static arteries such as the aortic arch (for diagnosis of coarctation) and the carotid arteries. It also has a limited role in determining the patency of coronary bypass grafts since these are not subject to the motion artefact of the native coronary system.

## *Interventional catheterization*

Interventional catheterization represents one of the most exciting fields in the treatment of cardiovascular disease and has found important application in paediatric and adult practice, often extending the role of the cardiologist into areas that were once exclusively surgical. The earliest example was the insertion of electrode-tipped catheters into the heart for pacing patients with bradyarrhythmias (see p. 219). Pacing technology has now reached a high level of sophistication and the interventional management of arrhythmias has expanded to include treatment of resistant tachyarrhythmias by overdrive pacing and, more recently, by the electrical ablation of conducting tissue with catheters placed strategically within the heart (see p. 249). Balloon angioplasty is a catheter technique used widely for treatment of coronary artery disease (see p. 115), particularly when medical treatment fails to control symptoms. Balloon valvuloplasty has found more limited application in adult cardiology, but in paediatric practice is the treatment of choice for congenital pulmonary stenosis (see p. 318). The insertion of obstructors for closure of patent ductus arteriosus, using specially adapted catheters, represents a recent advance that is reducing the requirement for surgery in young children (see p. 310), while in neonates with transposition of the great arteries the emergency Rashkind procedure is potentially life-saving (see p. 320).

## Intracardiac pressure measurement

Cardiac catheterization for measurement of blood flow and pressure within the heart and great vessels is used widely both for diagnostic purposes and to guide treatment (Fig. 3.17). The fluid-filled catheter is attached to a pressure transducer, which converts the pressure waves into electrical signals. For measurement of right-sided pressures, the catheter is directed by the venous route into the right atrium and then advanced through the right ventricle into the pulmonary artery. For measurement of left-sided pressures, the catheter is directed by the arterial route into the ascending aorta and advanced retrogradely through the aortic valve into the left ventricle. Because access to the left atrium is technically difficult,

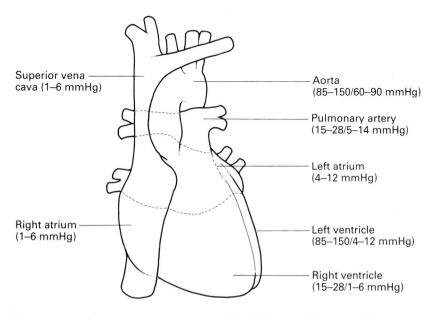

Superior vena cava (1–6 mmHg)

Aorta (85–150/60–90 mmHg)

Pulmonary artery (15–28/5–14 mmHg)

Left atrium (4–12 mmHg)

Right atrium (1–6 mmHg)

Left ventricle (85–150/4–12 mmHg)

Right ventricle (15–28/1–6 mmHg)

**Fig. 3.17** Normal pressure measurements within the heart and great vessels.

left atrial pressure is usually measured indirectly using the pulmonary artery wedge pressure. The pulmonary artery wedge pressure is obtained during the right heart catheterization by advancing the catheter distally into the pulmonary arterial tree until the tip wedges in a small branch. Alternatively, a catheter with a preterminal balloon (Swan–Ganz catheter) may be used. Inflation of the balloon in the pulmonary artery causes the catheter tip to be carried with blood flow into a more distal branch, which becomes occluded by the balloon. Regardless of which method is used, the wedge pressure recorded at the catheter tip is a more or less accurate measure of the left atrial pressure, transmitted retrogradely through the pulmonary veins and capillaries.

## Haemodynamic evaluation of valvular stenosis

In the normal heart there is no pressure gradient across an open valve. Such a gradient usually indicates valvular stenosis (Fig. 3.18) and, as stenosis worsens, the pressure gradient increases. This therefore provides a useful index of the severity of stenosis. However, it must be recognized that the pressure gradient is itself influenced by the flow through the valve. For example, if output is very low, the gradient may be small despite the presence of severe stenosis. This applies particularly to the aortic valve because flow velocity is normally high.

## Haemodynamic evaluation of intracardiac shunts

Left-to-right intracardiac shunts through atrial or ventricular septal defects introduce 'arterialized' blood into the right side of the heart. This results in an abrupt increase or step-up in the oxygen saturation of venous blood at the level of the shunt, which can be detected by right heart catheterization. Thus, by drawing serial blood samples for oxygen saturation from

**Table 3.1**  Oxygen saturation within the heart and great vessels. Representative values for the normal heart and for patients with a left-to-right shunt are shown

|  | Normal (%) | Sinus venosus defect (%) | Secundum atrial septal defect (%) | Ventricular septal defect (%) | Patent ductus arteriosus (%) |
|---|---|---|---|---|---|
| SVC | 75 | 85 | 75 | 75 | 75 |
| RA | 75 | 85 | 85 | 75 | 75 |
| IVC | 75 | 75 | 75 | 75 | 75 |
| RV | 75 | 85 | 85 | 85 | 75 |
| PA | 75 | 85 | 85 | 85 | 85 |
| LV | 95 | 95 | 95 | 95 | 95 |

SVC, superior vena cava; RA, right atrium; IVC, inferior vena cava; RV, right ventricle; PA, pulmonary artery; LV, left ventricle

the pulmonary artery, right ventricle, right atrium and venae cavae, the shunt may be localized to the site at which the step-up in oxygen saturation occurs (Table 3.1). The magnitude of the step-up is related to the size of the shunt but precise quantification of the shunt requires measurement of pulmonary and systemic blood flow. The extent to which the pulmonary–systemic flow ratio exceeds 1 is a measure of the size of the shunt.

## Measurement of cardiac output

Cardiac output is usually measured by application of the Fick principle. A Swan–Ganz catheter with a right atrial portal and a terminal thermistor is positioned in the pulmonary artery. A known volume of cold saline (usually 10 ml) is injected into the right atrium and the temperature reduction in the pulmonary artery is recorded at the thermistor. The contour of the cooling curve is dependent upon cardiac output, which is calculated by measurement of the area under the curve, using a bedside computer.

A relatively simple non-invasive measure of cardiac output can be obtained by Doppler echocardiography, using the 'area–length' method. Thus, the length of the column of blood ejected by the left ventricle during a single beat is obtained by multiplying the Doppler aortic flow velocity (cm/sec) by the ejection time (sec). The length of the column of blood is then multiplied by the echocardiographic cross-sectional area of the aorta to yield stroke volume (ml/beat). Cardiac output is the product of stroke volume and heart rate.

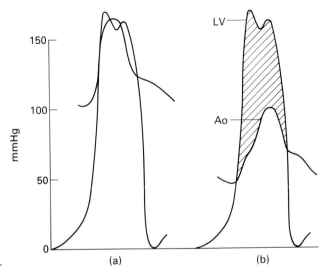

**Fig. 3.18** Valvular stenosis. Simultaneous measurements of the aortic and left ventricular pressure signals are shown. Note that during systole there is no pressure gradient across the normal aortic valve (a) and the pressure signals are superimposed. Aortic stenosis (b) causes a pressure gradient (shaded area) across the aortic valve throughout systole.

## Further reading

Anonymous. Thallium scintigraphy for diagnosis and risk assessment in coronary artery disease. *Lancet* 1991, **338**, 1424–5

Brundage B.H. (ed.). *Comparative Cardiac Imaging: Function, Flow, Anatomy, and Quantitation*. Rockville, Maryland, Aspen, 1990.

Hart G. Biomagnetometry: imaging the heart's magnetic field. *Br. Heart J.* 1991, **65**, 61–2.

Matsuzaki M., Toma Y. and Kusukawa R. Clinical applications of transesophageal echocardiography. *Circulation* 1990, **82**, 709–22.

Mendel D. and Oldershaw P. (eds). *A Practice of Cardiac Catheterisation*, 3rd edn. Oxford, Blackwell Scientific Publications, 1986.

Monaghan M.J. and Mills P.G. Doppler colour flow mapping: technology in search of an application. *Br. Heart J.* 1989, **61**, 133–8.

Pearlman A.S. Transesophageal echocardiography: sound diagnostic technique or two-edged sword. *N. Engl. J. Med.* 1991, **324**, 841–3.

Pohost G.M. and Henzlova M.J. The value of thallium-201 imaging. *N. Engl. J. Med.* 1990, **323**, 190–2.

Popp R.L. Medical progress: echocardiography. *N. Engl. J. Med.* 1990, **323**, 101–9 and 179–83.

Ritter S.B. Transesophageal echocardiography in children: new peephole to the heart. *J. Am. Coll. Cardiol.* 1990, **16**, 447–50.

Rubens M.B. Chest X-ray in adult heart disease. In Julian D.G., Camm A.J., Fox K.M., Hall R.J.C. and Poole-Wilson P.A. (eds), *Diseases of the Heart*. London, Baillière Tindall, 1989, pp. 254–87.

Simpson I.A. and Camm A.J. Colour Doppler flow mapping. *Br. Med. J.* 1990, **300**, 1–2.

Van der Wall E.E., de Roos A., van Voorthuisen A.E. and Bruschke A.V.G. Magnetic resonance imaging: a new approach for evaluating coronary artery disease? *Am. Heart J.* 1991, **121**, 1203–20.

# 4 Heart Failure

## Summary

Heart failure, in which cardiac output is inadequate for the perfusion requirements of metabolizing tissues, usually reflects left ventricular disease caused by previous myocardial infarction or hypertension. Compensatory physiological responses, directed at maintaining cardiac output and blood-pressure, include activation of the sympathoadrenal and renin–angiotensin systems and left ventricular (LV) dilatation and hypertrophy. In acute heart failure, only sympathoadrenal mechanisms are available to support the circulation, and sharp increments in atrial pressures and reductions in output commonly lead to pulmonary oedema and peripheral hypoperfusion. Chronic heart failure advances more slowly, providing time for compensatory ventricular dilatation and hypertrophy. It is characterized by fluid retention and peripheral hypoperfusion, expressed clinically as oedema, exertional dyspnoea and fatigue. Diagnosis is usually clear on clinical grounds, but identification of the underlying cause often requires additional tests, of which the echocardiogram is most useful. Treatment is aimed at reversing the underlying cause, correcting symptoms and improving prognosis. Diuretics are the first-line drugs but, as dyspnoea and fatigue get worse, addition of an angiotensin-converting enzyme (ACE) inhibitor helps control symptoms and may also improve prognosis. Digoxin controls the ventricular rate in atrial fibrillation but for patients in sinus rhythm is now only recommended if heart failure is severe and unresponsive to diuretics and ACE inhibitors. Once heart failure has become this severe, however, prognosis is poor and heart transplantation becomes the only treatment likely to provide long-term benefit.

## Introduction

Heart failure is a syndrome in which a cardiac disorder prevents the delivery of sufficient output to meet the perfusion requirements of metabolizing tissues. This definition is not all-embracing, but it serves to emphasize that the role of the heart is to drive the circulation. Any disturbance of ventricular function that undermines this role may result in heart failure.

Heart failure is common, with an estimated prevalence in the UK of at least 0.4%, rising to nearly 3% in those aged over 65. It is an important cause of morbidity and mortality, accounting for 5% of all adult hospital

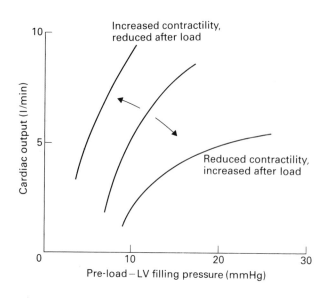

**Fig. 4.1**  Ventricular function curves. These are Starling curves, which define the relation between preload and cardiac output. Because changes in contractility and afterload have an independent influence on ventricular function, a 'family' of Starling curves may be constructed, as shown in this figure. Note that as ventricular function improves in response to increments in contractility or reductions in afterload the contour of the function curve becomes steeper. Deteriorating ventricular function, on the other hand, is associated with a flatter ventricular function curve such that changes in preload have a relatively small effect on cardiac output.

admissions and carrying a 2-year mortality of between 20 and 75%, depending on its severity.

## Determinants of ventricular function

Cardiac output is the product of heart rate and stroke volume. Heart rate is under autonomic control and reflects the balance of sympathetic and parasympathetic influence on the sinus node. Stroke volume is determined by the interaction of preload, afterload and contractility (Fig. 4.1).

### *Preload*

Changes in ventricular preload produce directionally similar changes in stroke volume. Preload refers to the passive stretch (or tension) of the ventricular myocardium at end-diastole and is equivalent to end-diastolic volume. Because end-diastolic volume is largely pressure-dependent, ventricular end-diastolic pressure or atrial pressure (collectively termed ventricular filling pressures) is widely used as a measure of preload. The curvilinear relation between preload and stroke volume (as described by Starling) provides a useful means of evaluating ventricular function (Fig. 4.1).

Although ventricular filling pressures provide a convenient measure of preload, the effect of compliance must not be overlooked. Thus, the hypertrophied non-compliant ventricle requires a higher filling pressure to produce the same end-diastolic volume (or preload) as the normally compliant ventricle (Fig. 4.2).

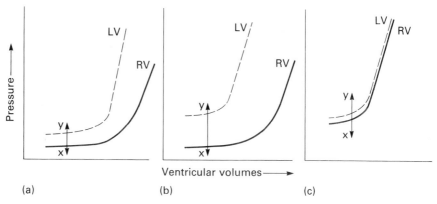

Pressure→

Ventricular volumes→

(a)        (b)        (c)

**Fig. 4.2**   Ventricular pressure–volume ('compliance') curves. (a) The normal heart. The RV curve lies below the LV curve because the pressure X required to fill the thin-walled RV in diastole is considerably lower than the pressure Y required to fill the thick-walled LV to the same volume. (b) Reduced LV compliance. This is usually caused by LV hypertrophy in patients with hypertension, aortic stenosis or hypertrophic cardiomyopathy. The LV diastolic pressure Y must rise considerably to maintain adequate filling. RV diastolic pressure is unaffected. (c) Reduced LV and RV compliance. Tamponade, constrictive pericarditis or restrictive cardiomyopathy usually impedes the diastolic filling of both ventricles equally. Thus, diastolic pressures of both ventricles (X and Y) rise and equilibrate to maintain adequate filling.

## Afterload

Changes in ventricular afterload produce directionally opposite changes in stroke volume (Fig. 4.1). Afterload is the systolic wall tension developed by the ventricle to expel blood against vascular resistance. It is a function of ventricular pressure and volume and is defined by the law of Laplace:

Ventricular wall tension = ventricular pressure × ventricular radius

Clinically, afterload is equated with systolic pressure, but the contribution of ventricular radius should not be overlooked. Thus, as the failing heart dilates, afterload (as well as preload) increases.

## Contractility

Changes in ventricular contractility produce directionally similar changes in stroke volume (Fig. 4.1). Contractility is not easily measured and the term is usually used qualitatively to describe the inherent force and velocity of ventricular contraction, independent of preload and afterload.

## Measurement of ventricular function

### Ejection fraction

Left ventricular function is usually assessed qualitatively by observation of wall motion and cavity size during dynamic imaging. Any of the major imaging techniques, e.g. echocardiography, radionuclide angiography, contrast ventriculography, are suitable for this purpose. These techniques may also be used for the quantitative assessment of left ventricular function by measurement of the ejection fraction, the fraction of left ventricular blood volume expelled per beat:

$$\text{Ejection fraction} = \frac{\text{end-diastolic volume} - \text{end-systolic volume}}{\text{end-diastolic volume}}$$

At rest, the lower limit of normal for the left ventricular ejection fraction is 55%, but during exercise it increases considerably and may exceed 90%. Failure of the ejection fraction to increase normally dur-

**Table 4.1**  Causes of heart failure

| Ventricular pathophysiology | Clinical examples | Ventricle predominantly affected | | |
|---|---|---|---|---|
| | | Left | Right | Both |
| **1** Restricted filling | Mitral stenosis | ● | | |
| | Tricuspid stenosis | | ● | |
| | Constrictive pericarditis | | ● | |
| | Tamponade | | ● | |
| | Restrictive cardiomyopathy | | | ● |
| | Hypertrophic cardiomyopathy | ● | | |
| **2** Pressure loading | Hypertension | ● | | |
| | Aortic stenosis | ● | | |
| | Coarctation of the aorta | ● | | |
| | Pulmonary vascular disease | | ● | |
| | Pulmonary embolism | | ● | |
| | Pulmonary stenosis | | ● | |
| **3** Volume loading | Mitral regurgitation | ● | | |
| | Aortic regurgitation | ● | | |
| | Pulmonary regurgitation | | ● | |
| | Tricuspid regurgitation | | ● | |
| | Ventricular septal defect | ● | | |
| | Patent ductus arteriosus | ● | | |
| **4** Contractile impairment | Coronary artery disease | ● | | |
| | Dilated cardiomyopathy | | | ● |
| | Myocarditis | | | ● |
| **5** Arrhythmia | Severe bradycardia | | | ● |
| | Severe tachycardia | | | ● |

ing exercise indicates left ventricular impairment, usually caused by ischaemia or by an intrinsic defect of contractile function. Thus, exercise stress may be used as a provocative test to unmask left ventricular impairment in the patient with a normal resting ejection fraction. Exercise stress is usually applied during radionuclide angiography, which allows sequential measurements of the ejection fraction following a single injection of isotope.

## Starling relation

Measurement of left atrial pressure (as reflected by pulmonary artery wedge pressure) and cardiac output provides a simple means of evaluating left ventricular function, and is widely used in the intensive care unit. Abnormal elevation of the wedge pressure with a normal or low cardiac output indicates downward displacement of the Starling curve and left ventricular dysfunction. However, these measurements do not define the cause of left ventricular dysfunction, which may result from restricted filling, excessive afterload or myocardial contractile impairment.

## Aetiology

### Low-output heart failure

Cardiac disorders produce heart failure by one or more of the following mechanisms (Table 4.1):
1   Restriction of ventricular filling.
2   Imposition of excessive load on the ventricle (volume or pressure).
3   Impairment of myocardial contractile function.

*Restriction of ventricular filling* is the principal cause of heart failure in mitral stenosis, where the left ventricle itself is entirely normal. It is also important in hypertrophic and restrictive cardiomyopathy and constrictive pericarditis, where there may be no intrinsic impairment of systolic function, but diastolic filling (or preload) is impaired by the stiff non-compliant ventricle (cardiomyopathy) or the diseased pericardium (constriction), resulting in depressed cardiac output (Fig. 4.2).

*Excessive loading* may be caused by pressure or volume, which have their major effects on afterload and preload, respectively. It is important to distinguish between the effects of acute and chronic loading. In acute pressure loading (e.g. pulmonary embolism), heart failure is a direct result of the sudden increase in afterload, which depresses stroke volume. Similarly, acute volume loading (e.g. valvular regurgitation in endocarditis) produces heart failure by overwhelming the Starling reserve of the ventricle. However, in chronic pressure or volume-loading compensatory mechanisms may protect against heart failure for prolonged periods (see below). Finally, myocardial contractile function deteriorates to the point that the ventricle can no longer tolerate the extra load.

*Ventricular contractile dysfunction* is the primary cause of heart failure in dilated cardiomyopathy. The Starling curve is displaced downwards and is flattened in contour, such that changes in filling pressure produce relatively small changes in cardiac output (see Fig. 4.1). In myocardial infarction, regional loss of contractile tissue reduces effective muscle mass, which has a similar effect on the Starling curve, and the dyskinetic ventricular contraction pattern further reduces pump efficiency. Chronic pressure and volume-loading ultimately lead to ventricular contractile dysfunction, as compensatory mechanisms fail to preserve cardiac output.

## High-output heart failure

In certain situations, the perfusion requirements of tissue metabolism cannot be met, despite considerable increments in cardiac output above the normal range. This is termed high-output heart failure. There are three major causes:

**1**  Chronic elevation of metabolic rate, e.g. thyrotoxicosis.
**2**  Reduced oxygen-carrying capacity of the blood, e.g. anaemia.
**3**  Arteriovenous shunting, which reduces the fraction of cardiac output delivered to the tissues, e.g. arteriovenous fistula, beriberi, Paget's disease.

Heart failure is a rare consequence of these disorders and, when it occurs, the mechanisms are often complex. Nevertheless, chronic volume

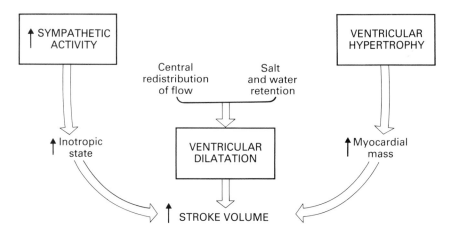

**Fig. 4.3**  Compensatory physiology in heart failure.

overload is an important factor because of the long-term requirement for increased output.

## Pathophysiology

### *Compensatory mechanisms*

Compensatory mechanisms in heart failure attempt to maintain cardiac output and blood pressure in the face of abnormal loading and contractile impairment. There are three major mechanisms (Fig. 4.3):

1  Neurohumoral activation.
2  Ventricular dilatation.
3  Ventricular hypertrophy.

The principal neurohumoral response is sympathoadrenal activation. This is immediately available when ventricular pump function is threatened, but ventricular dilatation and hypertrophy take longer to develop. Thus, an acute cardiac lesion is less well tolerated than a lesion of similar severity that has developed slowly. Nevertheless, even in chronic disease, the mechanisms that protect against heart failure are of limited potential and do not always prevent decompensation occurring.

### *Neurohumoral activation*

#### Sympathoadrenal system

Sympathetic stimulation of cardiac beta-1-adrenoceptors improves ventricular function by increasing heart rate and contractility. In addition, constriction of venous capacitance vessels by adrenergic pathways redistributes flow centrally, and the increased venous return to the heart further augments ventricular function by the Starling mechanism. To some extent, these beneficial effects are modified by arteriolar constriction in the skin, gut and kidneys, the vascular beds that respond most vigorously to sympathetic stimulation. Although this helps maintain blood-pressure, the increase in afterload tends to depress ventricular function. Moreover, the responsiveness of the heart to chronic adrenergic stimulation becomes attenuated due to reduction in both the density of cardiac adrenoceptors and their sensitivity to catecholamines (*receptor down-regulation*). Depletion of cardiac noradrenaline stores contributes to this process.

#### Renin–angiotensin system

Activation of the renin–angiotensin system may be trivial in mild heart failure, but in moderate to severe disease it plays an important role.

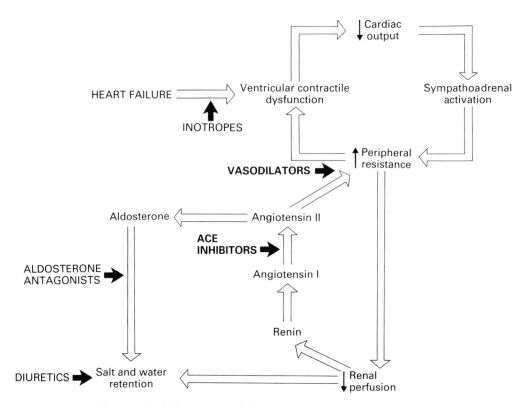

**Fig. 4.4** The kidney in heart failure. Note the vicious circle of falling cardiac output, increasing peripheral resistance and stimulation of angiotensin secretion. The effects of specific anti-failure treatment are shown. Only ACE inhibitors and vasodilators, however, have the potential to break the vicious circle.

Reduced renal perfusion and heightened sympathetic activity are the major stimuli for renin release from the juxtaglomerular apparatus of the kidney, although additional stimulus is provided by some of the drugs commonly used to treat heart failure, particularly diuretics and vasodilators. Renin is the rate-limiting enzyme in the synthesis of angiotensin II, a potent vasoconstrictor, which also stimulates aldosterone secretion from the adrenal gland. Angiotensin II-mediated vasoconstriction helps support the blood-pressure, while the action of aldosterone on the distal nephron stimulates salt and water retention, which further increases ventricular filling and maintains cardiac output by the Starling mechanism. However, the compensatory potential of the renin–angiotensin system is limited. Vasoconstriction adds significantly to left ventricular afterload, exacerbating contractile dysfunction. This further reduces renal perfusion, thereby establishing a vicious circle of increasing renin–angiotensin II production and deteriorating ventricular function (Fig. 4.4). Moreover, as salt and water retention increases, peripheral and pulmonary congestion cause oedema and contribute to dyspnoea.

**Antidiuretic hormone (vasopressin)**

Circulating levels of this vasoconstrictor are also increased in heart failure. Compensatory benefits of blood-pressure support and increased ventricular filling must be set against the long-term adverse effects of increased afterload, renal hypoperfusion and fluid retention.

**Atrial natriuretic peptide**

Circulating levels of this recently identified peptide are increased in heart failure, although its precise role remains uncertain. Nevertheless, it has potentially useful properties, including vasodilatation, salt and water diuresis and inhibition of renin and aldosterone secretion. Thus, it has the potential to modify the adverse consequences of renin–angiotensin activation.

## Ventricular dilatation

When the heart is volume-loaded, it dilates and ventricular contraction increases by the Starling mechanism. Thus, the dilatation that occurs in valvular incompetence allows 'forward' output to be maintained, despite the regurgitant volume of blood. Dilatation also occurs in myocardial disease, due to central redistribution of venous blood and expansion of plasma volume. The increase in preload helps maintain stroke volume. Once heart failure is established, the compensatory effects of cardiac dilatation become limited by associated increments in afterload (law of Laplace) and by the flattened contour of the Starling curve, which diminishes the responsiveness of the ventricle to increasing preload. Ultimately, rising left ventricular filling pressure may lead to pulmonary oedema, further destabilizing the circulation.

## Ventricular hypertrophy

Excessive ventricular loading stimulates myocardial hypertrophy, which augments the mass of contractile tissue and enables the heart to sustain the extra burden. Hypertrophy is most marked in the pressure-loaded ventricle (e.g. hypertension, aortic stenosis), when additional sarcomeres are laid down in parallel, producing significant increments in wall thickness. Nevertheless, hypertrophy also occurs in the volume-loaded ventricle (e.g. valvular regurgitation), but additional sarcomeres are laid down in series as the ventricle dilates, so that wall thickness remains close to normal, despite an overall increase in myocardial mass. Hypertrophy takes time to develop and acute overloading is not well tolerated. Moreover, in established myocardial hypertrophy, there is an intrinsic defect in ventricular function, affecting both systole and diastole, and, as loading increases, pump function deteriorates. Thus, like all the major compensatory mechanisms, hypertrophy has only limited potential to protect against the development of heart failure.

### The kidney in heart failure (Fig. 4.4)

The kidney plays a central role in the salt and water retention characterizing congestive heart failure. A significant reduction in glomerular filtration occurs early during heart failure, often before symptoms develop. This is caused by constriction of the preglomerular arterioles in response to increased sympathetic activity and angiotensin II production. The reduction in glomerular filtration inevitably reduces sodium delivery to the nephron, but this provides only a partial explanation for salt and water retention in heart failure. Increased sodium reabsorption from the nephron is the more important factor. This occurs particularly in the proximal tubule in the early stages of the heart failure, but, as failure worsens, the effects of aldosterone on sodium reabsorption in the distal nephron predominate. Ultimately, feedback regulation of salt and water balance breaks down completely, due to suppression of atrial natriuretic peptide and inappropriate antidiuretic hormone secretion. This produces intractable plasma volume overload and dilutional hyponatraemia.

### Oedema in heart failure

In heart failure, oedema is the result of increased capillary hydrostatic pressure. This drives fluid into the interstitial space at a rate which exceeds the combined effects of osmotic reabsorption and the clearing capacity of the lymphatic system.

#### Pulmonary oedema

Pulmonary oedema occurs in left heart failure. The pulmonary veins and capillaries are in continuity with the left atrium and therefore increments in left atrial pressure produce a similar increase in pulmonary capillary pressure. As left atrial pressure rises above 18–20 mmHg, pulmonary oedema develops. In acute left heart failure, the increase is due largely to sympathetically mediated central redistribution of flow. However, in chronic left heart failure, plasma volume overload secondary to salt and water retention is the more important mechanism.

#### Systemic oedema

This occurs in right heart failure and always reflects plasma volume overload secondary to salt and water retention. The effect of gravity on capillary hydrostatic pressure ensures that dependent parts of the body are particularly prone to oedema formation. With worsening plasma volume overload, oedema of the abdominal viscera and ascites develop. Hepatic engorgement may lead to impaired synthesis of plasma proteins, which exacerbates oedema formation by reducing capillary osmotic pressure.

## Clinical manifestations

Minor impairment of cardiac function may remain asymptomatic but, as compensatory mechanisms become overwhelmed, the clinical manifestations of heart failure emerge. These relate principally to the consequences of elevated atrial pressures and reduced cardiac output, expressed clinically as congestion and peripheral hypoperfusion, respectively. Increased sympathetic activity also plays an important role. Manifestations of left and right heart failure are conveniently considered separately, although they often occur together, resulting in *congestive heart failure.*

### *Acute left heart failure*

This is a medical emergency, usually caused by myocardial infarction, although other causes include acute aortic and mitral regurgitation, fulminant myocarditis and mitral stenosis. Pulmonary oedema and systemic hypoperfusion are invariable and the patient becomes abruptly dyspnoeic and may expectorate pink, frothy oedema fluid. Central cyanosis, hypotension and oliguria occur and in severe cases cardiogenic shock develops (see p. 97).

### *Chronic left heart failure*

This is usually the result of left ventricular failure caused by ischaemic, hypertensive, cardiomyopathic or valvular disease. In mitral stenosis, however, left ventricular contractile function is normal and heart failure is due to impaired left ventricular filling. Elevated left atrial pressure produces orthopnoea and, in advanced cases, paroxysmal nocturnal dyspnoea (see p. 3). More troublesome is exertional dyspnoea, causes of which are complex but include exertional elevations of left atrial pressure, respiratory muscle fatigue and metabolic factors, such as acidosis. Muscular fatigue, due to impaired cardiac output, also occurs during exercise.

The physical examination reveals signs of low cardiac output and reflex sympathetic stimulation, which include tachycardia, cool skin and peripheral cyanosis. Auscultation at the lung bases reveals inspiratory crackles, reflecting pulmonary congestion; signs of pleural effusion may also be present. Of greater diagnostic significance is the third heart sound, which produces a characteristic gallop rhythm. It is associated with rapid ventricular filling in early diastole and therefore never occurs when filling is impeded by mitral stenosis. In severe failure, left ventricular dilatation may stretch the mitral valve ring, producing 'functional' regurgitation, manifested by a pansystolic apical murmur. An alternating pulse also occurs in severe failure (see Fig. 1.6).

### Acute right heart failure

This is a medical emergency, seen in pulmonary embolism and, less commonly, in right ventricular infarction. Signs are those of critically reduced cardiac output and include cool skin, systemic hypotension and peripheral cyanosis. The jugular venous pulse is usually elevated (see also p. 137).

### Chronic right heart failure

This is usually the result of chronically elevated pulmonary artery pressure in patients with left heart failure or pulmonary disease. In these cases, dyspnoea is always prominent, but the effects of low cardiac out-put, elevated right atrial pressure and salt and water retention are also important. Fatigue is invariable, and congestion of the liver and gastro-intestinal tract causes abdominal discomfort and loss of appetite. The jugular venous pulse is elevated and in severe cases a giant 'v' wave indicates 'functional' tricuspid regurgitation, due to right ventricular dilatation. Peripheral oedema may be severe and visceral congestion produces enlargement of the liver and spleen; in long-standing disease, hepatic dysfunction results in jaundice and impaired protein synthesis. Auscultation at the lower left sternal edge reveals a pansystolic murmur if tricuspid regurgitation is present.

### Complications

Cardiac arrhythmias occur commonly in heart failure, particularly atrial fibrillation, which produces variable haemodynamic deterioration; ventricular arrhythmias are more sinister and an important cause of sudden death. Deep venous thrombosis (the result of sluggish flow in the veins of the legs and pelvis) may lead to pulmonary embolism, which may also cause sudden death; thrombosis within the dilated cardiac chambers may cause both systemic and pulmonary embolism. Chronic pulmonary congestion in left heart failure predisposes to chest infection.

Major organ failure is an inevitable consequence of advanced heart failure. Hypoperfusion in the kidney may lead to worsening renal failure.

Liver failure, with jaundice and elevation of liver enzymes, is usually reversible, following correction of visceral congestion, but in long-standing right heart failure cardiac cirrhosis develops, characterized by centrilobular necrosis and fibrosis ('nutmeg liver').

## Diagnosis

Heart failure can usually be recognized on clinical grounds, but full diagnosis demands identification of its cause.

### *Electrocardiogram (ECG)*

This is usually abnormal in heart failure, but the changes are non-specific. Most common are T-wave inversion, bundle branch block and atrial fibrillation. ECG abnormalities pointing to an aetiology include pathological Q waves in ischaemic disease and left ventricular hypertrophy in hypertensive and aortic valve disease.

### *Chest X-ray*

Cardiac enlargement is the most consistent finding and, in left-sided failure, this may be associated with pulmonary venous dilatation or pulmonary oedema (Fig. 4.5). In mitral stenosis, pulmonary congestion may occur without cardiac enlargement, though signs of left atrial dilatation are usually present. Cardiac enlargement without pulmonary congestion is seen in tamponade and primary right-sided failure.

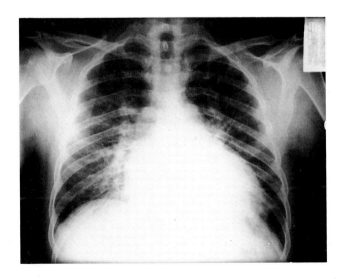

**Fig. 4.5** Left ventricular failure. The chest X-ray shows cardiac enlargement, dilatation of the upper-lobe veins and interstitial pulmonary oedema. Kerley B lines are seen in the right costophrenic angle.

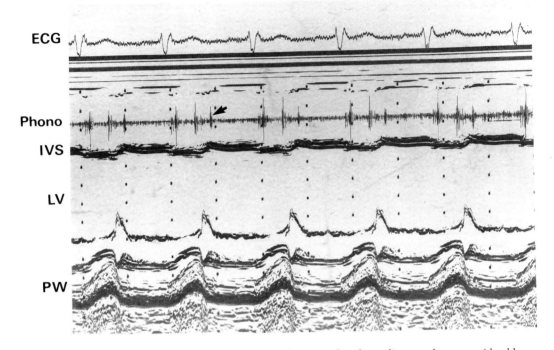

ECG

Phono

IVS

LV

PW

**Fig. 4.6**   Left ventricular failure. This M-mode echocardiogram shows considerable dilatation of the left ventricle (the vertical dots are a 1-cm scale). Note that the interventricular septum (IVS) is almost akinetic, but the posterior wall (PW) is contracting normally. Regional contractile impairment of this type indicates coronary artery disease and must be distinguished from the global contractile impairment which occurs in cardiomyopathy. The phonocardiogram recorded simultaneously shows normal first and second heart sounds and also a third heart sound (arrowed).

## Non-invasive imaging

The echocardiogram is potentially diagnostic of many of the cardiac defects that lead to heart failure. Left ventricular dilatation and *regional* contractile impairment indicate ischaemic disease (Fig. 4.6), whilst four-chamber dilatation and *global* contractile impairment indicate dilated cardiomyopathy (see Fig. 6.1). Heart failure due to valvular disease and tamponade is readily apparent (see Figs 7.5 and 9.10). Simultaneous Doppler studies permit identification of regurgitant jets through incompetent valves and shunting through septal defects.

Radionuclide ventriculography provides an alternative way of examining left ventricular cavity size and wall motion abnormalities. It is particularly useful for quantitating ejection fraction and for identifying early ventricular impairment by application of provocative tests.

## Cardiac catheterization

Right heart catheterization is occasionally of diagnostic value in acute myocardial infarction, particularly for identification of relative hypovolaemia, when low cardiac output is associated with an inappropriately low wedge pressure (see p. 60). Its principal value, however, is for monitoring responses to therapy.

Left heart catheterization rarely provides diagnostic information which cannot be obtained by non-invasive means. Nevertheless, in patients with surgically correctable disease (e.g. ventricular aneurysm, valvular disease), the surgeon usually requires precise definition of the lesion, with haemodynamic measurements and angiography.

## Differential diagnosis

Acute left heart failure must be distinguished from other causes of acute-onset dyspnoea, including bronchial asthma, pneumothorax and pulmonary embolism. In none of these conditions, however, does the chest X-ray demonstrate pulmonary oedema.

The differential diagnosis of chronic heart failure includes other causes of dyspnoea and peripheral oedema.

## Obstructive pulmonary disease

In bronchitis, a history of winter cough and sputum can usually be obtained. Although typical orthopnoea is unusual, nocturnal symptoms may interrupt sleep if diaphragmatic excursion is restricted by the weight of the abdominal viscera or nocturnal wheezing occurs. Respiratory function tests are usually diagnostic in these patients and non-invasive imaging will rule out important heart-disease.

## Dependent oedema of the elderly

This is common in sedentary patients and is caused by venostasis in the legs, which results from inactivity of the muscle pump, varicose veins and gravitational pooling of blood. Treatment with support stockings and elevation of the legs is usually effective.

## Treatment of acute left ventricular failure (LVF)

### General measures

The patient should be nursed in the head-up position. Urgent correction of arrhythmias and hypertension is essential. Treatment of hypoxaemia is directed at maintaining an arterial oxygen tension of at least 7 kPa; if this cannot be achieved despite high concentrations of inhaled oxygen, positive-pressure ventilation may be necessary.

**Table 4.2**  Medical treatment of acute left ventricular failure

| Drug | Action | Indication | Dose | Note |
|---|---|---|---|---|
| *Diuretics* | | | | |
| Frusemide | Diuresis | Pulmonary oedema | 40–80 mg | Often unhelpful in severe low-output states |
| *Opiates* | | | | |
| Morphine | Venodilatation Respiratory suppression Relief of anxiety | Pulmonary oedema | 5–10 mg | Use cautiously in patients with associated respiratory disease |
| *Vasodilators* | | | | |
| Glyceryl trinitrate | Venodilatation | Pulmonary oedema | 0.2–2.0 µg/kg/min | Contraindicated if systolic blood-pressure is < 90 mmHg |
| Nitroprusside | Arteriolar and venodilatation | Pulmonary oedema/ low output | 0.2–2.0 µg/kg/min | |
| *Inotropes* | | | | |
| Dobutamine | Positive intropism | Severe low output with hypotension | 2.0–10.0 µg/kg/min | Usually only indicated in severe low-output states or cardiogenic shock |
| Dopamine | Positive inotropism and renal arteriolar dilatation (low dose) Generalized arteriolar constriction (high dose) | Severe low output with oliguria | 1.0–5.0 µg/kg/min | Avoid high doses of dopamine |

## *Medical therapy* (Table 4.2)

Intravenous *opiates* and *diuretics* are the first-line agents. Morphine 10 mg or diamorphine 5 mg relieves dyspnoea by a combination of vasodilatation, respiratory depression and relief of anxiety. Loop diuretics (e.g. frusemide 40 mg) initiate a prompt diuresis, which reduces left atrial pressure, but, because diuretic activity depends largely on adequate renal perfusion, these drugs are of less value in severe low-output states.

## *Vasodilators and inotropes*

If opiates and diuretics are not rapidly effective, treatment should be directed at improving left ventricular function with vasodilators and inotropes. Responses are best monitored by measurement of pulmonary artery wedge pressure (indirect left atrial pressure), using a Swan–Ganz catheter. A thermodilution device permits simultaneous measurement of cardiac output, though urine output and skin temperature provide a more convenient index of peripheral perfusion. Agents with a short plasma half-life for intravenous infusion should be chosen. In this way infusion rates can be rapidly adjusted, with the aim of improving urine flow and skin temperature, and reducing pulmonary artery wedge pressure to between 15 and 20 mmHg — the level at which pulmonary oedema begins to clear. Further reductions in wedge pressure should be avoided because the reduction in preload lowers cardiac output.

*Glyceryl trinitrate* and *nitroprusside* are widely used vasodilators. Glyceryl trinitrate is predominantly a venodilator but nitroprusside also dilates arterioles. Both agents reduce venous return to the heart and lower left atrial pressure. The arteriole-dilating property of nitroprusside, however, produces greater increments in cardiac output, by lowering blood-pressure and afterload, but systolic blood-pressure must not be allowed to fall below 90 mmHg because of the risk to vital organ perfusion. Vasodilators are contraindicated in patients who are already hypotensive.

*Dobutamine* and *dopamine* are widely used inotropic agents with sympathomimetic activity: stimulation of cardiac beta-1-adrenoceptors enhances contractility and cardiac output. Dopamine (unlike dobutamine) also has important peripheral vascular effects: low doses (up to 5 μg/kg/min) selectively dilate the renal arterioles and improve renal perfusion but high doses produce widespread alpha-adrenoceptor-mediated arteriolar constriction. This improves blood-pressure but further depresses left ventricular function by increasing afterload. Thus, dopamine is best used at low dose for its renal action, whilst dobutamine produces dose-related increments in cardiac output without adverse peripheral vascular effects.

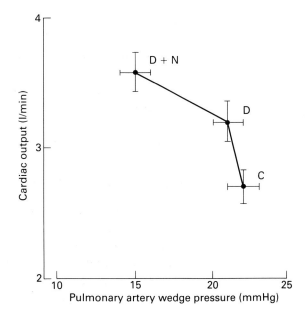

**Fig. 4.7**  Combination therapy in acute left ventricular failure. The points and bars are mean values (± standard error) for a group of 10 patients with acute left ventricular failure complicating myocardial infarction. Before treatment (C) the cardiac output was low despite very high pulmonary artery wedge pressure. Treatment with dobutamine (D) improved cardiac output, but had little effect on the pulmonary artery wedge pressure. The addition of nitroprusside (N), however, caused a further increase in cardiac output and a pronounced reduction in pulmonary artery wedge pressure. Thus, combination therapy with dobutamine and nitroprusside had a beneficial effect on left ventricular function, improving peripheral perfusion and correcting pulmonary oedema.

Combination therapy with dobutamine and low-dose dopamine is particularly useful for improving both cardiac output and renal perfusion.

Inotropic agents rarely produce significant reductions in left atrial (pulmonary artery wedge) pressure. Thus, simultaneous treatment with diuretics and vasodilators is often necessary for correction of pulmonary oedema (Fig. 4.7). The risk of cardiac arrhythmias during inotropic therapy demands careful ECG monitoring.

### *Intra-aortic balloon pump* (Fig. 4.8)

This device may be used to provide temporary support in acute LVF. A catheter with a terminal sausage-shaped balloon is introduced into the femoral artery and the tip is positioned in the thoracic aorta, just below the left subclavian branch. Pumping is synchronized with the ECG. The balloon inflates in early diastole, thereby augmenting pressure in the aortic root and improving coronary flow; it deflates immediately prior to ventricular systole, producing an abrupt fall in pressure, which reduces afterload and improves cardiac output.

Despite the short-term value of the intra-aortic balloon, it is often impossible to wean patients off the device. This limits its clinical application to patients with a surgically correctable cardiac lesion (e.g. ventricular

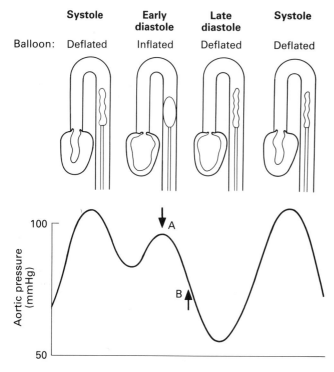

Fig. 4.8  Intra-aortic balloon pump and simultaneous aortic pressure signal. Balloon inflation in early diastole augments pressure in the ascending thoracic aorta (A). Deflation in late diastole leads to an abrupt fall in pressure (B).

septal defect, acute valvular incompetence) or to patients with a temporarily 'stunned' ventricle following heart surgery. In both groups, the device provides valuable haemodynamic support pending corrective surgery or spontaneous recovery of contractile function.

Complications include balloon rupture, peripheral embolism and trauma to the aorta and iliofemoral vessels, with varying degrees of arterial insufficiency.

## *Surgical therapy*

Emergency surgery is potentially life-saving when an acute mechanical cardiac lesion produces LVF without substantial myocardial damage. Any delay may cause irrecoverable loss of ventricular contractile function, following which results are less favourable. Thus, endocarditis complicated by LVF is usually an indication for urgent valve replacement. Similarly, papillary muscle or septal rupture following myocardial infarction usually requires immediate surgical correction.

## Treatment of congestive heart failure

Although the cause of congestive heart failure can usually be identified, its correction is not always feasible — particularly when ventricular contractile impairment is established. Thus, treatment is usually directed towards controlling symptoms and slowing the progression of disease. Although general measures, including arrhythmia and blood-pressure control, are important, most patients require a diuretic as the first-line drug. If dyspnoea and oedema persist despite treatment with frusemide 40–80 mg daily, an angiotensin-converting enzyme inhibitor such as captopril should be added. This often corrects symptoms and may also slow the progression of disease, thereby improving prognosis. In intractable heart failure, the addition of digoxin may be helpful in some cases, but, at this stage, prognosis is poor and heart transplantation becomes the only treatment likely to work.

## *General measures*

Simple measures, including control of cardiac arrhythmias, hypertension and anaemia, are important. Atrial fibrillation is particularly common and, if resistant to electrical cardioversion, can usually be controlled by digitalis, which slows the ventricular response and improves stroke volume. Treatment of hypertension improves left ventricular function by reducing afterload, and correction of anaemia improves oxygen delivery to metabolizing tissues.

Salt and water retention provides a rationale for limiting salt intake

**Table 4.3** Medical treatment of congestive heart failure

| Drug | Daily oral dose (mg) |
|---|---|
| *Thiazide diuretics* | |
| Bendrofluazide | 2.5–10.0 |
| Cyclopenthiazide | 0.25–1.0 |
| *Loop diuretics* | |
| Frusemide | 40–500 |
| Bumetanide | 0.5–5.0 |
| Ethacrynic acid | 25–150 |
| *Potassium-sparing diuretics* | |
| Spironolactone | 100–200 |
| Amiloride | 5–20 |
| Triamterene | 100–200 |
| *Angiotensin-converting enzyme inhibitors* | |
| Captopril | 25–150 |
| Enalapril | 5–40 |
| *Vasodilators* | |
| Isosorbide mononitrate | 40–80 |
| Prazosin | 4–20 |
| Hydralazine | 50–200 |

but, with the availability of potent diuretics, this is rarely necessary in practice.

## *Medical therapy* (Table 4.3)

Diuretics remain the most useful drugs. Angiotensin-converting enzyme inhibitors also play an important role but other vasodilators and inotropic agents are of less value.

## *Diuretics*

These promote salt and water excretion, which lowers atrial pressures and corrects pulmonary and systemic congestion. The associated reduction in body-weight provides a useful clinical yardstick of the diuretic response. Diuretics do not improve ventricular function; rather, by reducing preload, they tend to have the reverse effect and over-diuresis must therefore be avoided.

Thiazides increase sodium excretion in the distal renal tubule. They are mild diuretics and, in severe heart failure, the more potent loop diuretics are more effective. These inhibit sodium reabsorption in the ascending loop of Henle, thereby removing the osmotic gradient in the renal medulla and preventing concentration of the urine. In the very oedematous patient, drug absorption from the bowel is unreliable and parenteral administration may be required.

Diuretics increase the sodium concentration in the distal nephron for aldosterone-mediated exchange with potassium. This predisposes to hypokalaemia, with the attendant risk of cardiac arrhythmias. Hypokalaemia can be avoided by potassium supplementation or, preferably, by simultaneous prescription of a potassium-sparing diuretic. Spironolactone, an aldosterone inhibitor, is the most effective but, because it causes gastrointestinal side-effects and gynaecomastia, amiloride is usually preferred.

Dilutional hyponatraemia during diuretic therapy is caused by profound natriuresis without equivalent loss of water, and usually responds to fluid restriction (less than 1 litre daily). A serum sodium concentration below 115 mmol/litre, however, requires treatment with hypertonic saline, because of the risk of cerebral oedema, convulsions and death.

## Angiotensin-converting enzyme (ACE) inhibitors

These block the renin-induced conversion of angiotensin I to angiotensin II. Removal of angiotensin II has two important effects: producing vasodilatation, which increases cardiac output by reducing blood-pressure (afterload), and removing the major stimulus for aldosterone secretion, thereby enhancing the renal excretion of salt and water. Thus, by increasing cardiac output and promoting salt and water excretion, ACE inhibitors improve both peripheral perfusion and the congestive manifestations of heart failure.

Because ACE inhibitors are potent vasodilators they can produce profound hypotension in susceptible patients. Thus, careful monitoring of blood-pressure and serum biochemistry is essential early in the course of treatment to guard against prerenal failure. Reductions in diuretic therapy are often required as the ACE inhibitor is introduced, to maintain adequate plasma volume. ACE inhibitors, by reducing aldosterone secretion, conserve potassium, so that potassium supplements or potassium-sparing diuretics are not usually necessary.

## Vasodilators

Drugs with venodilator (e.g. nitrates), arteriolar dilator (e.g. hydralazine) or both properties (e.g. prazosin) have been widely used in the treatment of congestive heart failure. Venodilatation causes pooling of blood in the abdominal capacitance vessels, which reduces venous return to the heart and lowers atrial pressure (preload). Arteriolar dilatation improves cardiac output by reducing blood-pressure (afterload). This can improve both pulmonary congestion and peripheral perfusion.

Vasodilator therapy is certainly beneficial in acute heart failure (see p. 88) but efficacy is often short-lived and not all patients experience long-term symptomatic improvement. Drug tolerance is an important factor, particularly during nitrate therapy; in addition, the reflex sympathetic response to vasodilators and the direct activation of the renin–angiotensin system combine to produce a vasoconstrictor stimulus which may attenuate treatment effects. Conventional vasodilator therapy now plays only a limited role in the management of congestive heart failure.

## Inotropic agents

Digoxin is the only orally active inotropic agent licensed for clinical use. Like all other inotropes, it increases the availability of intracellular calcium to the myocardial contractile proteins and increases the force of contraction. However, its inotropic properties are mild and the therapeutic range narrow, increasing the risk of side-effects. The major indication for digoxin is to control the ventricular response in atrial fibrillation, a common arrhythmia in congestive heart failure. For the patient in sinus rhythm, digoxin is now only recommended if heart failure is severe and unresponsive to diuretics and ACE inhibitors, when it will sometimes produce limited clinical improvement.

## Other medical measures

Pleural effusions usually respond well to diuretics but, when large, they should be aspirated, particularly if the patient is severely dyspnoeic. Severe oedema, unresponsive to full medical therapy, can be corrected by ultrafiltration, when body water is selectively removed by passing the blood across a highly permeable membrane.

Preliminary work has shown a paradoxically beneficial response to beta-blocker therapy in certain patients with advanced congestive heart failure. These drugs have the potential to protect against myocardial adrenoceptor down-regulation (see p. 79) and restore responsiveness to catecholamines. Nevertheless, they are negatively inotropic and potentially dangerous in heart failure, and at present are not recommended for clinical use.

## Surgical therapy

Heart failure caused by valvular disease, left ventricular aneurysm or certain congenital defects is potentially correctable by surgery. However, in the majority of patients, heart transplantation is the only option, although it is only appropriate in advanced left ventricular disease resistant to all medical therapy. The orthotopic procedure is favoured in most transplant centres. The diseased heart is subtotally excised with preservation of the posterior atrial wall, and suturing of recipient–donor atria to atria and great vessels to great vessels is then undertaken. The operative risk is small compared with the hazards of organ rejection and immunosuppressive therapy. These hazards are greatest during the first year following surgery, but thereafter the threat of accelerated coronary atherosclerosis (the cause of which is unknown) becomes increasingly important. Due largely to advances in the early recognition and treatment of rejection, the results of heart transplantation have improved rapidly and there is now an 80% 2-year survival rate. The results of heart–lung transplantation (in patients with intractable right-sided failure caused by advanced pulmonary vascular disease) are also improving.

Undoubtedly the major limitation of heart transplantation is the lack of donor organs, which ensures that many patients referred for this procedure die on the waiting-list before a suitable heart can be found. Recently a totally artificial heart driven by an external power source, has been developed to provide temporary circulatory support for patients awaiting transplantation. This may permit survival for several weeks pending definitive surgery.

Cardiomyoplasty is another new surgical technique, in which an electrically stimulated skeletal muscle autograft (usually latissimus dorsi) is applied to the ventricular wall to assist contractile function in advanced heart failure. Early results have looked promising, but the long-term tolerance of skeletal muscle to continuous work remains uncertain.

## Prognosis

Heart failure resulting from a surgically correctable lesion may have an excellent prognosis following definitive treatment. In the majority of cases, however, left ventricular contractile impairment is irreversible and the outlook is poor (Fig. 4.9). Survival is closely related to the severity of disease, whether assessed symptomatically, haemodynamically, functionally or by its association with arrhythmias. In the most advanced cases (New York Heart Association (NYHA) functional classification III and IV), annual mortality approaches 50%. Specific neurohumoral antagonists may improve survival in these high-risk patients. Evidence is best for ACE inhibitors, which, when added to diuretics, cause a small but significant reduction in mortality, perhaps through interruption of the vicious circle illustrated in Fig. 4.3. More substantial benefit would be expected to derive from introduction of ACE inhibitors earlier in the course of heart failure, before ventricular function becomes severely depressed. In end-stage disease, heart transplantation is the only treatment likely to provide a substantial prognostic benefit.

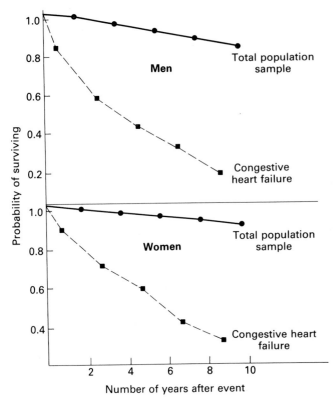

**Fig. 4.9**  Survival of men and women after the onset of heart failure in the Framingham study. (Reproduced with permission from McKee *et al.*, *N. Engl. J. Med.* 1971, **285**, 1441.)

## Shock

Shock is a syndrome of critically impaired vital organ perfusion, which, if not rapidly corrected, leads to irreversible cell damage with multiple organ failure and death. It is usually caused by severe heart failure (cardiogenic shock), hypovolaemia or septicaemia. The pathogenesis is complex and poorly understood, involving a combination of haemo-dynamic and toxic factors. Widespread capillary damage intensifies the tissue perfusion deficit, threatening vital organs, including the heart. As myocardial perfusion deteriorates, a vicious circle of falling cardiac output and worsening end-organ damage becomes established.

Clinically the patient is cold, clammy and cerebrally obtunded, with tachycardia, hypotension and oliguria. If urine flow cannot be maintained with volume replacement, inotropic drive, low-dose dopamine and frusemide, tubular damage leads to oliguric renal failure, requiring dialysis. Pulmonary oedema is common, even when shock is non-cardiac in origin, and results from capillary damage, which allows protein-rich fluid to leak into the lung (adult respiratory distress syndrome). Hypoxaemia requires mechanical ventilation, although the increase in intrathoracic pressure reduces venous return to the heart and exacerbates the critical haemodynamic state. Heart failure may respond to inotropic support (intra-aortic balloon pumping is inappropriate in the absence of a surgically correctable lesion), but the improvement is usually only temporary and the prognosis remains very poor, with a mortality greater than 80%.

## Cardiogenic shock

Any cause of heart failure with severe reduction in cardiac output may lead to cardiogenic shock. The majority of cases, however, are the result of acute myocardial infarction, involving damage to at least 40% of the left ventricle. Physiological responses directed at maintaining left ventricular pump function include elevation of left atrial pressure and catecholamine drive. Nevertheless, although these responses help maintain cardiac output by the Starling mechanism and inotropic stimulation, respectively, they also lead to pulmonary oedema and peripheral vasoconstriction, which exacerbate hypoxaemia, left ventricular dysfunction and the vital organ perfusion deficit. Treatment is aimed at improving left ventricular function with intravenous inotropic agents, which may be given in combination with vasodilators if blood-pressure is adequately maintained (see Fig. 4.7).

Pulmonary artery pressure monitoring with a Swan–Ganz catheter is recommended in these critically ill patients. Arterial oxygen tension should also be monitored and, if this cannot be maintained above 7 kPa with inhaled oxygen, mechanical ventilation is necessary. When cardiogenic shock is the result of a surgically correctable lesion (e.g. mitral regurgitation, ventricular septal defect), intra-aortic balloon pumping provides useful haemodynamic support, but surgery should not be delayed in these cases.

## Hypovolaemic shock

This is usually the result of haemorrhage but may also occur in extensive burn injury and severe vomiting or diarrhoea (particularly in children). Important iatrogenic causes include inappropriate diuretic therapy and inadequate fluid replacement following surgery. Modest reductions in blood volume (less than 500 ml) elicit an acute sympathoadrenal response, which increases heart rate and peripheral resistance so that blood-pressure is maintained. Thereafter, increased secretion of antidiuretic hormone and aldosterone encourages salt and water retention, which restores the volume deficit. When reductions in blood volume exceed 20% of normal (more than 1 litre), cardiac output falls abruptly and sympathoadrenal responses are inadequate to maintain blood-pressure, despite intense vasoconstriction. The patient becomes agitated and pale, with tachycardia, tachypnoea, diaphoresis and oliguria. At this stage there is no compensatory reserve and any further volume loss leads inexorably to severe shock, with life-threatening reductions to cardiac output, blood-pressure and tissue perfusion. Physiologically, therefore, the condition resembles cardiogenic shock except that atrial pressures are low. Thus, the JVP is not elevated and pulmonary oedema does not develop acutely. These patients are nevertheless prone to adult respiratory distress syndrome if not treated promptly with plasma volume replacement. This should be titrated against the JVP, but in patients with left ventricular disease pulmonary artery pressure monitoring provides a better guide to volume requirements.

## Septicaemic shock

This is usually caused by Gram-negative organisms, particularly *Escherichia coli*, and species of *Klebsiella* and *Pseudomonas*. Less commonly, Gram-positive infection with *Pneumococcus* or *Streptococcus* is responsible. In Gram-negative septicaemia, the shock syndrome is the result of endotoxins, which cause cell damage directly and also indirectly, by stimulating release of lysosomal enzymes from leucocytes and activating the complement cascade. Severe capillary injury and tissue anoxia are invariable. Haemodynamic changes are complex and difficult to predict. Cutaneous vasodilatation may cause a warm skin, although sequestration of venous blood and capillary damage, with loss of plasma protein, ensure that cardiac output and vital organ perfusion are critically impaired. Myocardial contractile function is often depressed, not only by coronary hypoperfusion but also by the direct effects of toxaemia. The JVP may be low or elevated and does not usually provide a useful guide to volume requirements, which should be titrated against pulmonary artery wedge pressure, measured with a Swan–Ganz catheter. Metabolic changes are also complex, ranging from hyperventilation and respiratory alkalosis in early shock to profound lactic acidaemia and metabolic acidosis as the condition deteriorates. Adult respiratory distress syndrome and disseminated intravascular coagulation, with consumption of clotting factors, commonly accompany the progression of the illness. Treatment is with circulatory and respiratory support and usually requires plasma volume adjustment, inotropic drive and mechanical ventilation. Intravenous antibiotics via a central line are essential and should be started as soon as blood samples for bacteriological culture have been obtained. Ampicillin (6–12 g/day) and gentamicin (titrated against blood levels) provide broad-spectrum cover against most Gram-negative organisms and provide initial therapy pending the blood culture result. A penicillinase-resistant penicillin (e.g. flucloxacillin 6–12 g/day) should also be prescribed to cover staphylococcal infection. Glucocorticoids continue to be widely used but are of no proven clinical value.

## Further reading

Braunwald E. ACE inhibitors: a cornerstone of the treatment of heart failure. *N. Engl. J. Med.* 1991, **325**, 351–3.

Burnett J.C. Atrial natriuretic factor: is it physiologically important? *Circulation* 1990, **82**, 1523–4.

Cheng T.O. Cardiac failure in coronary heart disease. *Am. Heart J.* 1990, **120**, 396–412.

Cohn J.N. Inotropic therapy for heart failure: paradise postponed. *N. Engl. J. Med.* 1989, **320**, 729–31.

Curfman G.D. Inotropic therapy for heart failure — an unfulfilled promise. *N. Engl. J. Med.* 1991, **325**, 1509–10.

Fowler M.B. Exercise intolerance in heart failure. *J. Am. Coll. Cardiol.* 1991, **17**, 1073–4.

Francis G.S. The relationship of the sympathetic nervous system and the renin–angiotensin system in congestive heart failure. *Am. Heart J.* 1989, **118**, 642–8.

Gottlieb S.S. The use of antiarrhythmic agents in heart failure: implications of CAST. *Am. Heart J.* 1989, **118**, 1074–7.

Grossman W. Diastolic dysfunction in congestive heart failure. *N. Engl. J. Med.* 1991, **325**, 1557–64.

Millner R.W.J. and Pepper J.R. Cardiomyoplasty. *Br. Med. J.* 1991, **302**, 1353–4.

Packer M. What causes tolerance to nitroglycerin? The 100 year old mystery continues. *J. Am. Coll. Cardiol.* 1990, **16**, 932–5.

Schofield P.M. Indications for heart transplantation. *Br. Heart J.* 1991, **65**, 55–6.

Sutton G.C. Epidemiologic aspects of heart failure. *Am. Heart J.* 1989, **120** (suppl. 6), 1538–46.

Timmis A.D. Modern treatment of heart failure. *Br. Med. J.* 1988, **297**, 83–4.

Timmis A.D. A new look at digoxin in congestive heart failure and sinus rhythm. *Postgrad. Med. J.* 1989, **65**, 715–17.

# 5 Coronary Artery Disease

## Summary

Coronary artery disease is the most common cause of premature death in the UK. Its cause is unknown but a number of risk factors have been identified, including cigarette smoking, hypertension and hypercholesterolaemia, correction of which may protect against the development or progression of disease. It is characterized pathologically by the atheromatous plaque which may stenose the coronary arterial lumen sufficiently to cause exertional myocardial ischaemia, experienced by the patient as angina. Plaque rupture provides a focus for platelet deposition and thrombosis, and may result in unstable angina or myocardial infarction, depending on whether the thrombus is sub-occlusive or occludes the coronary lumen completely.

*Angina* is best diagnosed from a careful clinical history concentrating on the character, location, radiation and duration of the pain and its relation to provocative stimuli, particularly exertion. It often responds to treatment with nitrates, beta-blockers and calcium antagonists. In cases of diagnostic uncertainty, stress testing (exercise ECG, thallium perfusion scintigram) is helpful and may also provide useful prognostic information. In young patients and those with symptoms inadequately controlled by medical treatment, coronary revascularization by angioplasty or bypass surgery should be considered.

*Myocardial infarction* is fatal in about 40% of cases, often as a result of ventricular fibrillation before hospital admission. In hospital, however, where ventricular fibrillation can be corrected by electrical cardioversion, left ventricular failure due to extensive infarction is the most important cause of death. Thus, significant reductions in mortality can be achieved by rapid transfer to hospital (ensuring early access to a defibrillator) and by specific treatment with thrombolytic drugs and aspirin, which restore coronary patency and reduce the extent of infarction. Before discharge from hospital, steps should be taken to protect against recurrent myocardial infarction and death. Patients with continuing chest pain or an ischaemic predischarge stress test are at increased risk and require coronary arteriography with a view to revascularization. Correction of established risk factors and long-term treatment with beta-blockers and aspirin are recommended for all patients.

## What is coronary heart disease?

Every year in the UK, coronary artery disease causes more than 50 000 premature deaths in people aged under 70, and is responsible for the loss of 25 million working-days. Recent data have shown a downward trend in mortality during the last 10 years, probably caused by a decline in both incidence and case fatality rate. A similar, though considerably more substantial, trend became established in the United States more than 20 years ago, since when mortality has fallen by over 30%. It is still not known whether the decline in the UK will continue, but it seems certain to remain a major social and medical challenge in the foreseeable future.

## Aetiology

Coronary artery disease is nearly always caused by atherosclerosis; indeed, the two terms are often used synonymously. Other causes of coronary artery disease, listed in Table 5.1, are rare. Thus, a middle-aged or elderly patient with polyarteritis nodosa or syphilis is as likely to have atherosclerosis causing angina as arteritic or syphilitic involvement of the coronary circulation.

**Table 5.1**  Causes of coronary artery disease

1  *Atherosclerosis*

2  *Arteritis*
Systemic lupus erythematosus
Polyarteritis nodosa
Rheumatoid arthritis
Ankylosing spondylitis
Syphilis
Takayasu disease

3  *Embolism*
Infective endocarditis
Left atrial/ventricular thrombus
Left atrial/ventricular tumour
Prosthetic valve thrombus
Complication of cardiac catheterization

4  *Coronary mural thickening*
Amyloidosis
Radiation therapy
Hurler's disease
Pseudoxanthoma elasticum

5  *Other causes of coronary luminal narrowing*
Aortic dissection
Coronary spasm

6  *Congenital coronary artery disease*
Anomalous origin from pulmonary artery
Arteriovenous fistula

The cause of atherosclerosis is unknown. Epidemiological evidence points to a complex interaction of genetic and environmental influences, the relative importance of which remains speculative. Although the cause of the disease is unknown, a number of risk factors have been identified which, though associated with coronary artery disease, are not essential for its development. Conversely, the absence of risk factors in an individual does not confer immunity against the disease.

## Reversible risk factors

These are particularly important because their avoidance or correction may protect against the development or progression of coronary artery disease. Most important of these are cigarette smoking, hypertension and hypercholesterolaemia. It is now widely accepted that control of these risk factors, particularly in young adults, provides the most important weapon against the continuing high prevalence of coronary artery disease in the UK. Risk factor control should also receive priority in the treatment of patients with established disease.

### Cigarette smoking

The risk of coronary artery disease rises in proportion to the number of cigarettes smoked. Stopping smoking reduces the risk, though recent evidence indicates that it remains higher than in individuals who have never smoked.

### Hypertension

The risk rises in proportion to the level of both systolic and diastolic blood-pressure. Thus, systolic and diastolic pressures greater than, or equal to 160 and 95 mmHg, respectively, increase risk by two to three times. Whether treatment of hypertension reduces the risk remains uncertain, though recent evidence provides grounds for optimism. Nevertheless, the main benefit of treatment is reduction in the incidence of stroke and heart failure.

### Hypercholesterolaemia

Risk rises in proportion to the total blood cholesterol level. For example, at levels of 6.5 and 7.8 mmol/litre, the risk rises to two and four times that seen at 5.2 mmol/litre. Low-density lipoprotein is the major component of total cholesterol and is particularly atherogenic; high-density lipoprotein, on the other hand, protects against the disease. In hypercholesterolaemic patients (arbitrarily defined as greater than 6.5 mmol/litre), reducing total cholesterol levels and simultaneously increasing the ratio of high- to low-density lipoproteins reduces risk. Treatment may also slow the progression of established coronary artery disease and in some cases lead to regression of atheromatous plaques.

Hypertriglyceridaemia is not usually regarded as a risk factor for coronary artery disease; however, it is often accompanied by low levels of high-density lipoproteins and may cause a small increase in risk, particularly in women.

## Lipoprotein a

This lipoprotein is produced in the liver; blood concentrations above 0.3 g/litre are associated with an increased risk of coronary artery disease. To date, there is no effective treatment for reducing raised blood concentrations.

## Obesity

The increased risk of coronary artery disease in obese individuals is largely due to associated hypertension, hypercholesterolaemia and diabetes.

## Physical inactivity

A considerable body of evidence links regular exercise to a reduced risk of coronary artery disease. Nevertheless, the effect is not large and is probably mediated indirectly through the beneficial effects of exercise-induced increases in high-density lipoproteins and reductions in resting blood-pressure.

## Irreversible risk factors

### Age

The risk of coronary artery disease rises progressively with increasing age.

### Male sex

The risk is low in young women but, after the age of 60, comes to equal that of men.

### Family history

Although the familial incidence of coronary artery disease is largely the result of genetic predisposition to hypertension, hypercholesterolaemia and diabetes, it is now well established that family history is itself an independent predictor of increased risk.

### Diabetes mellitus

This increases the risk in both men and women.

### Personality type

Although the type A personality (chronic sense of time urgency) has been associated with an increased risk compared with the more placid type B personality, the evidence remains inconclusive.

## Pathology

The heart is essentially an obligate aerobic organ: without oxygen, energy production fails within seconds and contraction ceases. The capacity of the heart to extract arterial oxygen, though high (75%), is relatively fixed. Thus, under circumstances of increased myocardial oxygen demand (e.g. exercise), oxygen delivery must be increased. This can only be achieved through an increase in coronary flow (Fig. 5.1). Appropriately, therefore, myocardial oxygen demand is the principal regulator of coronary flow: increments in demand stimulate coronary arteriolar dilatation and flow increases accordingly. Coronary artery disease, however, restricts flow and deprives the heart of its primary metabolic substrate, undermining its capacity to function. The left ventricle is particularly vulnerable because

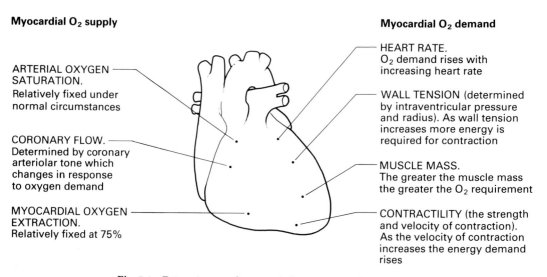

**Myocardial O$_2$ supply**

ARTERIAL OXYGEN SATURATION.
Relatively fixed under normal circumstances

CORONARY FLOW.
Determined by coronary arteriolar tone which changes in response to oxygen demand

MYOCARDIAL OXYGEN EXTRACTION.
Relatively fixed at 75%

**Myocardial O$_2$ demand**

HEART RATE.
O$_2$ demand rises with increasing heart rate

WALL TENSION (determined by intraventricular pressure and radius). As wall tension increases more energy is required for contraction

MUSCLE MASS.
The greater the muscle mass the greater the O$_2$ requirement

CONTRACTILITY (the strength and velocity of contraction).
As the velocity of contraction increases the energy demand rises

**Fig. 5.1**   Determinants of myocardial oxygen supply and demand.

its oxygen requirement is greater than any of the other cardiac chambers, reflecting its muscle mass and wall tension, both of which are major determinants of oxygen demand. Thus, while coronary artery disease may affect oxygen delivery to any part of the heart, the left ventricle (particularly the subendocardium) is worst affected.

The proximal 6 cm of the coronary arteries are usually involved, with relative sparing of the smaller distal vessels. The disease is characterized pathologically by the *atherosclerotic plaque*, a focal proliferation of smooth muscle cells, collagen and cholesterol esters lying within the intimal and medial layers of the arterial wall. The plaque is usually endothelialized but, as it increases in size, it may ulcerate and rupture, providing a focus for platelet deposition and thrombosis.

### Clinicopathological correlates

Coronary atherosclerosis is often asymptomatic. The development of symptoms is closely related to the pathology of the atherosclerotic plaque. Four symptom complexes (syndromes) are recognized, each associated with characteristic coronary pathology: stable angina, variant angina, unstable angina and myocardial infarction.

### Stable angina

This is associated with a smooth, endothelialized coronary plaque causing luminal stenosis. Stenosis in excess of 70% of the coronary luminal diameter may restrict flow to the extent that myocardial oxygen delivery fails to meet demand. This produces myocardial ischaemia, experienced by the patient as angina.

### Variant angina

This unusual syndrome is associated with a smooth, endothelialized coronary plaque, which may be small, causing only trivial luminal stenosis. In up to 30% of cases the artery is normal. However, unprovoked increments in coronary tone (*spasm*) restrict coronary flow sufficiently to cause myocardial ischaemia, experienced by the patient as angina.

### Unstable angina

This is provoked by the abrupt rupture of an atheromatous plaque, exposing its contents and providing a focus for platelet deposition and thrombosis. In unstable angina the thrombus is subocclusive but causes intense myocardial ischaemia. Progression to thrombotic coronary occlusion and myocardial infarction occurs in up to 30% of cases.

## *Myocardial infarction*

The pathological process is identical to unstable angina, except that the thrombus completely occludes the coronary artery. This usually produces myocardial infarction in the territory subtended by the occluded artery. Nevertheless, a well-developed collateral supply or early spontaneous recanalization may modify the evolution of the infarct, restricting damage to the vulnerable subendocardial layer (see p. 125).

## Clinical manifestations

The major clinical manifestations of coronary artery disease are angina, myocardial infarction and sudden death, which are discussed in this chapter. Others include heart failure and cardiac arrhythmias and are discussed elsewhere.

## *Angina*

Angina, the pain that occurs during periods of myocardial ischaemia, is usually a manifestation of coronary artery disease. However, any other cause of imbalance between myocardial oxygen supply and demand may also cause angina indistinguishable from that associated with coronary artery disease (Table 5.2). Three anginal syndromes are recognized:

1   Stable angina.
2   Variant angina.
3   Unstable angina.

The commonest of these is stable angina.

## *Stable angina*

### Clinical manifestations

Angina consists of a retrosternal constricting discomfort, which may radiate to either arm, the throat or the jaw, and may be associated with

**Table 5.2**   Causes of angina

| |
|---|
| *Reduced myocardial oxygen supply* |
| Coronary artery disease (see Table 5.1) |
| Severe anaemia |
| |
| *Increased myocardial oxygen demand* |
| Left ventricular hypertrophy — hypertension |
| aortic stenosis |
| aortic regurgitation |
| hypertrophic cardiomyopathy |
| Rapid tachyarrhythmias |

shortness of breath. Typically it is provoked by exertion and relieved within 2–10 min by rest; other precipitating factors are emotion and sexual intercourse. Symptoms are usually worse after a heavy meal and in cold weather. Surprisingly, the severity of symptoms is not closely related to the extent of coronary artery disease; indeed, extensive disease is sometimes entirely asymptomatic, although episodes of 'silent' myocardial ischaemia can often be detected by special techniques.

Some patients with coronary artery disease experience angina predominantly at night, although typical exercise-related symptoms are usually also present. Tachycardia during dreaming has been blamed but a more plausible explanation relates to the dynamics of coronary arterial tone. An increase in tone reduces coronary luminal diameter and accentuates the stenosis caused by an atheromatous plaque. If this leads to a critical reduction in flow, the patient will experience angina. Coronary arterial tone is at its height in the early morning, the time when nocturnal angina is most frequent.

The examination is usually normal. Nevertheless, elevated blood-pressure and evidence of other major risk factors should be noted. Hypercholesterolaemia is associated with tendon xanthomas but ocular manifestations, including corneal arcus and xanthelasma, are relatively non-specific, particularly in the elderly. In diabetes, retinopathy and neuropathy are often present. Patients with signs of peripheral vascular disease (e.g. absent pulses, arterial bruits) have associated coronary artery involvement in at least 75% of cases.

### Complications

Angina is a symptom and does not itself produce complications. Nevertheless, patients with angina are at risk of all the other manifestations of coronary artery disease, including myocardial infarction and sudden death.

### Diagnosis

Figure 5.2 summarizes diagnostic strategy for the evaluation of the patient with chest pain. A careful history — emphasizing the location of the pain, its character and relation to provocative stimuli — provides the most useful information. If the history is *typical*, the probability of coronary artery disease is high, rising to above 90% in men over 40 years of age and women over 60. If the history is *atypical*, the diagnostic probability is lower, falling below 10% in men under 30 and women under 40. In patients where the history, age and sex indicate an intermediate probability (10–90%) of coronary artery disease, stress testing helps to confirm or refute the diagnosis. However, it is not an infallible technique,

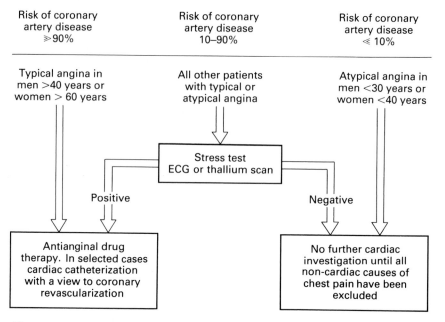

**Fig. 5.2**  Diagnostic strategy in chronic stable angina.

and Bayes' theory of diagnostic probability states that the predicted accuracy of a positive test will vary according to the probability of coronary heart disease in the population under study. Thus, stress testing is generally unhelpful in patients with a very low risk (less than 10%), because misleading false positive results are common in this group; also, in patients with a very high risk (more than 90%), a positive result — whilst strongly predicting coronary heart disease — can hardly increase the diagnostic probability further. For these reasons, stress testing is best reserved for patients in whom the history, age and sex indicate an intermediate probability of coronary heart disease.

### Stress testing

*Exercise electrocardiogram (ECG)* (Fig. 5.3)   This is one of the most widely used tests for evaluating the patient with chest pain. The patient is usually exercised on a treadmill, the speed and slope of which can be adjusted to increase the workload gradually. The exercise ECG provides important diagnostic and prognostic information.

   *Diagnostic information.*   The resting ECG is often normal in the patient with coronary artery disease, but, as heart rate and blood-pressure increase during exercise, myocardial oxygen demand may rise sufficiently to cause ischaemia. Exercise-induced horizontal (planar) or down-sloping ST segment depression is strongly suggestive of myocardial ischaemia —

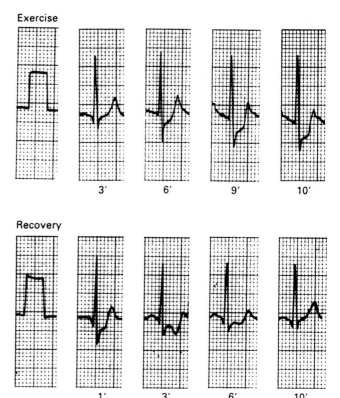

**Fig. 5.3**  Stress testing — exercise ECG (lead V4). Note the progressive planar depression of the ST segment during exercise. During recovery the ECG slowly reverts to normal after a period of 10 min.

particularly when associated with typical chest pain. Other causes of ST depression unassociated with coronary disease are shown in Fig. 2.13. Note that ST segment changes are usually impossible to interpret in the presence of left bundle branch block, digitalis therapy or paced rhythms, any of which effectively contraindicates the exercise ECG for diagnostic purposes.

*Prognostic information.*  Diagnostic ST segment depression at a low workload usually indicates very severe coronary artery disease and a poor prognosis. Exercise-induced ventricular arrhythmias or a paradoxical fall in blood-pressure is also a bad prognostic sign, sometimes reflecting extensive coronary artery disease but more commonly advanced left ventricular dysfunction.

*Exercise thallium-201 myocardial perfusion scintigraphy* (see p. 61)  The resting myocardial perfusion scintigram may be normal in coronary artery disease, but exercise-induced ischaemia produces a regional perfusion defect, which reverses during rest. Reversible perfusion defects of this type are strongly suggestive of myocardial ischaemia caused by coronary artery disease, and must be distinguished from fixed perfusion defects

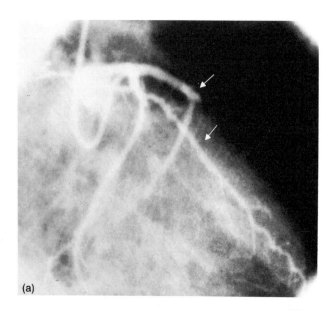

(a)

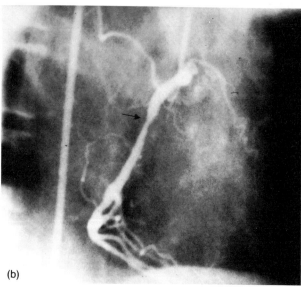

(b)

Fig. 5.4  Coronary arteriography. Left (a) and right (b) coronary arteriograms are shown. The left anterior descending coronary artery is occluded after the first septal branch (arrowed) and there is diffuse disease in the obtuse marginal branch of the circumflex artery (arrowed). The right coronary artery has a tight narrowing in its mid portion (arrowed).

(present at rest and during exercise), which are caused by an area of myocardial infarction. In general, the larger the area of hypoperfusion (fixed or reversible) the worse the prognosis.

*Stress radionuclide angiography* (see p. 61)   In practice, peripheral cold stress (cold pressor test) is used more commonly than exercise during radionuclide angiography. In patients with coronary artery disease, stress-

**Table 5.3**    Indications for coronary arteriography

1  Severe angina unresponsive to medical treatment
2  Angina in patients aged under 50
3  Unstable angina
4  Myocardial infarction in patients aged under 50
5  Angina or a positive exercise test following myocardial infarction
6  Cardiac arrhythmias when there is clinical suspicion of underlying coronary artery disease
7  Preoperatively in patients requiring valve surgery when advanced age (>40) or angina suggests a high probability of coronary artery disease

induced myocardial ischaemia produces regional abnormalities of left ventricular wall motion, which reverse following withdrawal of the stress.

### Coronary arteriography (see p. 68)

This is the definitive diagnostic test (Fig. 5.4). The technique is invasive and not without risk (mortality below 0.1%) and is not appropriate in every patient. It is usually reserved for patients being considered for coronary artery bypass grafting or coronary angioplasty (Table 5.3).

### Differential diagnosis

Careful consideration of the differential diagnosis is essential in the patient with chest pain. Angina is a term which jeopardizes insurance and career prospects and may condemn someone to a life of needlessly restricted activity.

*Neuromuscular disorders*    Chest wall pain from the costochondral junctions or the muscular insertions on the ribs and sternum is common. The pain is usually sharp and localized and may be provoked by coughing or isometric stress such as pushing or pulling.

*Upper gastrointestinal disorders*    Oesophageal pain caused by acid reflux is retrosternal but, unlike angina, has a burning quality and is provoked by stooping or lying flat, particularly after a meal. Peptic ulceration occasionally causes pain in the lower chest but the history will usually demonstrate a specific relation to eating. Importantly, upper gastrointestinal pain is not provoked by exertion and usually responds to antacids. Oesophageal spasm may be more difficult to distinguish from angina because the pain is retrosternal and may be relieved by glyceryl trinitrate. Nevertheless, symptoms are usually protracted and unrelated to exertion.

*Psychological disorders*    Neurotic anxiety that focuses on the heart is common and disabling. Symptoms, however, are rarely typical of angina:

stabbing pains in the left side of the chest are a common complaint and may be associated with hyperventilation. Time spent discussing the problem with the patient is more productive than extensive investigation, which only serves to reinforce fixed notions of underlying heart-disease.

*Syndrome X*   A number of patients have typical angina but normal coronary arteries and none of the conditions listed in Table 5.2. Definitive diagnosis requires the demonstration of normal angiographic anatomy by cardiac catheterization. The name, syndrome X, adequately describes the lack of understanding which surrounds this condition, although undoubtedly there is some heterogeneity with psychological chest pain. In some cases inadequate coronary vasodilator reserve may be the cause of ischaemia, but anti-anginal drugs are rarely effective. Nevertheless, as a group, patients with syndrome X have an excellent prognosis, comparable to that of the general population.

## Treatment

### General measures

The management of angina should include correction of established risk factors, particularly in young patients. Conditions which exacerbate angina (e.g. obesity, hypertension, arrhythmias, thyrotoxicosis, anaemia) require prompt attention. Exercise should be encouraged — within limits set by the severity of angina — because it enhances the sense of well-being and also has a training effect that leads to long-term improvement in functional capacity.

### Medical therapy (Table 5.4)

Drugs used to treat angina help correct the imbalance between myocardial oxygen supply and demand, most importantly by coronary vasodilatation. However, reductions in oxygen demand may be achieved by reducing heart rate, contractility or left ventricular wall tension as determined by blood-pressure. Nitrates and beta-blockers are usually used as first-line agents, with calcium antagonists as the second choice. In addition, low-dose aspirin (75–150 mg daily) is now recommended in patients with angina to protect against myocardial infarction.

*Nitrates*   These dilate the coronary arteries and peripheral circulation, improving the myocardial oxygen supply–demand ratio by increasing coronary flow and reducing left ventricular wall tension (blood-pressure). Sublingual glyceryl trinitrate, by tablet or spray, is rapidly absorbed through the buccal mucosa, providing relief within 3 min, and can also

**Table 5.4** Medical treatment of angina

| Drugs | Dose |
|---|---|
| *Nitrates* | |
| Glyceryl trinitrate | |
|    sublingual tablet | 0.3 mg as required |
|    aerosol spray | 0.4–0.8 mg as required |
|    cutaneous cream | 25–50 mg daily (only 5–10 mg absorbed) |
| Isosorbide mononitrate | 20 mg twice daily |
| *Beta-blockers* | |
| Metoprolol | 50–100 mg three times daily |
| Slow-release metoprolol | 200 mg daily |
| Atenolol | 50–100 mg once or twice daily |
| Bisoprolol | 5–10 mg once daily |
| *Calcium antagonists* | |
| Nifedipine | 5–10 mg three times daily |
| Slow-release nifedipine | 20 mg twice daily |
| Verapamil | 40–80 mg three times daily |
| Diltiazem | 60–120 mg three times daily |
| Amlodipine | 5–10 mg once daily |

be used prophylactically to prevent angina during vigorous exertion. Glyceryl trinitrate is now available as a cream for percutaneous absorption by application of an adhesive skin-patch. This provides sustained blood concentrations, which appear to encourage the development of nitrate tolerance in some patients. For this reason, responsiveness is variable and current recommendations are for the patch to be removed for periods of up to 12 hours each day, ensuring peaks and troughs of nitrate activity.

Long-term nitrates for regular oral administration are widely used. Isosorbide dinitrate undergoes considerable first-pass metabolism in the liver, unlike the more recently introduced mononitrate, which is now the preferred agent. A twice-daily regimen provides effective 24-hour cover (Table 5.4).

Nitrates are non-toxic and generally well tolerated. Side-effects caused by vasodilatation include headache and postural dizziness.

*Beta-blockers* These reduce myocardial oxygen demand by slowing the heart rate and reducing contractility and wall tension (blood-pressure). A wide variety of agents is available, all with similar anti-anginal efficacy; choice is largely determined by patient acceptability. In general, long-acting drugs such as atenolol are preferred for once- or twice-daily administration. Additional advantages of atenolol are its cardioselectivity and its lipid insolubility, which largely prevents entry into the central nervous system. Thus, non-cardiac effects of beta-blockade, including cold extremities and drowsiness, are less troublesome than with non-selective agents, such as propranolol. Beta-blockers, regardless of cardioselectivity, should never be used in patients with a history of bronchial asthma since they can precipitate severe bronchospasm. They should also be avoided in heart failure, because of their negative inotropic action.

*Calcium antagonists*   Like nitrates, these are vasodilators and improve myocardial oxygen balance by their effect on coronary flow and blood-pressure. They also cause variable reductions in contractility, particularly verapamil, which should be avoided in heart failure. Side-effects are related to vasodilatation and include facial flushing, headache, postural dizziness and mild ankle oedema.

### Revascularization procedures

These include coronary artery bypass surgery and balloon angioplasty. An essential prerequisite of both is coronary arteriography, in order to define the coronary anatomy and select the appropriate revascularization procedure.

*Coronary artery bypass surgery*   In patients with proximal coronary artery stenoses or occlusions, saphenous vein grafts applied to the ascending aorta may be inserted into the coronary arteries distal to the diseased segments. Alternatively, the internal mammary artery can be mobilized, for grafting. This produces a better long-term result, but the procedure is technically more demanding and is usually only practicable for left-anterior descending disease.

Coronary bypass surgery provides significant relief from angina in

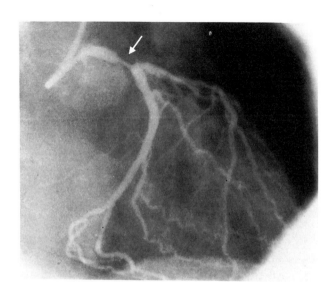

**Fig. 5.5**   Left main coronary artery disease. This left coronary arteriogram shows a very tight narrowing in the left main stem (arrowed).

over 80% of cases, and mortality is less than 2%, rising to between 5 and 10% for a second procedure. In addition to the symptomatic benefit, prospective studies of bypass surgery versus medical therapy have shown a clear prognostic benefit for surgery in certain subgroups with high-risk coronary anatomy, including patients with left main disease (Fig. 5.5) and patients with multi-vessel disease, particularly when the proximal left-anterior descending coronary artery is involved. The potential for prognostic benefit provides the rationale for offering coronary arteriography to all young patients (less than 50 years) with angina.

Saphenous vein grafts have a perioperative occlusion rate of up to 10%, depending largely on the adequacy of 'run-off', which determines flow within the graft. Anticoagulation with aspirin or warfarin helps preserve graft patency in the perioperative period, but late occlusion can be expected in many patients after 10–12 years, due to accelerated atherosclerotic disease. Internal mammary grafts, however, usually remain patent much longer than this.

*Coronary angioplasty* (Fig. 5.6)   This is being used increasingly for myocardial revascularization. A catheter with a terminal balloon is introduced percutaneously and directed into the diseased coronary artery over a fine guide-wire. Inflation of the balloon dilates the artery and restores normal flow. The technique is less invasive and less costly than bypass surgery and offers particular advantages to the patient, because hospitalization is brief and immediate return to normal activities is possible. However, only 33–50% of patients with symptomatic coronary artery disease are suitable candidates for angioplasty and results are best in patients with a proximal stenosis involving only one or two major vessels. Nevertheless, as experience increases, excellent results are being obtained in patients with more extensive disease. Coronary angioplasty provides effective relief from angina in over 80% of cases and carries a low mortality (less than 1.5%), although effects on prognosis will not be known until the results of randomized survival studies become available. The major disadvantage of coronary angioplasty is restenosis of the artery in 20–30% of cases, nearly always in the first 6 months. Prophylactic treatment with warfarin, aspirin or calcium antagonists has proved unhelpful. Repeat angioplasty is usually successful, but the recently introduced coronary stent (an expansile tubular wire-mesh device), designed to preserve luminal patency, may also find application in these cases. Recurrent angina beyond the first 6 months is more commonly the result of disease progression elsewhere in the coronary tree.

In complete coronary occlusion, conventional angioplasty is successful in only about 50% of cases. Drills and laser devices are being developed for these difficult cases but it remains uncertain whether they will play a useful clinical role.

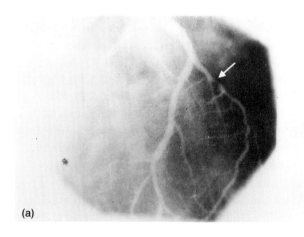

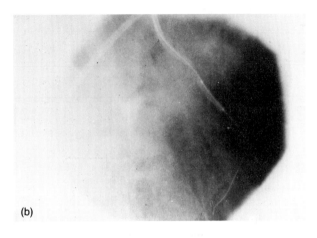

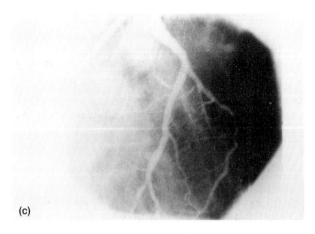

**Fig. 5.6** Coronary angioplasty. (a) A tight stenosis in the left anterior descending coronary artery is shown (arrowed). (b) During angioplasty. A balloon catheter has been positioned across the stenosis and inflated. (c) After angioplasty. The stenosis has been successfully dilated and the left anterior descending coronary artery is now widely patent.

## Prognosis

The natural history of coronary artery disease is summarized in Fig. 5.7. In individual patients with angina, the pattern of symptoms may show

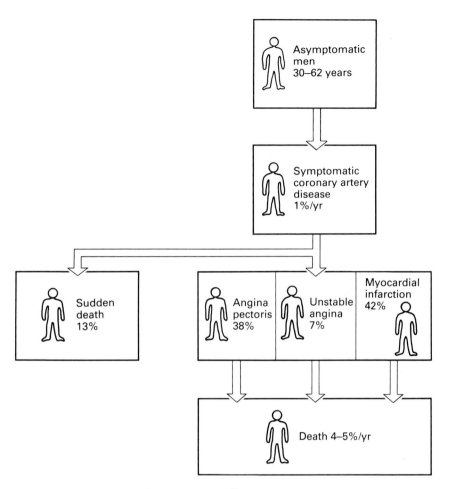

**Fig. 5.7**   Natural history of coronary artery disease.

little change over several years and may even improve as collateral vessels open up. More common is a gradual deterioration in symptoms, with an annual mortality of about 4%. Arteriographic findings permit a more precise prediction of prognosis with the annual mortality rising from less than 2% in single-vessel to 12% in multi-vessel disease.

## Variant angina

This unusual anginal syndrome was first described by Prinzmetal and is characterized by unprovoked episodes of chest pain, which may be associated with ST segment elevation on the ECG. Coronary artery disease is present in 70% of cases, but in the remainder the coronary arteries appear normal. An exaggerated increase in coronary arterial tone (spasm) has been demonstrated in these patients during attacks of angina.

The spasm is usually focal in distribution and even in the absence of coronary artery disease can restrict flow sufficiently to produce profound myocardial ischaemia. These patients are at risk of cardiac arrhythmias, and prolonged attacks of spasm may result in myocardial infarction. Calcium antagonists prevent spasm and are the treatment of choice. Nitrates are also beneficial, but beta-blockers are less so and may be detrimental if unopposed alpha-adrenergic stimulation further increases coronary tone.

### Unstable angina

This is caused by subocclusive coronary thrombosis, initiated by rupture of an atheromatous plaque. It presents with recurrent and usually prolonged episodes of angina, occurring on minimal exertion or at rest, and may be the first manifestation of coronary artery disease or may occur as an abrupt change in an established pattern of chronic stable angina. Attacks of pain are often associated with reversible ST segment depression on the ECG (Fig. 5.8).

Unstable angina is a medical emergency requiring management in the coronary care unit. Myocardial infarction or death occurs in between 5 and 30% of cases within 3 months. The antithrombotic effects of heparin infusion and aspirin (independently and in combination) have been shown to improve prognosis by preventing progression of the coronary thrombosis to complete occlusion. Patients should also receive glyceryl

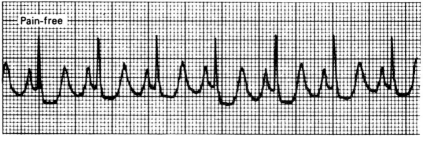

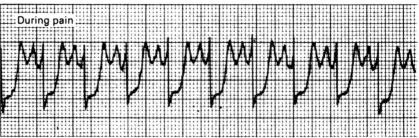

**Fig. 5.8** Unstable angina. During chest pain the heart rate increases and marked depression of the ST segment occurs; there is some loss of R-wave amplitude. These changes reverse as chest pain is relieved.

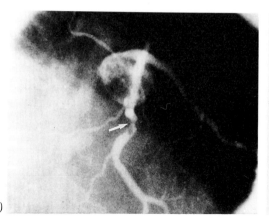
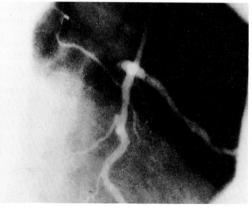

(a)                                    (b)

**Fig. 5.9** Unstable angina treated by coronary angioplasty. The patient had continuing severe chest pain despite medical treatment. Coronary arteriography showed a subocclusive thrombus, clearly visible as a filling defect in the circumflex coronary artery (arrowed). Angioplasty (right panel) restored arterial patency and relieved symptoms.

trinitrate infusion and beta-blockers to improve the myocardial oxygen supply–demand imbalance. Calcium antagonists are less helpful. Early coronary arteriography with a view to bypass surgery or angioplasty is usually recommended, particularly in younger patients and those in whom symptoms fail to settle promptly (Fig. 5.9).

## Myocardial infarction (MI)

This is caused by occlusive coronary thrombosis, initiated by rupture of an atheromatous plaque. It may be the first manifestation of coronary artery disease or may occur against a background of chronic stable angina, often with the recent development of unstable symptoms.

## Clinical manifestations

Clinical manifestations of acute myocardial infarction are largely attributable to the direct effects of ischaemic myocardial damage and to autonomic disturbance. The effects of complications are discussed on pp. 130–139.

### Myocardial damage

Chest pain is the most prominent manifestation of ischaemic myocardial damage. It is characteristically unprovoked, unaffected by glyceryl trinitrate and prolonged, often lasting several hours. Like angina, the pain has a band-like constricting quality, which is retrosternal and may radiate into the arms, neck and jaw. In an estimated 10% of cases, symptoms are so trivial that medical attention is not sought. Asymptomatic infarction of this type is more common in the elderly and in diabetic patients with autonomic neuropathy. Other manifestations of ischaemic myocardial damage include a palpable dyskinetic impulse over the left precordium (more common in anterior infarction) and a fourth heart sound. Pyrogens released from the damaged myocardium cause low-grade pyrexia for the first 3 days and during this period the white cell count and erythrocyte sedimentation rate (ESR) are commonly elevated.

### Autonomic disturbance

Manifestations of autonomic disturbance may include sweating, vomiting or syncope. Sympathoadrenal activation causes tachycardia and elevation of blood-pressure (these usually settle with pain relief), and also hyperglycaemia and hyperlipidaemia by stimulation of glycogenolysis and lipolysis. Hypokalaemia is also common and is caused by stimulation of sodium—potassium exchange at the cell membrane.

## Diagnosis

Early diagnosis of myocardial infarction is essential to allow prompt intervention with specific treatment to limit infarct size. In most cases the clinical history and the presenting ECG provide sufficient information. However, confirmation of the diagnosis requires documentation of the typical evolution of ECG and serum enzyme changes over a period of 2–3 days. Non-invasive imaging techniques are only rarely helpful.

### Electrocardiogram

This provides the most convenient and reliable method of early diagnosis. The typical evolution of changes is shown in Fig. 5.10. Peaking of the T wave and ST segment elevation occur within seconds of coronary occlusion and are often associated with reciprocal ST segment depression in the opposite ECG leads. These hyperacute changes resolve over a period of 18–24 hours, or much more rapidly if spontaneous or drug-induced coronary recanalization occurs. During this period a pathological Q wave (see p. 37) develops, which usually persists indefinitely and is pathognomonic of infarction. T-wave inversion may also occur at the time of Q-wave formation. Occasionally, changes are restricted to the ST segment and T wave without the development of a Q wave. Non-Q-wave infarction of this type often denotes more limited myocardial damage.

Because coronary occlusion affects different regions of the left ventricle, depending on the artery involved, the ECG provides a useful guide to infarct location. Left-anterior descending coronary occlusion causes

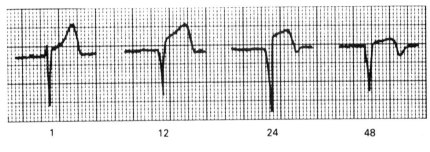

1    12    24    48

Hours after onset of chest pain

**Fig. 5.10** Evolution of ECG changes in acute myocardial infarction.

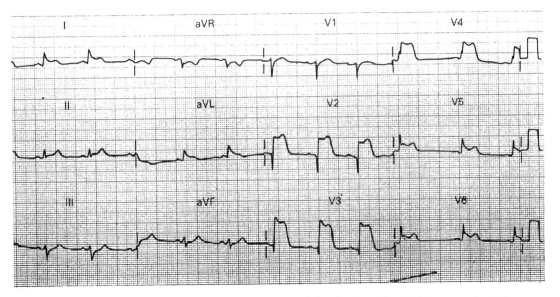

**Fig. 5.11** Acute anteroseptal myocardial infarction. The ECG shows marked ST segment elevation in leads V1–V3 with the development of pathological Q waves. There is also ST elevation in leads I, AVL and V4, indicating some lateral extension of the infarct. The ST depression in leads II, III and aVF is 'reciprocal'.

anterior infarction, with the characteristic evolution of changes in the anteroseptal (V1 to V3) or anterolateral (V1 to V6) leads, depending on the extent of damage (Fig. 5.11). The right coronary artery usually supplies the inferior wall of the ventricle by its posterior descending branch, and occlusion causes the characteristic evolution of ECG changes in leads II, III and aVF (Fig. 5.12). Circumflex occlusion causes lateral infarction with ECG changes in leads I, aVL and V6. It may also cause inferior damage in the 15% of people in whom the posterior descending artery arises from the circumflex rather than the right coronary artery. If the high posterior

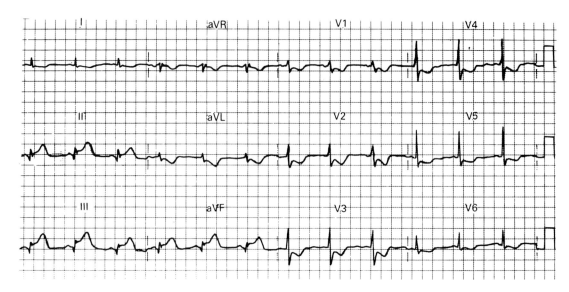

**Fig. 5.12** Acute inferoposterior myocardial infarction. ST segment elevation in leads II, III and aVF is associated with 'reciprocal' ST depression in leads I, aVL and V1–V4. Posterior extension of the infarct is indicated by the dominant R waves in leads V1 and V2.

wall of the ventricle is involved in the infarct, ECG changes may be difficult to detect but dominant R waves in leads V1 and V2 often develop (see Fig. 5.12).

The ECG is of little diagnostic value in patients with left bundle branch block or paced ventricular rhythms. Previous infarction with extensive Q waves and persistent ST segment changes may also make ECG interpretation difficult. Very occasionally patients with acute infarction present with a normal ECG, although serial recordings almost invariably reveal the development of diagnostic changes. A persistently normal ECG is rarely, if ever, consistent with the diagnosis of myocardial infarction.

## Serum enzymes

Electron microscopy has identified disruption of the sarcolemmal membrane as one of the earliest histological manifestations of myocardial infarction. Disruption allows intracellular enzymes to escape into the circulation for use as biochemical markers of infarction. Serial measurements are required to show diagnostic changes in blood concentrations (Fig. 5.13).

### Creatine kinase (CK)

Blood activities do not rise above normal until 6–10 hours after the onset of symptoms, peaking at 17–24 hours. This is earlier than other enzymatic

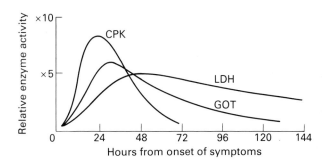

**Fig. 5.13** Serum enzyme activity (relative to normal values) in acute myocardial infarction.

tests but, nevertheless, limits its value for very early diagnosis. Skeletal-muscle CK may cause false-positive results in patients who have received intramuscular injections or external cardiac massage and, in difficult cases, the isoenzyme MB (specific for myocardial CK) can be measured.

### Glutamic oxaloacetic transaminase (GOT)

Serum levels peak on the second day. The enzyme, however, is non-specific, and liver, lung or brain disorders may give false-positive results.

### Lactic dehydrogenase (LDH)

Because serum levels remain elevated for 2 weeks, this is useful for patients who present late. Red cells are rich in LDH and traumatic vene-section or other causes of haemolysis may give false-positive results.

### Non-invasive imaging

Non-invasive imaging techniques require expensive equipment and are of limited diagnostic value. Echocardiography reliably identifies abnormal left ventricular wall motion in the zone of infarction, but the finding is not diagnostic because the same abnormality may reflect old infarction or acute ischaemia without irreversible damage. Radionuclide imaging with infarct-avid agents (usually technetium-99m pyrophosphate) is occasionally helpful in difficult cases (see Fig. 3.11). The isotope is taken up selectively in the zone of infarction, producing a 'hot spot' on the scintigram, but because uptake is rarely adequate until 24 hours after the onset of symptoms the method is of no value for early diagnosis. Moreover, false-positive results may occur in unstable angina. The role of immuno-scintigraphy with radio-labelled antimyosin antibody fragments is being investigated. These fragments adhere to myosin filaments through sarco-lemmal defects in necrotic cells and animal studies have detected infarction very early after interruption of coronary flow. Clinically, however, this technique looks less helpful because cardiac imaging cannot be done until 24 hours after the administration of antibody, to permit its clearance from the blood.

**Differential diagnosis**

Acute MI must be differentiated from other conditions presenting with chest pain and ECG changes, particularly pericarditis and pulmonary embolism. In these, however, the character of the chest pain is usually different and the typical ECG and enzyme changes do not occur. Aortic dissection may also cause ECG changes if the dissection occludes a coronary artery, producing coincidental MI.

## Treatment

The main aims of treatment are to correct symptoms, especially chest pain, and prevent death. Myocardial infarction has an estimated 35–40% mortality. About half of these deaths occur within 2 hours of the onset of symptoms, before hospital admission, and in most cases are the result of ventricular fibrillation, although myocardial rupture also contributes. In hospital, however, lethal arrhythmias can be corrected by defibrillation and the most important cause of death is left ventricular failure due to extensive infarction. Patients with large infarcts are also at increased risk of death in the year following hospital discharge. Thus, significant reductions in the mortality from acute myocardial infarction can be achieved by ensuring early access to a defibrillator and by intervention with specific drugs to prevent myocardial rupture and reduce infarct size.

**General measures**

Early access to a defibrillator prevents death from ventricular fibrillation. This requires prompt hospital admission and patients with unrelieved cardiac chest pain should be encouraged to call an ambulance immediately. Some centres have special resuscitation ambulances or helicopters, which save lives by providing access to a defibrillator during transfer to hospital. Following admission, the patient should be managed in the coronary care unit, where facilities are available for continuous ECG monitoring and cardiopulmonary resuscitation. Pain relief and sedation with intravenous (IV) diamorphine (2.5–5.0 mg) are essential, and drug-induced nausea and vomiting is prevented by IV prochlorperazine (25–50 mg). Anticoagulation with heparin is recommended, not only as an adjunct to thrombolytic therapy (see below), but also to guard against thromboembolism by preventing deep venous thrombosis and mural thrombosis within the left ventricle. If the early course is uncomplicated, the patient should be transferred to the general ward after 24 hours and mobilized, with a view to discharge within 7–10 days.

### Treatment to prevent myocardial rupture

Hypertensive patients appear to be at special risk of myocardial rupture in the first 24 hours. Early treatment with an IV beta-blocker reduces hospital mortality by about 15%, possibly because reductions in left ventricular wall tension and the force of contraction reduce the risk of rupture. Current recommendations are for IV metoprolol or atenolol (5 mg) in patients with a systolic blood-pressure of greater than 160 mmHg. The dose should be repeated every 15 min and titrated against the blood-pressure and heart rate responses. Treatment is contraindicated in patients with asthma, severe bradycardia (less than 60 beats/min) or left ventricular failure.

### Treatment to reduce infarct size

Myocardial infarction is a dynamic process and, although the subendocardium infarcts within 30 min, outward extension to involve the full thickness of the left ventricular wall may take several hours. If dissolution of the occlusive thrombus (thrombolysis) occurs before the transmural spread of infarction is complete, reperfusion and salvage of the threatened myocardium may reduce eventual infarct size. Spontaneous thrombolysis and coronary recanalization occur in about 15% of cases, accounting for many of the small non-Q-wave infarcts encountered in clinical practice. Thrombolytic therapy, however, increases the recanalization rate to 60–70% and can reduce mortality by up to 50% if given within 6 hours of the onset of chest pain; some benefit can still be demonstrated in patients treated within 24 hours (Fig. 5.14). Aspirin also reduces mortality, probably because its effects on platelet function favour coronary patency (Fig. 5.15). Current recommendations are for IV infusion of streptokinase (1.5 million units over 1 hour) and oral aspirin (75–150 mg) to be given as soon as possible after admission. Concurrent heparin infusion (1000 units/hour) may help maintain coronary patency after successful thrombolysis, and is usually continued until the patient starts to mobilize, with maintenance aspirin treatment thereafter. Contraindications to thrombolytic therapy include active peptic ulceration, prolonged resuscitation and surgery or stroke within the previous 4 weeks.

Streptokinase is antigenic and elicits an antibody response, which, in the event of re-exposure to the drug, neutralizes its thrombolytic activity and predisposes to anaphylaxis. Thus, patients with acute myocardial infarction who have received streptokinase in the previous 12 months should be treated with alteplase, an alternative, more expensive but

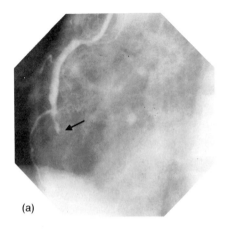

(a)

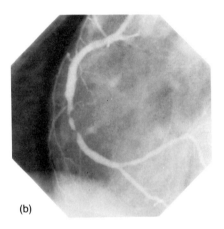

(b)

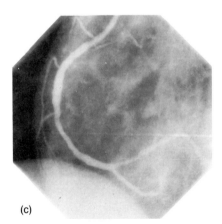

(c)

**Fig. 5.14** Thrombolytic therapy in acute myocardial infarction. (a) Before thrombolytic therapy. The right coronary artery is occluded (arrowed). (b) After intravenous streptokinase 1.5 million units. The coronary artery has recanalized, but there remains a very tight stenosis in its mid portion. (c) After coronary angioplasty. In order to prevent coronary reocclusion the stenosis has been successfully dilated.

equally effective thrombolytic agent. Alteplase is not antigenic because it is synthesized by recombinant deoxyribonucleic acid (DNA) technology to resemble the tissue plasminogen activator normally secreted by human endothelial cells.

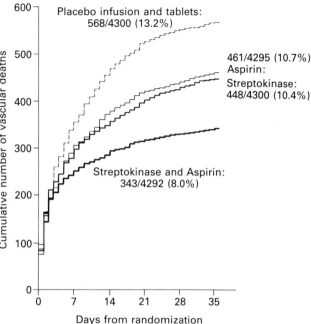

**Fig. 5.15**  ISIS-2 Study: randomized study of streptokinase and aspirin versus placebo in acute myocardial infarction. Treatment was given within 24 hours of the onset of chest pain. More than 17 000 patients were randomized in this study, which showed a >20% mortality reduction at 5 weeks for patients who received either streptokinase or aspirin as monotherapy. The beneficial effects of these drugs were additive, and patients who received both agents showed >40% mortality reduction. (Reproduced with permission from *Lancet* 1988, **ii**, 349–61.

Other drugs that may also reduce hospital mortality by limiting infarct size include glyceryl trinitrate and magnesium, although further studies are necessary to determine whether their use in combination with thrombolytic therapy should be adopted as standard practice.

**Secondary prevention**

In the year after MI, recurrent infarction or sudden death occurs in 10–15% of cases. Only stopping cigarette smoking, and therapy with beta-blockers (timolol, atenolol, metoprolol) has been shown unequivocally to reduce the incidence. Nevertheless, there is now increasing evidence that daily aspirin is beneficial, and also treatment to lower blood cholesterol in patients with hypercholesterolaemia. Recurrent infarction is more common following successful thrombolytic therapy because of the risk of coronary reocclusion. Daily aspirin may reduce that risk, but to date there is no evidence that revascularization by angioplasty or surgery is helpful. Revascularization is only recommended in patients with continuing chest pain or evidence of residual ischaemia during exercise stress testing. This has led to a policy of early ECG exercise testing at the time of hospital discharge in all uncomplicated cases (Fig. 5.16). Patients who develop ST segment depression suggestive of ischaemia or ventricular arrhythmias undergo cardiac catheterization with a view to bypass surgery or angioplasty. Cardiac catheterization is also recommended in patients of less

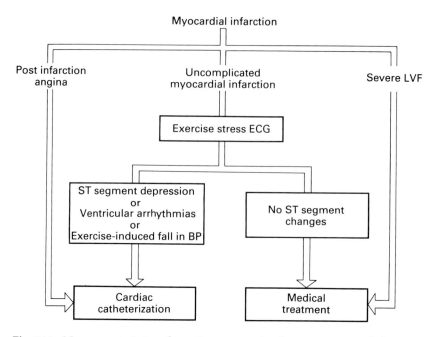

**Fig. 5.16**   Management strategy for patients recovering from acute myocardial infarction.

than 50 years of age in order that those with high-risk coronary anatomy (see p. 115) can be identified and offered revascularization for prognostic reasons.

### Rehabilitation treatment

Rehabilitation services after acute myocardial infarction vary from centre to centre, some offering none at all, others issuing simple advice on healthy living and a few providing a combination of health education and supervised physical training. Many patients find the psychological benefits of rehabilitation treatment invaluable, but it has been difficult to identify significant benefit in terms of secondary prevention. Nevertheless, at the very least, patients recovering from acute infarction should be advised about the risks of continued smoking and those who are hypertensive should be treated, ideally with a beta-blocker. In addition, cholesterol screening should be undertaken at 4–6 weeks (blood levels may be spuriously elevated before this), values above 6.3 mmol/litre requiring treatment by dietary restriction, with the addition of cholesterol-lowering drugs if this fails to reduce blood levels. Most patients can return to work after 2–3 months and meanwhile should be encouraged to undertake a programme of gradually increasing gentle exercise (walking, golf or swimming are ideal). Activities such as driving and sexual intercourse can usually be resumed 4 weeks after discharge from hospital.

## *Prognosis*

MI is fatal in approximately 40% of cases.

### Pre-hospital mortality (20%)

This is due to primary ventricular fibrillation (VF) in an estimated 75% of cases, with fulminant left ventricular failure (LVF) and myocardial rupture accounting for the remainder. Primary VF does not necessarily reflect extensive infarction and the prognosis for those patients who are successfully resuscitated is only slightly worse than for other early survivors.

### Hospital mortality (10–12%)

This is closely related to infarct size and with the introduction of thrombolytic and aspirin therapy has fallen from 15–25% to between 10 and 12%. Nevertheless, when infarction is sufficiently extensive to cause LVF, mortality exceeds 30%, rising to 80% for cardiogenic shock. Other factors, in addition to overt heart failure, are also predictive of a poor prognosis (Table 5.5), but, apart from advanced age, these are all variably related to extensive myocardial damage, emphasizing the important relation between infarct size and prognosis.

### Post-hospital mortality (10% in first year)

Prognosis after discharge is also influenced by infarct size, and patients with poor left ventricular function have a considerably higher 1-year mortality. Recent evidence indicates that treatment with ACE inhibitors reduces the mortality in this group of patients. Ventricular arrhythmias, particularly those occurring later than 36 hours after infarction, are often associated with extensive myocardial damage and are predictive of sudden death in the year after hospital discharge. Patients at high risk can be identified by electrophysiological stimulation studies (see p. 43), those with inducible ventricular arrhythmias being susceptible to sudden death. Less invasive methods can also identify patients at risk. These include the

**Table 5.5**  Adverse prognostic features in MI

Advanced age
Left ventricular failure (cardiomegaly, pulmonary congestion)
Systolic hypotension
Anterior full-thickness infarction
Left bundle branch block
History of previous myocardial infarction
Complex ventricular arrhythmias (particularly those occurring late (>36 h) after MI

**Table 5.6**  Arrhythmogenic factors in MI

Myocardial ischaemia/infarction
Heightened sympathoadrenal activity
   pain
   anxiety
   heart failure
Metabolic abnormalities
   hypoxaemia — pulmonary congestion
   acidosis — low cardiac output
   hypokalaemia — diuretics
   hypomagnesaemia — diuretics
Drugs
   sympathomimetic agents
   digitalis
   beta-adrenergic blockers

signal-averaged ECG, in which late potentials are a poor prognostic sign, and reduced vagal tone, as evidenced by reductions in heart rate variability (see p. 45). Unfortunately, however, there is no evidence that treatment of high-risk individuals affects outcome.

## Complications

### Arrhythmias

Patients with acute MI are at high risk of cardiac arrhythmias. Arrhythmia provocation is enhanced by autonomic responses, metabolic abnormalities and drug actions (Table 5.6). Management must include modification of these provocative factors, but specific treatment is usually only required if the arrhythmia intensifies ischaemia or embarrasses left ventricular function.

### *Atrial arrhythmias*

Abnormalities of sinus rhythm rarely require specific treatment. Severe *sinus bradycardia* my occur in inferior infarction and, if associated with low cardiac output, usually responds to intravenous atropine (0.3–0.6 mg). Treatment of *sinus tachycardia* should be directed at the underlying cause, particularly unrelieved pain, anxiety and heart failure.

*Atrial premature beats* occur commonly and require no treatment. *Atrial fibrillation* affects up to 15% of patients in the first 24 hours. Untreated, it usually reverts spontaneously to sinus rhythm but, meanwhile, the ventricular rate should be controlled with digoxin. There is no evidence that therapeutic doses of digoxin increase the risk of ventricular arrhythmias, but amiodarone is sometimes preferred for patients in whom ventricular arrhythmias have been troublesome.

### Ventricular arrhythmias

*Ventricular premature beats* occur in all patients after myocardial infarction. Considerable importance has been attached to certain patterns of ectopy as predictors of ventricular fibrillation:
1  Ectopic beat frequency greater than 5/min.
2  Very early 'R on T' ectopic beats.
3  Coupled ectopic beats.
4  Multifocal ectopic beats.
5  Runs of two or more consecutive ectopic beats.
It has been regular practice to treat these 'warning arrhythmias' with lignocaine and to ignore other patterns of ectopy. However, there is no evidence that this affects prognosis and the current view is that ventricular ectopic beats require no treatment, unless they are so frequent that they cause significant impairment of left ventricular function.

*Ventricular tachycardia (VT)* is defined as three or more consecutive ventricular premature beats at a rate in excess of 100 beats/min. It occurs in up to 40% of patients with acute MI and is associated with increased mortality. If VT complicates an excessively slow heart rate, atropine or pacemaker therapy is indicated; otherwise, paroxysmal attacks require suppression with lignocaine or amiodarone. Sustained VT usually produces severe hypotension and requires urgent direct-current cardioversion followed by lignocaine infusion. In most patients, antiarrhythmic therapy can be safely discontinued during mobilization on the ward. However, 'late' VT (more than 24 hours after admission) usually reflects extensive infarction and is a poor prognostic sign. Prophylactic antiarrhythmic treatment is not always helpful, and the pro-arrhythmic effects of some drugs may adversely affect prognosis (see p. 244). Amiodarone is preferred, but patients with troublesome late arrhythmias should undergo electrophysiological studies to provoke the arrhythmia and to test the efficacy of treatment before discharge from hospital (see p. 43).

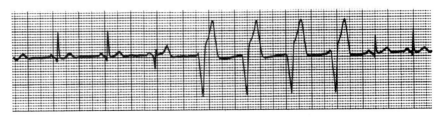

**Fig. 5.17** Idioventricular rhythm. After the second sinus beat there is a fusion beat (part sinus, part ventricular in origin) followed by a short four-beat run of accelerated idioventricular rhythm before the sinus node re-establishes itself.

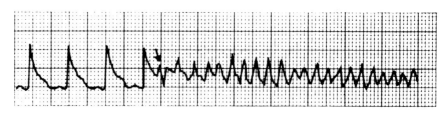

**Fig. 5.18** Primary ventricular fibrillation. The first four complexes are sinus beats with marked ST segment elevation indicating acute myocardial infarction. A very early ('R on T') ventricular premature beat (arrowed) initiates ventricular fibrillation.

*Accelerated idioventricular rhythm* (rate 60–100 beats/min) commonly complicates acute MI, particularly after thrombolytic therapy, but is rarely seen in other contexts (Fig. 5.17). The accelerated ventricular ectopic focus is usually in continuous competition with the sinus node, such that the idioventricular rhythm is typically intermittent, alternating with episodes of sinus rhythm. Treatment is unnecessary because the ventricular rate is, by definition, slow and haemodynamic stability is usually well maintained.

*Ventricular fibrillation* (Fig. 5.18) may be a primary electrical event (occurring within the first 24–48 hours of infarction) or may be secondary to severe left ventricular dysfunction (often occurring late after infarction). Urgent direct-current cardioversion is mandatory to prevent death. Primary VF affects up to 15% of patients in the coronary care unit and it is now clear that those patients successfully resuscitated have only a slightly increased risk of in-hospital and late mortality. It is generally accepted that the increased mortality risk is not sufficient to warrant prophylactic antiarrhythmic therapy. On the other hand, secondary VF predicts a very high incidence of sudden death during early follow-up, and prophylactic antiarrhythmic treatment is mandatory. The choice of prophylactic treatment is influenced by the same considerations as for 'late' VT (see above).

**Table 5.7** Indications for pacemaker therapy in MI

| |
| --- |
| Third-degree (complete) AV block complicating inferior MI and any of the following if unresponsive to atropine: |
|     rate <40/min |
|     low-output state |
|     unreliable escape rhythm |
|     bradycardia-dependent ventricular arrhythmias |
| Third-degree or Mobitz type II second-degree block complicating anterior infarction |
| Bifascicular block |

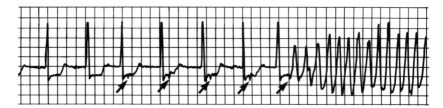

**Fig. 5.19**  Fixed-rate ventricular pacing early after myocardial infarction (VOO). The potential danger of using a pacemaker that is not inhibited by ventricular activation is illustrated here. The fixed-rate pacing artefact (arrowed) is seen early after each QRS complex, when the ventricle is refractory and unresponsive. However, electrical stimulation in this 'vulnerable period' of the cardiac cycle is dangerous and eventually triggers rapid ventricular tachycardia. This would not have happened if a ventricular-inhibited pacemaker (VVI) had been used.

### Heart block

MI may damage the specialized conducting tissues, causing an excessively slow heart rate, and pacemaker therapy may be necessary (Table 5.7). A temporary pacemaker is used in the first instance, which must be of the ventricular-inhibited demand type (VVI, see p. 220) because, in acute ischaemia, delivery of electrical stimuli during the vulnerable period of the cardiac cycle (T wave) may trigger lethal ventricular arrhythmias (Fig. 5.19).

#### *Atrioventricular (AV) nodal block*

This is usually a complication of inferior MI, resulting from inflammation and oedema around the AV node. Treatment, if necessary, is nearly always a temporary measure and recovery of normal conduction can be expected within 10 days. First-degree AV block, characterized by prolongation of the PR interval (greater than 0.20 sec), requires no treatment. Second-degree AV block is nearly always Mobitz type I (Wenckebach), in which successive sinus impulses find the AV node increasingly refractory

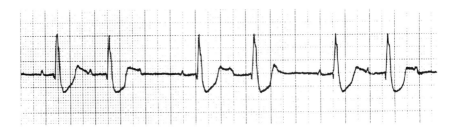

**Fig. 5.20**  Mobitz type I (Wenckebach) second-degree heart block in acute myocardial infarction. The patient has suffered a recent inferior infarct. Three Wenckebach cycles are shown, in each of which progressive prolongation of the PR interval culminates in a dropped beat.

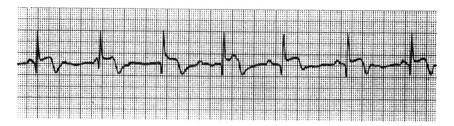

**Fig. 5.21**  Third-degree (complete) AV block. The lead is aVF and shows changes consistent with acute inferior myocardial infarction. There is complete failure of AV conduction, evidenced by the dissociation of the P waves and QRS complexes. The block is at the level of the AV node and a junctional focus has taken over pacemaker activity. Thus, the QRS complexes are narrow and the rate is well maintained.

until AV conduction fails (Fig. 5.20). No treatment is necessary unless the ventricular rate is very slow, when atropine will increase AV conduction. In third-degree (complete) AV block, complicating inferior infarction, a junctional pacemaker (low AV node, bundle of His) takes over in most instances (Fig. 5.21). The escape rhythm is usually reliable and cardiac output is well maintained, so that treatment is required only if the ven-

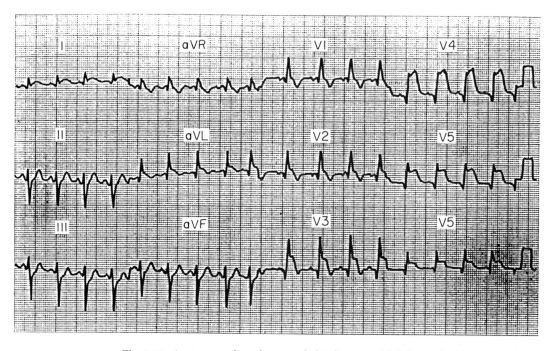

**Fig. 5.22**  Acute anterolateral myocardial infarction with bifascicular block. Note ST segment elevation in leads I, aVL and V1–V6. The rSR configuration in lead V1 indicates right bundle branch block. In addition there is marked left axis deviation, indicating damage to the anterior division of the left bundle branch. AV conduction is dependent upon the posterior division of the left bundle.

tricular rate is very slow. Junctional pacemakers often respond to atropine but, if this fails to increase the heart rate, temporary pacing is indicated until recovery of AV conduction occurs.

When AV block complicates anterior MI, damage is always extensive and mortality high. Block is usually below the bundle of His, involving both bundle branches, and, whether it is intermittent (Mobitz type II) or complete, the ventricular rate is usually slow and there is a significant risk of prolonged asystole. Temporary pacing is mandatory and, because recovery of normal AV conduction does not always occur, a permanent pacemaker may be required in the long term.

### *Bundle branch block*

Left or right bundle branch block complicating MI is an adverse prognostic sign but requires no specific treatment. Similarly, left or right axis devia-tion (indicating selective damage to the anterior or posterior divisions of the left bundle, respectively) requires no specific treatment. But, when axis deviation (hemiblock) and right bundle branch block occur together (bifascicular block), AV conduction is dependent upon the remaining division of the left bundle (Fig. 5.22). The risk of progression to com-plete heart block is considerable and temporary prophylactic pacing is indicated.

### Heart failure

Heart failure is the principal cause of death in the coronary care unit. It used to affect up to 50% of all patients admitted to hospital with MI but has become less common since the advent of thrombolytic and aspirin therapy to reduce infarct size. Because right ventricular damage is rarely

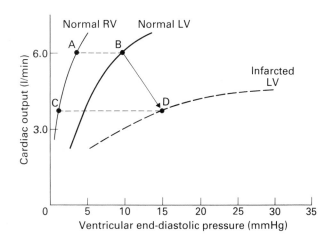

**Fig. 5.23**   Left ventricular function in acute myocardial infarction.

severe, LVF usually dominates and the function curve shifts downwards, with reduction in cardiac output (Fig. 5.23). However, the output of the two ventricles must remain equal and the ventricles, which previously operated on the horizontal line A–B, must now operate on the line C–D. This involves little change in right ventricular (RV) diastolic pressure, but left ventricular (LV) diastolic pressure increases considerably to maintain output. Thus, in acute myocardial infarction (AMI), the discrepancy between diastolic pressures in the right and left ventricles is variable (depending on the relative degrees to which the function curves are depressed) and measurement of central venous pressure is unhelpful for assessing left-sided filling pressure, which, if necessary, must be obtained by measurement of the pulmonary artery wedge pressure (see p. 70).

### Left ventricular failure

The severity is closely related to infarct size. When about 40% of the left ventricle is damaged, cardiogenic shock develops, characterized by cold, clammy skin, tachycardia, hypotension and oliguria. The principal clinical manifestations of LVF are pulmonary oedema and peripheral hypoperfusion, caused by elevated left atrial pressure and reduced cardiac output, respectively. Pulmonary oedema occurs when left atrial pressure rises above 18 mmHg and is best assessed by observation of the chest X-ray. Peripheral hypoperfusion occurs when cardiac output falls below 3.5 litres/min and is best assessed by measurement of urine output and skin

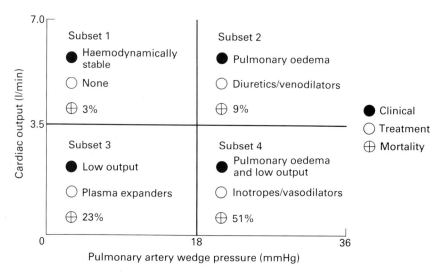

**Fig. 5.24** Haemodynamic subsets in acute myocardial infarction. The clinical, therapeutic and prognostic correlates of subset classification are demonstrated.

temperature. Four subsets of patients have been identified based on these clinical observations and defined by a left atrial (pulmonary artery wedge) pressure of 18 mmHg and a cardiac output of 3.5 litres/min (Fig. 5.24):

**1** Well-preserved left ventricular function requiring no specific therapy.

**2** Dominantly 'backwards' failure with pulmonary oedema but well-maintained cardiac output. Treatment with morphine and diuretics is usually effective.

**3** Dominantly 'forwards' failure without pulmonary oedema. Left atrial (pulmonary artery wedge) pressure is inappropriately low and oliguria and hypotension may be corrected by infusion of a plasma volume expander (e.g. blood, plasma), which increases cardiac output by the Starling mechanism. Careful monitoring of pulmonary artery wedge pressure, using a Swan–Ganz catheter, is recommended to prevent overloading the circulation. Pulmonary oedema develops if the wedge pressure rises above 18 mmHg.

**4** Low cardiac output and pulmonary oedema occurring together. Treatment must be directed towards improving left ventricular function with vasodilators and inotropes, which should be given by controlled intravenous infusion, to reduce pulmonary artery wedge pressure and improve cardiac output. Responses are best monitored with a Swan–Ganz catheter (see p. 70).

Subset classification provides not only a useful basis for therapeutic decision-making but also a means of predicting prognosis. Mortality rises from less than 5% in subset 1 to greater than 50% in subset 4.

### Right ventricular failure (RVF)

When right coronary occlusion causes inferior infarction, it is occasionally associated with variable right ventricular damage, which, if severe, may produce significant RVF with low cardiac output. The right ventricular function curve is displaced downwards (see Fig. 5.23), and the right atrial and jugular venous pressures are elevated. Useful increments in cardiac output can be achieved by further increasing right atrial pressure with infusion of a plasma volume expander, which increases the output of the right ventricle by the Starling principle. During the infusion, monitoring of the pulmonary artery wedge pressure with a Swan–Ganz catheter is recommended to guard against overloading the circulation and precipitating pulmonary oedema.

### Myocardial rupture

This is an important cause of death early after myocardial infarction, but may occur any time during the first 10 days. When rupture involves the free wall of the left ventricle, it produces severe tamponade, which is

**Table 5.8**  Differential diagnosis of ventricular septal defect and papillary muscle rupture

|  | Ventricular septal defect | Papillary muscle rupture |
|---|---|---|
| Murmur | Left sternal edge | Apex |
| Heart failure | Dominantly right-sided — often with minimal pulmonary oedema | Dominantly left-sided — always with severe pulmonary oedema |
| Infarct location | Anterior or inferior | Inferior |
| Right heart catheter | 'Step-up' in oxygen saturation in RV | Dominant 'v' wave in pulmonary artery wedge pressure trace |
| Echocardiography | Permits direct visualization of defect in some cases | Demonstrates flail valve leaflet |
| Doppler study | Demonstrates high-velocity jet across defect | Demonstrates high-velocity regurgitant jet |

nearly always rapidly fatal. Sudden haemodynamic deterioration, associated with the development of a pansystolic murmur, is caused by rupture of either the interventricular septum or a papillary muscle. This results in a ventricular septal defect or torrential mitral regurgitation, respectively. Clinically they are difficult to distinguish (Table 5.8) but accurate differential diagnosis is possible with colour-flow Doppler imaging, which identifies the high-velocity jet from left to right across the septum or backwards through the mitral valve, depending on the lesion. In most cases, however, urgent cardiac catheterization is required to define both the lesion and the coronary anatomy to assess the potential for surgical correction. Mortality is high and, although temporary haemodynamic support can be provided with the intra-aortic balloon pump, surgery should not be delayed unduly.

### Thromboembolism

Deep venous thrombosis and intracardiac mural thrombosis (overlying the infarcted ventricular myocardium) are potential sources of pulmonary and systemic thromboembolism, respectively. Heparin should be used prophylactically (see p. 124).

### Pericarditis

Pericarditis is a common cause of persistent chest pain the first 3 days following full-thickness myocardial infarction. It is a direct consequence of the underlying muscle damage and usually resolves within a week. During this period, the temperature may remain elevated and a pericardial friction rub is intermittently audible. Pericarditic pain can usually be distinguished from ongoing ischaemic pain by its sharp quality and its relation to deep inspiration, coughing or changes in posture. Anti-inflammatory analgesics such as aspirin or indomethacin provide effective symptomatic relief.

### Dressler's syndrome

About 40% of patients develop a pyrexial illness, often with pericarditis and pleurisy, 2–12 weeks after myocardial infarction. A similar illness is sometimes seen following heart surgery (post-cardiotomy syndrome). The cause is uncertain but autoimmune mechanisms seem likely: elevation of the ESR and leucocytosis occur in most cases. Anti-inflammatory analgesics are effective and, in severe cases, corticosteroids may shorten the course of the illness. Relapses may occur up to 2 years after MI.

### Left ventricular aneurysm

Following acute infarction, shrinkage and scarring of the damaged myocardium is usually complete within 6 weeks. In about 10% of cases, however, the healing process is inadequate and a thin-walled ventricular aneurysm develops. This may be associated with persistent ST segment elevation on the ECG. The risk of rupture is negligible and in many cases the aneurysm is of little consequence. However, left ventricular aneurysm can be a cause of cardiac arrhythmias, heart failure or clot embolization. If these complications cannot be controlled medically, excision of the aneurysm may be required.

### Sudden death

The majority of sudden deaths in the community occur in association with coronary artery disease and are presumed due to VF. The coronary artery disease usually involves all three major vessels and myocardial scars indicating old infarction may be present. In many cases, death occurs as a result of the abrupt rupture of an atheromatous plaque and coronary thrombosis. However, when successful resuscitation is achieved there is often no evidence of fresh infarction, indicating that severe ischaemia is the mechanism responsible for VF in many cases.

Following successful resuscitation, the patient requires full in-hospital investigation. This will usually involve cardiac catheterization with a view to myocardial revascularization (bypass surgery, angioplasty) or aneurysmectomy, if appropriate. Programmed electrical stimulation studies using intracardiac electrode catheters, in order to provoke the ventricular arrhythmia and to test the efficacy of antiarrhythmic therapy, may also be necessary (see p. 43). Only when a treatment regimen has been selected to protect against dangerous ventricular arrhythmias should the patient be discharged from hospital.

# Further reading

## *Prevalence, risk factors and secondary prevention*

Anonymous, Secondary prevention of coronary artery disease with lipid lowering drugs. *Lancet* 1989, **i**, 473–4.

Blackburn H. and Jacobs D.R. Physical activity and the risk of coronary artery disease. *N. Engl. J. Med.* 1988, **319**, 1217–19.

Davies M.J., Krikler D.M. and Katz D. Atherosclerosis: inhibition or regression as therapeutic possibilities. *Br. Heart J.* 1991, **65**, 302–10.

Fuster V., Cohen M. and Halperin J. Aspirin in the prevention of coronary disease. *N. Engl. J. Med.* 1989, **321**, 183.

Kannel W.B. Update on the role of cigarette smoking in coronary artery disease. *Am. Heart J.* 1981, **101**, 319–28.

Loscalzo J. Regression of coronary atherosclerosis. *N. Engl. J. Med.* 1990, **323**, 1337–9.

MacMahon S., Peto R., Cutler J. *et al.* Blood pressure, stroke and coronary heart disease. Part 1. Prolonged differences in blood pressure: prospective observational studies corrected for regression dilution balance. *Lancet* 1990, **335**, 765–74.

Myers R.H., Kiely D.K., Cupples L.A. and Kannel W.B. Parental history is an independent risk factor in coronary artery disease: the Framingham Study. *Am. Heart J.* 1990, **120**, 963–9.

Norwegian Multicenter Study Group. Timolol: timolol-induced reduction in mortality and reinfarction in patients surviving acute myocardial infarction. *N. Engl. J. Med.* 1981, **304**, 801–7.

Ross R. Pathogenesis of atherosclerosis: an update. *N. Engl. J. Med.* 1986, **314**, 488–99.

Scott J. Lipoprotein (a). *Br. Med. J.* 1991, **303**, 663–4.

Simpson R.J. and White A. Getting a handle on the prevalence of coronary heart disease. *Br. Heart J.* 1990, **64**, 291–2.

Tunstall Pedoe D.S. Exercise and heart disease: is there still a controversy? *Br. Heart J.* 1990, **64**, 293–4.

Wilson P.W.F., Cupples A. and Kannel W.B. Is hyperglycemia associated with cardiovascular disease? The Framingham Study. *Am. Heart J.* 1991, **121**, 586–90.

## *Angina*

Anonymous. Thallium scintigraphy for diagnosis and risk asessment of coronary artery disease. *Lancet* 1991, **338**, 786–8.

Block P.C. Coronary artery stents and other endoluminal devices. *N. Engl. J. Med.* 1991, **324**, 52–4.

Borow R.O. Prognostic applications of exercise testing. *N. Engl. J. Med.* 1991, **325**, 887–8.

Bourassa M.G. Fate of venous grafts: the past, the present and the future. *J. Am. Coll. Cardiol.* 1991, **17**, 1081–4.

Brady A.J.B. and Warren J.B. Angioplasty and restenosis. *Br. Med. J.* 1991, **303**, 729–30.

Cameron E.W.J. and Walker W.S. Coronary artery bypass surgery. *Br. Med. J.* 1990, **300**, 1219–20.

Campbell S. Silent myocardial ischaemia. *Br. Med. J.* 1988, **297**, 751–2.

Cannon R.O. Chest pain with normal coronary angiograms: is the heart innocent or guilty? *J. Am. Coll. Cardiol.* 1990, **16**, 596–8.

Detre K., Holubkov K., Kelsey S. *et al.* Percutaneous transluminal coronary angioplasty in 1985–1986 and 1977–1981: the National Heart, Lung, and Blood Institute Registry. *N. Engl. J. Med.* 1988, **318**, 265–70.

Gershlick A.H. and de Bono D.P. Restenosis after angioplasty. *Br. Heart J.* 1990, **64**, 351–3.

Helfant R.H. Stable angina pectoris: risk stratification and therapeutic options. *Circulation* 1990, **82** (suppl. II), 66–74.

Jones E.L. Multivessel coronary angioplasty. *J Am. Coll. Cardiol.* 1990, **16**, 1103.

Killip T. Twenty years of coronary bypass surgery. *N. Engl. J. Med.* 1988, **319**, 366–8.

Maseri A. Syndrome X: still an appropriate name. *J. Am. Coll. Cardiol.* 1991, **17**, 1471–2.

Petch, M.C. Coronary bypasses 10 years on. *Br. Med. J.* 1991, **303**, 661–2.

Selwyn A.P. and Ganz P. Myocardial ischemia in coronary artery disease. *N. Engl. J. Med.* 1988, **318**, 1058–60.

Sigwart U. Percutaneous transluminal coronary angioplasty: what next? *Br. Heart J.* 1990, **63**, 321–2.

Timmis A.D. Probability analysis in the diagnosis of coronary artery disease. *Br. Med. J.* 1985, **291**, 1443–4.

## *Acute ischaemic syndromes*

Anonymous. Twenty-five years of coronary care. *Lancet* 1988, **ii**, 830–1.

Anonymous. Non-Q-wave myocardial infarction. *Lancet* 1989, **ii**, 899–900.

Anonymous. Magnesium for acute myocardial infarction. *Lancet* 1991, **338**, 667–8.

Anonymous. Predictors of sudden death after myocardial infarction. *Lancet* 1991, **338**, 727–8.

Braunwald E. Optimizing thrombolytic therapy of acute myocardial infarction. *Circulation* 1990, **82**, 1510–13.

Byimgton R.P. and Furberg C.D. Beta blockers during and after acute myocardial infarction. In Francis G.S. and Alpert J.S. (eds), *Modern Coronary Care*. Boston, Little, Brown and Co., 1990, pp. 511–39.

Coplan N.L. Evolving management strategy for managing patients following thrombolytic therapy. *Am. Heart J.* 1990, **120**, 464–6.

Davies M.J. and Thomas A.C. Plaque fissuring — the cause of acute myocardial infarction, sudden ischaemic cardiac death, and crescendo angina. *Br. Heart J.* 1985, **53**, 363–73.

Forrester J.S., Diamond G.A., Chatterjee K. and Swan H.J.C. Medical therapy of acute myocardial infarction by application of hemodynamic subsets. *N. Engl. J. Med.* 1976, **295**, 1356 and 1404.

Fuster V., Cohen M., Stein B., Israel D.H. and Chesebro J.H. Anticoagulant and platelet inhibitor agents for myocardial infarction. In Francis G.S. and Alpert J.S. (eds), *Modern Coronary Care*. Boston, Little, Brown and Co., 1990, pp. 511–39.

Geltman E.M. Conservative management after thrombolysis: the strategy of choice. *J. Am. Coll. Cardiol.* 1990, **16**, 1535–7.

Goldstein S. Toward a new understanding of the mechanism and prevention of sudden death in coronary heart disease. *Circulation* 1990, **82**, 284–8.

Julian D.G., Pentecost D.L. and Chamberlain D.A. A milestone for myocardial infarction. *Br. Med. J.* 1988, **297**, 497–8.

Keung E.C. Antiarrhythmic treatment and myocardial infarction. *J. Am. Coll. Cardiol.* 1990, **16**, 1719–21.

Lamas G.A. and Pfeffer M.A. Left ventricular remodeling after acute myocardial infarction: clinical course and beneficial effects of angiotensin-converting enzyme inhibition. *Am. Heart J.* 1991, **121**, 1194–1202.

Lipkin D.P. Is cardiac rehabilitation necessary? *Br. Heart J.* 1991, **65**, 237–8.

Lubsen J. Medical management of unstable angina: what have we learnt from the randomized trials? *Circulation* 1990, **82** (suppl. II), 82–7.

Martin G.V. and Ritchie J.L. Thrombolysis: evidence for infarct size reduction. *J. Am. Coll. Cardiol.* 1991, **17**, 1458–60.

Peter C.T. and Helfant R.H. Postinfarction ventricular tachycardia and fibrillation: reassessing the role of drug therapy and approach to the high risk patient. *J. Am. Coll. Cardiol.* 1990, **16**, 531–2.

Rossouw, J.E., Lewis B. and Rifkind B.M. The value of lowering cholesterol after myocardial infarction. *N. Engl. J. Med.* 1990, **323**, 1112–19.

Schoenfeld M.H. Sustained ventricular arrhythmias after infarction: when should the worrying begin? *J. Am. Coll. Cardiol.* 1991, **17**, 327–9.

Theroux P., Ouimet H., McCans J. *et al.* Aspirin, heparin, or both to treat unstable angina. *N. Engl. J. Med.* 1988, **319**, 1105–11.

Timmis A.D. Post myocardial infarction syndrome. *Br. Med. J.* 1984, **289**, 636–7.

Timmis A.D. Early diagnosis of acute myocardial infarction. *Br. Med. J.* 1990, **301**, 941–2.

Wenger N.K. Rehabilitation of the coronary patient. *Prog. Cardiovasc. Dis.* 1986, **29**, 181–204.

White H. Thrombolytic therapy for recurrent myocardial infarction. *Br. Med. J.* 1991, **302**, 429–30.

Wilcox R.G. Coronary thrombolysis: round two and beyond *Br. Heart J.* 1991, **65**, 175–6.

Yusuf S., Sleight P., Held P. and McMahon S. Routine medical management of acute myocardial infarction: lessons from overviews of recent randomized controlled trials. *Circulation* 1990, **82** (suppl. II), 117–34.

# 6 Cardiomyopathy and Specific Heart Muscle Disorders

## Summary

Cardiomyopathy is defined as chronic heart muscle disease of unknown cause. *Dilated cardiomyopathy* is characterized by ventricular dilatation and hypertrophy with global impairment of systolic function and presents with the symptoms and signs of congestive heart failure. The chest X-ray and echocardiogram help confirm the diagnosis and treatment is the same as for other causes of heart failure. *Hypertrophic cardiomyopathy* is a familial disorder characterized anatomically by left ventricular hypertrophy, histologically by myocyte disarray and physiologically by impaired diastolic relaxation. The echocardiogram is usually diagnostic. Hypertrophic cardiomyopathy may cause dyspnoea or angina, requiring treatment with beta-blockers, but in many cases it presents with sudden death, caused by ventricular arrhythmias. Thus, all patients should undergo ambulatory electrocardiogram (ECG) monitoring and those with arrhythmias should be protected with amiodarone. *Restrictive cardiomyopathy* is rare in the UK and is characterized by endomyocardial fibrosis, often associated with hypereosinophilia. Physiologically it resembles constrictive pericarditis and differential diagnosis may require endomyocardial biopsy. It usually presents with symptoms of heart failure, requiring treatment with diuretics. Steroids may improve prognosis, particularly in patients with hypereosiniphilia.

Cardiomyopathy must be distinguished from those specific heart muscle diseases with an identifiable cause, such as viral infection, chronic alcohol abuse or daunorubicin toxicity. In all these examples the myocardial lesion and clinical presentation may be indistinguishable from dilated cardiomyopathy. Nevertheless, the differential diagnosis is important because in some cases correction of the underlying disorder prevents progression of the myocardial disease.

## Cardiomyopathy

The cardiomyopathies are a group of chronic heart muscle disorders of unknown cause, excluding those that are secondary to coronary artery disease, valvular disease, hypertension or other systemic disorders. Three types of cardiomyopathy are recognized: dilated, hypertrophic and restrictive.

## Dilated cardiomyopathy

Dilated cardiomyopathy is characterized by ventricular dilatation and hypertrophy associated with impaired systolic function. It occurs more commonly in 'developing' countries than in Western countries.

### Aetiology

The cause of dilated cardiomyopathy is, by definition, unknown but some evidence exists for an infectious–immune aetiology related to myocarditis. Heart-reactive antibodies and other serological markers of auto-immunity can occasionally be demonstrated in dilated cardiomyopathy. Moreover, myocardial biopsy specimens show histological features typical of myocarditis in over 15% of cases; in some of these, antibody tests for Coxsackie B virus are positive. Thus, it is possible that in certain cases abnormal immunological responses to common viral infections result in myocardial damage, leading to dilated cardiomyopathy.

### Pathophysiology

In dilated cardiomyopathy, the relative degree of left and right ventricular impairment is variable but in advanced cases severe biventricular failure is usually present. Enhanced sympathoadrenal activity is a hallmark of the disease and may be regarded as a compensatory phenomenon directed at maintaining systolic function and increasing ventricular filling by central redistribution of flow. Nevertheless, the inotropic responsiveness of the failing heart diminishes progressively, possibly as a result of adrenoceptor down-regulation (see p. 79). As cardiac output and renal perfusion deteriorate, secondary aldosteronism leads to salt and water retention, which not only further increases ventricular filling but also causes worsening systemic and pulmonary congestion.

Thus, the heart is exposed to a considerably exaggerated volume load. This results in progressive dilatation, hypertrophy and fibrosis of all the cardiac chambers. Atrial fibrillation (AF) commonly supervenes and stretching of the atrioventricular valve rings can lead to functional incompetence of the mitral and tricuspid valves, which causes additional impairment of ventricular function.

### Clinical manifestations

Dilated cardiomyopathy often remains asymptomatic in its early stages, but, with progression of the disease, symptoms and signs of congestive heart failure develop, particularly effort-related fatigue and dyspnoea. Orthopnoea and peripheral oedema develop later in the course of the illness. At this stage, tachycardia and signs of cardiac enlargement are invariably present. The jugular venous pulse (JVP) is elevated, often with a giant 'v' wave, due to tricuspid regurgitation. Auscultation reveals a third heart sound; pansystolic murmurs of mitral and tricuspid regurgitation may also be present.

## Complications

Cardiac arrhythmias are common in dilated cardiomyopathy, particularly AF and ventricular premature beats. More complex ventricular arrhythmias account for the significant incidence of sudden death in this condition. Systemic and pulmonary thromboembolism, arising from the dilated left- and right-sided cardiac chambers, may also occur (Fig. 6.1).

## Diagnosis

The ECG is invariably abnormal in dilated cardiomyopathy but the changes are non-specific and may include arrhythmias (see above), bundle branch block and T-wave flattening or inversion. The chest X-ray (CXR) shows cardiac enlargement with dilated upper-lobe veins, progressing to pulmonary oedema. The echocardiogram is the most useful diagnostic investigation and shows four-chamber dilatation and global left ventricular contractile impairment (Fig. 6.1). Doppler studies often reveal mitral and tricuspid regurgitation.

### Differential diagnosis

The differential diagnosis includes all causes of specific heart muscle disease. Coronary artery disease, valvular disease, hypertension and

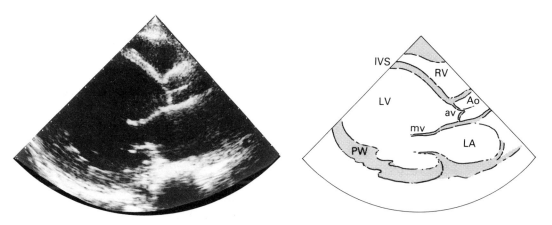

**Fig. 6.1** Dilated cardiomyopathy. Echocardiogram. Note the severe left ventricular dilatation with global contractile impairment.

alcohol abuse are the most important because heart failure is potentially preventable. Coronary artery disease is suggested by a history of angina or myocardial infarction (MI), associated with pathological Q waves on the ECG. Valvular disease can usually be diagnosed by echocardiography, although mitral regurgitation can present difficulties as it can be both the cause and the result of left ventricular failure (LVF). In hypertensive and alcoholic heart-disease, the history is often helpful and the examination may reveal other non-cardiac manifestations of end-organ injury.

## Treatment

Management is the same as that of congestive heart failure (see p. 91). Angiotensin-converting enzyme (ACE) inhibitors may slow the progression of left ventricular disease and should be introduced early in the course of the illness, together with diuretics.

Prophylactic anticoagulation with warfarin is necessary for patients in atrial fibrillation, because the risk of thromboembolism is greatest in this group. Anticoagulation is mandatory for patients who have already had a thromboembolic event, so long as there are no specific contraindications.

Ventricular arrhythmias — particularly ventricular tachycardia — should be suppressed with an appropriate agent, although it is not known whether this prevents sudden death. Amiodarone is the drug of choice because it is less negatively inotropic. Treatment should be monitored by ambulatory ECG monitoring (see p. 40).

## Prognosis

The prognosis in dilated cardiomyopathy is variable, depending upon the degree of left ventricular dysfunction and the incidence of ventricular arrhythmias. Once symptoms of heart failure develop, the average five-year survival is less than 50%.

## Hypertrophic cardiomyopathy

Hypertrophic cardiomyopathy is known by a variety of other names (e.g. hypertrophic obstructive cardiomyopathy, idiopathic hypertrophic sub-aortic stenosis, asymmetric septal hypertrophy), all of which should now be discarded since they make inaccurate assumptions about the nature of the disease. Hypertrophic cardiomyopathy is characterized *anatomically* by ventricular hypertrophy of unknown cause, usually with disproportionate involvement of the interventricular septum. *Physiologically* the disorder is one of impaired diastolic relaxation of the non-compliant ventricles; systolic function is well preserved and usually hyperdynamic.

*Pathologically* there is extensive disarray and disorganization of cardiac myocytes.

## Aetiology

It shows an autosomal dominant pattern of inheritance, although family studies have shown that the expression of disease within the family is very variable. The disease has protean manifestations and it is now uncertain whether there is one genetic abnormality or several, all of which produce abnormal left ventricular hypertrophy. The difficulties of producing a unifying genetic aetiology are heightened by the observation that in some patients the disease is present from a very young age while in others, born with apparently normal hearts, it does not develop until adulthood. Further complexity is introduced by recent autopsy findings

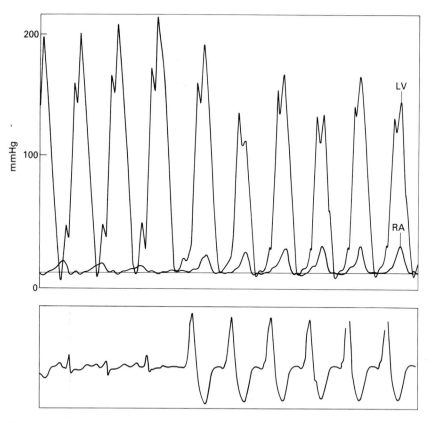

**Fig. 6.2** Hypertrophic cardiomyopathy — ventricular pacing. Simultaneous recordings of the ECG and left ventricular (LV) and right atrial (RA) pressure signals are shown. Ventricular pacing produces a broad-complex rhythm with AV dissociation. The loss of synchronized atrial contraction at end-diastole impairs LV filling and causes abrupt deterioration in function, evidenced by pulsus alternans, a fall in LV pressure and a rise in RA pressure.

in young, previously healthy, patients who died suddenly and whose families were known to have hypertrophic cardiomyopathy. There was the extensive myocardial disarray typical of the disease without evidence of hypertrophy. Whether these patients would have gone on to develop the morphological features of hypertrophic cardiomyopathy is unknown.

## Pathophysiology

Disordered diastolic function is the principal pathophysiological feature. The hypertrophic, non-compliant ventricle exhibits profoundly impaired diastolic relaxation (see Fig. 4.2). Thus, adequate ventricular filling is dependent upon high diastolic pressure. Atrial systole is particularly important for maintaining adequate filling and the development of AF (or atrioventricular (AV) dissociation) can produce abrupt deterioration in cardiac output (Fig. 6.2).

Systolic function is always vigorous in hypertrophic cardiomyopathy and the left ventricular ejection fraction is usually in excess of 90%. Ventricular emptying is not only more complete than in the normal ventricle, it is also more rapid. Thus, 80% of the stroke volume is ejected in the first half of systole compared with 57% in the normal ventricle.

In the past, considerable importance has been attached to the subvalvular pressure gradient in the left ventricular outflow tract which can be demonstrated in some, but not all, patients (Fig. 6.3). The gradient is characteristically labile and can be provoked or exaggerated by a variety of physiological and pharmacological stimuli (Fig. 6.4). The concept has

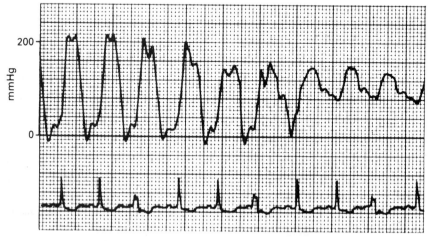

**Fig. 6.3** Hypertrophic cardiomyopathy — left ventricular outflow gradient. The catheter has been pulled back from the apex of the left ventricle into the aorta during simultaneous pressure recording. After the fourth beat there is an abrupt drop in left ventricular systolic pressure, representing a subvalvular gradient of about 50 mmHg. Note that there is no systolic pressure gradient across the aortic valve itself.

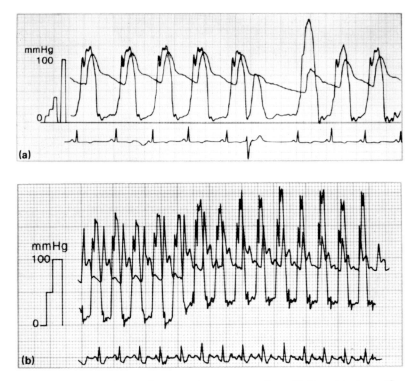

**Fig. 6.4** Hypertrophic cardiomyopathy — provocation of left ventricular outflow gradient. Simultaneous recordings of the left ventricular and aortic pressure signals are shown. (a) Ventricular premature beat. After the fifth sinus beat there is a ventricular extrasystole. Note that in the post-extrasystolic beat marked exaggeration of the subvalvular pressure gradient occurs. (b) Valsalva manoeuvre. During Valsalva (evidenced by the rise in left ventricular diastolic pressure) there is a progressive increase in the subvalvular pressure gradient.

arisen of *dynamic* left ventricular outflow obstruction, which must be distinguished from the *fixed* outflow obstruction of aortic stenosis. The dynamic obstruction in hypertrophic cardiomyopathy has been attributed to the hypertrophied septum and to the mitral valve leaflets, which show a characteristic forward movement into the left ventricular outflow tract during systole (Fig. 6.5).

The importance of the subvalvular pressure gradient in hypertrophic cardiomyopathy may have been exaggerated. The obstruction caused by the anterior motion of the mitral valve leaflets occurs too late to impede left ventricular ejection, 80% of which is complete by mid-systole. Although symptoms may be improved by surgical debulking of the interventricular septum, this is as likely to reflect improved diastolic relaxation as relief of outflow obstruction. Importantly, neither symptoms nor prognosis is related to the presence or severity of the subvalvular pressure gradient.

## Clinical manifestations

Hypertrophic cardiomyopathy is often asymptomatic. The most common complaint is exercise-related dyspnoea, due to the elevated left atrial pressure required to fill the stiff, non-compliant ventricle. In advanced cases, frank congestive heart failure occasionally develops. Angina, due to the excessive oxygen demand of the hypertrophied ventricle, may also be troublesome.

Examination reveals a jerky carotid pulse, due to forceful ejection early in systole. The apical impulse is forceful and often has a double thrust, due to a palpable fourth heart sound. Auscultatory features include the fourth heart sound and a mid-systolic murmur in the aortic area, due to turbulent flow in the left ventricular outflow tract. Mitral regurgitation affects nearly 50% of cases, causing an apical pansystolic murmur.

## Complications

Cardiac arrhythmias are the major complication. AF causes abrupt clinical deterioration (see above). Paroxysmal ventricular arrhythmias produce dizziness and syncope (Stokes–Adams attacks) and herald sudden death.

## Diagnosis

In the majority of patients, the ECG shows ventricular hypertrophy with prominent voltage deflexions in the chest leads (see Fig. 12.1). A broad-notched P wave reflects left atrial enlargement. Q waves unrelated to infarction are found in up to 30% of cases, usually in the inferolateral leads. The chest X-ray is normal.

The echocardiogram is usually diagnostic (Fig. 6.5) and shows left ventricular hypertrophy, often with disproportionate involvement of the interventricular septum (*asymmetric septal hypertrophy*). The two-dimensional recording is required for accurate assessment of the extent and distribution of left ventricular hypertrophy (Fig. 6.5). Other echocardiographic manifestations of hypertrophic cardiomyopathy include systolic obliteration of the left ventricular cavity, systolic anterior motion (SAM) of the mitral valve and mid-systolic closure of the aortic valve.

In difficult cases, cardiac catheterization is necessary. The left ventricular angiogram shows a hypertrophic ventricle with systolic cavity obliteration. Haemodynamic studies may demonstrate the pressure gradient in the left ventricular outflow tract.

### Differential diagnosis

The symptoms, signs and ECG findings in hypertrophic cardiomyopathy resemble those in aortic stenosis, although the character of the carotid

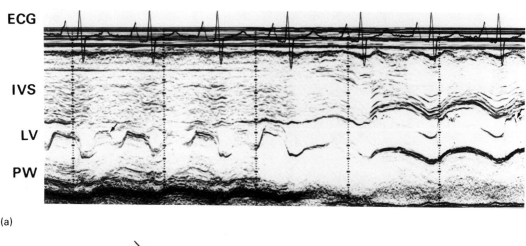

ECG

IVS

LV

PW

(a)

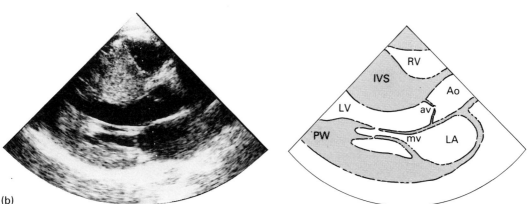

RV
IVS
Ao
LV
av
PW
mv
LA

(b)

**Fig. 6.5** Hypertrophic cardiomyopathy — echocardiogram. The M-mode recording (a) shows marked hypertrophy of the interventricular septum with a normal posterior wall. Systolic anterior motion of the mitral valve and early closure of the aortic valve are indicated by the arrows. A better appreciation of the septal hypertrophy is provided by the two-dimensional recording (b).

pulse is different (jerky versus slow-rising). The echocardiogram is particularly helpful and, in aortic stenosis, shows a thickened valve associated with left ventricular hypertrophy but not with other features of hypertrophic cardiomyopathy.

Other important differential diagnoses are coronary artery disease and hypertensive heart-disease. In patients with angina, exclusion of coronary artery disease may require coronary arteriography. Hypertensive heart-disease is suggested by a history of hypertension and by evidence of hypertensive injury elsewhere in the body, particularly the optic fundus and the kidneys.

## Treatment

No drugs have been shown to affect disease progression in hypertrophic cardiomyopathy; treatment is aimed toward correcting symptoms and preventing sudden death; beta-blockers (e.g. propranolol, atenolol) are first-line agents. By slowing the heart rate they control angina and improve diastolic filling of the noncompliant left ventricle. Calcium antagonists (e.g. verapamil) improve diastolic relaxation and are sometimes helpful in patients who fail to respond to beta-blockers.

Surgical procedures in which the hypertrophic myocardium is excised have been shown to correct symptoms (see above), but do not affect long-term prognosis and should be reserved for patients with intractable symptoms.

All patients with hypertrophic cardiomyopathy should undergo ambulatory ECG monitoring for at least 48 hours. If ventricular arrhythmias are detected, amiodarone is the drug of choice because preliminary evidence suggests that it may prevent sudden death. Because hypertrophic cardiomyopathy is inherited, the patient should receive genetic counselling and members of the family should be screened.

## Prognosis

Hypertrophic cardiomyopathy has an annual mortality of about 2.5% in adults, but the prognosis is worse in children, about 6% of whom die each year. The majority of deaths occur suddenly, presumably caused by ventricular fibrillation (VF).

## Restrictive cardiomyopathy

Restrictive cardiomyopathy is characterized by endomyocardial fibrosis with progressive obliteration of the ventricular cavities. Systolic function is normal but diastolic filling is restricted, due to reduced ventricular compliance (see Fig. 4.2). It is rare in the UK and is nearly always associated with cryptogenic hypereosinophilia. It occurs more commonly in the tropics but usually without hypereosinophilia.

## Aetiology

The cause of restrictive cardiomyopathy is, by definition, unknown. Endomyocardial damage induced by local release of eosinophilic granules has been postulated but this is unlikely to provide the full explanation since an identical cardiac lesion occurs in the tropical form of the disease without hypereosinophilia.

## Pathophysiology

The pathophysiology is almost identical to constrictive pericarditis, and resembles some cases of amyloid heart-disease and haemochromatosis

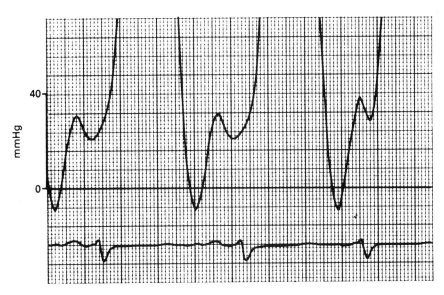

**Fig. 6.6** Restrictive cardiomyopathy — left ventricular pressure signal. The rapid rise in diastolic pressure is checked abruptly in mid-diastole by the restrictive effect of the left ventricle. This gives the diastolic pressure signal its characteristic dip-and-plateau contour.

(see Chapter 16). In all these conditions, the ventricle relaxes normally in early diastole but by mid-diastole becomes virtually indistensible. Thus, ventricular filling is at first rapid but is abruptly checked in mid-diastole, producing a characteristic dip-and-plateau configuration on the ventricular diastolic pressure recording obtained at cardiac catheterization (Fig. 6.6). With progression of endomyocardial fibrosis, ventricular filling deteriorates and elevation of atrial pressures, associated with reduced cardiac output, results in congestive heart failure. In restrictive cardiomyopathy, the normal differential between right- and left-sided filling pressures is occasionally preserved, such that right atrial pressure, though elevated, remains lower than left atrial pressure throughout the cardiac cycle. This is in contrast to constrictive pericarditis, in which equalization of the ventricular filling pressures on both sides of the heart always occurs (see Fig. 7.6). Nevertheless, the differential diagnosis may be very difficult and thoracotomy is sometimes required to rule out pericardial disease.

## Clinical manifestations

Restrictive cardiomyopathy presents with congestive heart failure. The patient complains of peripheral oedema and effort-related fatigue and dyspnoea. The JVP is elevated with an unusually dynamic waveform due to a prominent Y descent (rapid ventricular filling in early diastole), and

Kussmaul's sign is present. Auscultation reveals third or fourth heart sounds (see Chapter 1).

## Complications

Cardiac arrhythmias are less common than in other types of cardio-myopathy. Systemic and pulmonary thromboembolism from the affected ventricles may occur.

## Diagnosis

Laboratory investigations demonstrate hypereosinophilia in most cases of endomyocardial fibrosis seen in the UK. ECG abnormalities, including ST segment and T-wave changes, are non-specific. The CXR is usually normal but may show pulmonary infiltrates related to hypereosinophilia. The echocardiogram shows variable obliteration of the ventricular cavities, but this is rarely diagnostic. In most cases, confirmation of the diagnosis is dependent upon demonstration of typical restrictive physiology at cardiac catheterization (Fig. 6.6). Endomyocardial biopsy during the catheter procedure provides the histological diagnosis.

### Differential diagnosis

Constrictive pericarditis and amyloid heart-disease are the most important differential diagnoses. Demonstration of a calcified or otherwise thickened

**Table 6.1**  Common causes of specific heart muscle disease

| | |
|---|---|
| **1  Cardiovascular**<br>Coronary artery disease<br>Chronic valvular disease<br>Hypertension | **5  Toxic**<br>Alcohol<br>Doxorubicin<br>Cobalt |
| **2  Infective**<br>Viral, e.g. Coxsackie A and B, influenza,<br>  varicella, mumps, herpes simplex<br>Protozoal, e.g. trypanosomiasis (Chagas'<br>  disease) | **6  Connective tissue disease**<br>Polyarteritis nodosa<br>Systemic lupus erythematosus<br><br>**7  Neuromuscular disease**<br>Muscular dystrophy<br>Friedreich's ataxia |
| **3  Metabolic**<br>Thiamine deficiency (beriberi)<br>Kwashiorkor | |
| **4  Endocrine**<br>Thyrotoxicosis<br>Myxoedema<br>Diabetes mellitus | **8  Infiltrative**<br>Amyloidosis<br>Haemochromatosis<br>Sarcoidosis<br>Neoplastic<br><br>**9  Miscellaneous**<br>Peripartum cardiomyopathy<br>Obesity |

pericardium by conventional radiology or computed tomography indicates constriction. Haemodynamic studies usually show similar physiology in all these conditions. Endomyocardial biopsy is necessary to confirm cardiac amyloid.

### Treatment

In restrictive cardiomyopathy associated with hypereosinophilia, steroids or cytotoxic agents lower the eosinophil count. This may halt disease progression and produce significant symptomatic improvement. When symptoms continue to deteriorate, surgical excision of the ventricular endocardium is usually helpful, presumably because the reduction in myocardial mass improves diastolic relaxation.

Other measures include diuretic therapy for heart failure and anticoagulants to guard against thromboembolism.

### Prognosis

In patients who respond well to definitive medical and surgical treatment (see above) the prognosis is good. Progressive endomyocardial fibrosis, with worsening congestive heart failure, has a less favourable outlook.

## Specific heart muscle disease

The presence of an identifiable aetiological agent distinguishes specific heart muscle disease from cardiomyopathy, which is, by definition, idiopathic. Nevertheless, in most cases, the cardiac lesion in specific heart muscle disease is similar to and often indistinguishable from cardiomyopathy. A variety of systemic disorders affect the myocardium (Table 6.1), of which the most common are viral infection, alcohol and doxorubicin toxicity. Other disorders are discussed in Chapter 16.

### Viral myocarditis

Myocarditis occurs in a variety of infective disorders but viral disease is the most important cause in the UK. Although viruses have never been unequivocally recovered from human myocardium, serological studies have identified Coxsackie B as the most common. Others include influenza and herpes simplex.

Transient ECG changes (usually T-wave inversion) commonly occur during viral infection and probably reflect subclinical myocardial involvement. Occasionally symptoms and signs of congestive heart failure develop, usually while other signs of viral infection are subsiding. Cardiac arrhythmias and pericarditis may also occur. The CXR shows variable cardiac enlargement and the echocardiogram confirms ventricular dilatation and contractile impairment. In most cases there is complete recovery within a week but, rarely, fulminant heart failure and death occur. The relation between viral myocarditis and dilated cardiomyopathy remains speculative (see p. 144). Although endomyocardial biopsy by the transvenous route is potentially diagnostic in acute myocarditis, the findings do not influence management because no specific treatment is of proven value. Nevertheless, certain features of the illness suggest immunologically mediated damage, and the role of immunosuppressive therapy (steroids, azathioprine) is being investigated.

## Alcoholic myocardial disease

The acute and chronic effects of alcohol poisoning on the heart must be distinguished. Acutely, alcohol intoxication causes cardiac arrhythmia, usually atrial fibrillation, which reverts spontaneously to sinus rhythm as blood alcohol levels decline. Indeed, alcohol intoxication is probably the most common cause of atrial fibrillation in young adults. Much more serious is chronic alcohol abuse, which, over a period of 10 years or more, can lead to life-threatening myocardial disease. In some cases, nutritional deficiencies (e.g. thiamine) or toxic beer additives (e.g. cobalt) may contribute to myocardial damage. In the large majority of cases, however, the toxic effects of alcohol or its metabolites are directly responsible.

AF occurs more commonly in alcoholic myocardial disease than in dilated cardiomyopathy, but in all other respects cardiac manifestations are identical in the two conditions. A history of heavy alcohol consumption is highly suggestive of an alcoholic aetiology, particularly when other manifestations of alcohol abuse are present.

Abstinence may prevent progression of alcoholic myocardial disease and, in some cases, results in variable improvement; complete regression occasionally occurs if treatment is started early.

## Doxorubicin-induced myocardial disease

The myocardial toxicity of the cytotoxic drug doxorubicin (Adriamycin) is largely dose-related and rarely occurs if the total cumulative dose is less than $500\,mg/m^2$, a level normally achieved after 6–8 months of therapy. Children appear particularly susceptible, and even relatively small doses can lead to a lifelong reduction in myocardial mass that may result in decreased cardiac reserve. Other factors, such as mediastinal irradiation, may have synergistic cardiotoxic effects in patients receiving doxorubicin.

Myocardial disease usually presents acutely, with symptoms and signs of severe congestive heart failure. The response to anti-failure treatment is almost invariably unsatisfactory and death usually occurs within a few weeks of presentation. Once symptomatic heart failure is established, withdrawal of doxorubicin does not halt progression of the disease. Endomyocardial biopsy is the most sensitive means of identifying early doxorubicin toxicity but this is not feasible in most centres. Regular non-invasive monitoring by echocardiography or radionuclide ventriculography is recommended, with a view to doxorubicin withdrawal at the first sign of left ventricular dysfunction.

## Further reading

Anonymous. Cardiac biopsy in myocarditis. *Lancet* 1990, **336**, 283−4.

Anonymous. Dilated cardiomyopathy and enteroviruses. *Lancet* 1990, **336**, 971−3.

Braunwald E. Hypertrophic cardiomyopathy: continued progress. *N. Engl. J. Med.* 1989, **320**, 800−2.

Caforio A.L.P., Stewart J.T. and McKenna W.J. Idiopathic dilated cardiomyopathy. *Br. Med. J.* 1990, **300**, 890−1.

Chahine R.A. Surgical versus medical therapy of hypertrophic cardiomyopathy: is the perspective changing? *J. Am. Coll. Cardiol.* 1991, **17**, 643−5.

Davies M.J. Hyperytrophic cardiomyopathy: one disease or several? *Br. Heart J.* 1990, **63**, 263−4.

Diamond I. Alcoholic myopathy and cardiomyopathy. *N. Engl. J. Med.* 1989, **320**, 458−60.

Doroshow J.H. Doxorubicin-induced cardiotoxicity. *N. Engl. J. Med.* 1991, **324**, 843−5.

Nicod P., Polikar R. and Peterson K.L. Hypertrophic cardiomyopathy and sudden death. *N. Engl. J. Med.* 1988, **318**, 1255−7.

Oakley C.M. and Olsen E.G.J. Eosinophilic heart disease. *Br. Heart J.* 1977, **39**, 233−7.

O'Connell J.B. Immunosuppression for dilated cardiomyopathy. *N. Engl. J. Med.* 1989, **321**, 1119−21.

Parrillo J.E. Heart disease and the eosinophil. *N. Engl. J. Med.* 1990, **323**, 1560−1.

Peters N.S. and Poole-Wilson P.A. Myocarditis − continuing clinical and pathologic confusion. *Am. Heart J.* 1991, **121**, 942−7.

Rezkalla S.H. and Kloner R.A. Management strategies in viral myocarditis. *Am. Heart J.* 1989, **117**, 706−8.

Wilmshurst P.T. and Katritsis D. Restrictive cardiomyopathy. *Br. Heart J.* 1990, **63**, 323−4.

# 7 Pericardial Disease

## Summary

*Pericarditis*, the most common pericardial disorder, is usually idio-pathic or viral in origin, occasionally reflecting more serious systemic disease. It presents with typical chest pain, often associated with wide-spread concave ST elevation on the electrocardiogram (ECG). Treat-ment is with anti-inflammatory analgesics and recovery can normally be expected within a few days. Almost any cause of pericarditis can cause effusion, and *tamponade* may develop if the fluid collects rapidly, leading to critical elevation of pressure in the pericardial sac and restriction of ventricular filling. This is particularly common when malignant disease of the breast or lung invades the pericardium. In tamponade the diastolic filling pressures of both right and left ven-tricles rise and equilibrate, with loss of the normal differential. The patient presents with dyspnoea and hypotension; a paradoxical pulse is invariable, the jugular venous pulse (JVP) is elevated and Kussmaul's sign is commonly present. Treatment is by pericardiocentesis. When pericarditis leads to fibrosis and shrinkage of the pericardial sac, *constriction* may occur. This impedes diastolic relaxation and restricts ventricular filling, with physiology similar to that of tamponade. It is a chronic, debilitating illness, characterized by elevation of the JVP, a positive Kussmaul's sign and fluid retention, with oedema and ascites. Cardiac catheterization demonstrates elevation and equalization of the ventricular filling pressures, and computed tomography confirms thickening of the pericardium. Diuretics are sometimes helpful, but definitive treatment requires pericardiectomy.

## Introduction

The pericardium envelops the heart and the proximal portions of the great arteries and veins. The visceral pericardium is intimately attached to the epicardial surface of the heart and is separated from the parietal pericardium by the pericardial space, which is filled by the heart in diastole. Further dilatation of the heart is resisted by the relatively indis-tensible pericardial sac. The pericardium plays an important role in preventing rapid cardiac dilatation when ventricular diastolic pressures rise acutely, but, in contrast to its effect on diastolic function, does not influence the systolic function of the heart.

**Table 7.1** Causes of acute pericarditis

1  Idiopathic
2  Infective — viral (Coxsackie B, influenza, mumps, varicella)
              — bacterial (*Staphylococcus, Streptococcus, Mycobacterium tuberculosis*)
3  Connective tissue disease — systemic lupus erythematosus, rheumatoid arthritis
4  Myocardial infarction
5  Following myocardial infarction or cardiac surgery — Dressler's syndrome
6  Uraemia
7  Neoplastic disease — breast, lung, lymphoma, leukaemia
8  Radiation therapy

## Acute pericarditis

### Aetiology

Causes of pericarditis are listed in Table 7.1. Viral infection probably accounts for the majority of cases, including many of those idiopathic cases in which a specific cause cannot be positively identified. Purulent bacterial pericarditis (e.g. *Staphylococcus, Streptococcus*) has become considerably less common, as has tuberculous pericarditis. Pericarditis is a frequent complication of advanced renal failure and is not always prevented by regular dialysis; the cause is unknown. In acute myocardial infarction (MI), pericarditis usually denotes extensive full-thickness damage, but it may also occur late following infarction, when Dressler's syndrome is the likely diagnosis (see p. 139). Polyserositis involving the pericardium characterizes many connective tissue disorders, particularly rheumatoid disease and systemic lupus erythematosus. Patients with neoplastic disease may develop pericarditis, due either to cardiac metastases or to therapeutic irradiation of the chest. It is an inevitable consequence of opening the pericardial sac during heart surgery, and may also occur following accidental chest trauma.

### Clinical manifestations

In acute pericarditis, chest pain is the predominant symptom and commonly follows an upper respiratory tract infection in viral pericarditis. It is retrosternal in most cases but differs from the pain of MI by its sharp quality, aggravated by deep inspiration, coughing and changes in posture (particularly lying flat). Occasionally, the pain has an aching quality and radiates into the shoulders or arms, making it more difficult to distinguish from ischaemic cardiac pain. Auscultation of the heart typically, though not invariably, reveals a pericardial friction rub, which confirms the diagnosis. The rub has a high-pitched scratching quality and may be audible during any phase of the cardiac cycle. Its intensity is influenced by respiration and changes in posture.

## Complications

The major complication is pericardial effusion, which may cause tamponade. Pericarditis can also progress to pericardial constriction. Atrial arrhythmias are reported to occur commonly in pericarditis, but this has been difficult to confirm in prospective studies.

## Diagnosis

The chest X-ray (CXR) is usually normal in pericarditis, except when pericardial effusion produces cardiac enlargement. The ECG may also be normal, but in most cases there is ST segment elevation, reflecting epicardial injury (Fig. 7.1). The ST segment elevation affects any or all of the standard or precordial leads (except aVR), depending on the site of inflammation, and is characteristically concave upwards (unlike myocardial infarction), returning towards base-line as pericardial inflammation subsides. T-wave inversion is common, but the evolution of ST segment and T-wave changes seen in myocardial infarction does not occur. Importantly, Q waves never develop in pericarditis.

The aetiological diagnosis in viral pericarditis depends upon the demonstration of elevated viral antibody titres in acute serum samples, which decline during convalescence. Virus may sometimes be cultured from throat swabs and stools. In connective tissue disorders there is usually evidence of multisystem disease; specific serology, including rheumatoid or antinuclear factors, may be positive. Purulent pericarditis

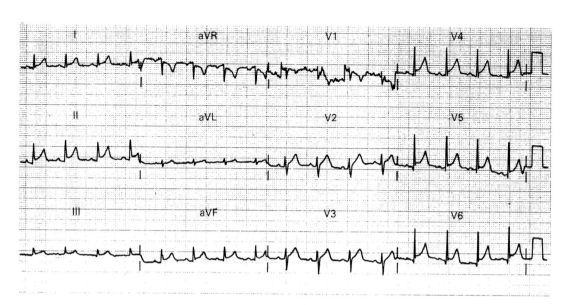

**Fig. 7.1** ECG in acute pericarditis. Note the concave ST segment elevation present in multiple leads.

is often associated with infective foci elsewhere in the body, particularly the lungs, and cultures of sputum and blood samples should be obtained. Recognition of tuberculous pericarditis is difficult if the CXR is normal. When the aetiology is doubtful, pericardial fluid (if present) may be aspirated for bacteriological, cytological and serological examination.

## Differential diagnosis

Important differential diagnoses in acute pericarditis are MI and pleurisy. The quality of pericarditic pain, the failure of Q waves to develop on the ECG and the absence of serum enzyme changes are usually sufficient to rule out MI. Pleuritic pain is similar in quality to pericarditis but its location is different: a pleural rub is often audible over the painful area and signs of pleural effusion may also be present. In making the differential diagnosis, remember that pericarditis may occur in association with both MI and pleurisy.

## Treatment

Treatment is directed at relieving chest pain and, if possible, correcting the underlying cause. Non-steroidal anti-inflammatory analgesics (e.g. aspirin, indomethacin) are drugs of choice for controlling symptoms. In viral pericarditis, no other treatment is necessary. Bacterial pericarditis requires vigorous antibiotic treatment, which in tuberculosis (TB) should be continued for at least a year.

Pericarditis may be recurrent, particularly in Dressler's syndrome, connective tissue disorders and idiopathic disease. When frequent and troublesome, low-dose steroid therapy offers effective prophylaxis.

**Table 7.2**   Causes of tamponade

---

1   *Pericarditis*
    Neoplastic disease
    Connective tissue disease (particularly rheumatoid)
    Any other cause of pericarditis when pericardial effusion is a complication (see Table 7.1)

2   *Haemopericardium*
    Heart surgery — postoperative haemorrhage
    Myocardial infarction — rupture of free wall of ventricle
    Aortic aneurysm — rupture into pericardial sac
    Aortic dissection — rupture into pericardial sac
    Chest trauma — penetrating or non-penetrating injury
    Anticoagulant therapy

3   *Chylopericardium*
    Idiopathic
    Heart surgery — postoperative accumulation of lymph
    Malignant disease — obstruction of lymphatics draining the heart

---

## *Prognosis*

Pericarditis is usually a benign disorder and the prognosis relates to the underlying cause. Nevertheless, any cause of pericarditis can lead to pericardial effusion and tamponade, which may be lethal if not corrected. Pericarditis can also progress to pericardial constriction and heart failure.

## Pericardial effusion and tamponade

## *Aetiology*

The major causes of cardiac tamponade are haemopericardium following heart surgery and pericardial effusion complicating neoplastic disease (Table 7.2). Nevertheless, almost any other causes of pericardial haemorrhage or effusion may lead to tamponade, depending principally on the rate of fluid accumulation within the pericardial sac.

## *Pathophysiology*

Gradual accumulation of fluid permits progressive stretching of the pericardial sac, such that a substantial effusion may develop without

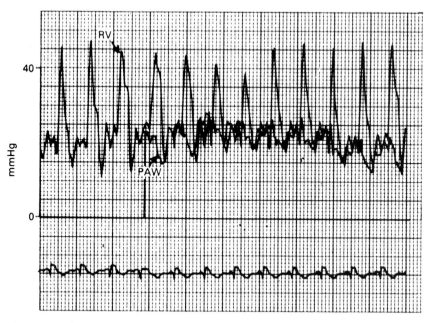

**Fig. 7.2**  Cardiac tamponade. Simultaneous recordings of the right ventricular (RV) and pulmonary artery wedge (PAW) pressure signals. Note that during diastole pressures are elevated and the recordings are effectively superimposed with loss of the normal differential. Equalization and elevation of the right- and left-sided ventricular filling pressures are characteristic of tamponade but also occur in constrictive pericarditis and restrictive cardiomyopathy.

significant elevation of intrapericardial pressure. However, rapid accumulation of fluid leads to critical elevation of pressure, which impedes diastolic relaxation of both ventricles equally. Thus, adequate ventricular filling depends on the end-diastolic pressures in both ventricles rising to equilibrate with the intrapericardial pressure. The normal differential between ventricular filling pressures is therefore lost and the filling pressure on the right side of the heart comes to equal that on the left (Fig. 7.2). As tamponade worsens, progressive increments in ventricular filling pressures become inadequate to maintain cardiac output.

## Clinical manifestations

Tamponade occurs abruptly following haemorrhage into the pericardial sac, but the onset is usually more gradual in patients with pericardial effusion. Shortness of breath and fatigue are the principal complaints.

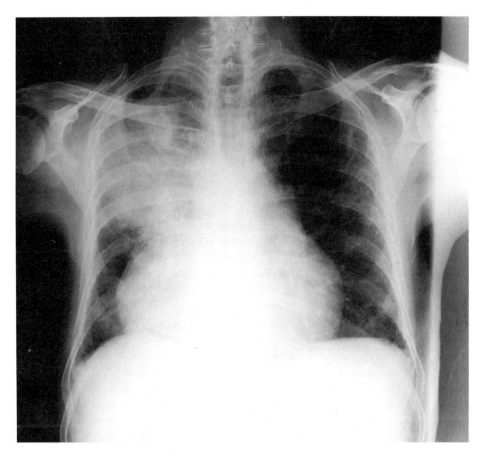

**Fig. 7.3** Cardiac tamponade. The CXR shows globular cardiac enlargement with segmental consolidation in the right upper lung field. Bronchoscopy confirmed a right hilar carcinoma which had infiltrated the pericardium, causing tamponade.

The examination reveals tachycardia, elevated JVP, hypotension and signs of reduced cardiac output; frank cardiogenic shock may occur. A paradoxical pulse is almost invariable in cardiac tamponade and in many patients Kussmaul's sign also occurs (see Fig. 1.7). The waveform of the JVP is unusually dynamic, due to an exaggerated X descent (see p.16). Auscultation reveals faint heart sounds.

## *Diagnosis*

Pericardial effusion produces globular enlargement of the cardiac silhouette (Fig. 7.3). The diagnosis should always be considered if an abrupt increase in heart size is demonstrated on serial CXRs (see Fig. 16.2). The ECG shows diminished voltage deflexions and electrical alternans may be present (Fig. 7.4). Echocardiography confirms pericardial effusion (Fig. 7.5). In difficult cases, right heart catheterization is helpful, which demonstrates equilibration of the right- and left-sided filling pressures, as reflected by the right ventricular diastolic and pulmonary capillary wedge pressures, respectively (Fig. 7.2).

## *Differential diagnosis*

Tamponade must be differentiated from other causes of low cardiac output and shock, including MI, pulmonary embolism and septicaemia.

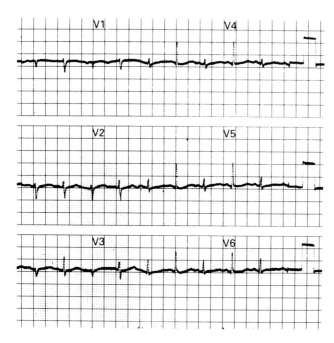

**Fig. 7.4** Acute tamponade. The ECG shows diminished voltage deflexions and also electrical alternans — beat-to-beat variation in R-wave amplitude, most prominent in leads V4–V6.

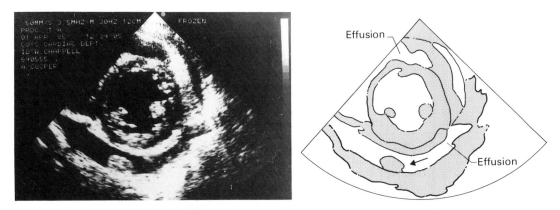

**Fig. 7.5** Pericardial effusion. Two-dimensional echocardiogram, short-axis view. The effusion produces an echo-free space around the heart. The patient had chicken-pox (a rare cause of pericardial effusion) and a pox lesion (arrowed) is visible on the parietal layer of the pericardium.

This is not difficult if pulsus paradoxus and pericardial effusion can be demonstrated.

## *Treatment*

Pericardiocentesis should be undertaken at the earliest opportunity in order to decompress the heart. This is best performed by the subxiphisternal route while the patient reclines at 45°. Following infiltration of local anaesthetic, a needle is introduced into the angle between the xiphisternum and the left costal margin, and is advanced beneath the costal margin towards the left shoulder. Continuous suction applied to the syringe ensures that pericardial fluid is aspirated as the needle enters the effusion. The effusion is then aspirated to dryness.

When pericardial effusion is the result of neoplastic infiltration of the pericardium, fluid commonly reaccumulates following pericardiocentesis. In order to prevent reaccumulation, a drainage catheter can be left in the pericardial sac, pending definitive treatment. The catheter is usually introduced over a guide-wire, which can be inserted through the lumen of the aspiration needle. If cytotoxic therapy fails to prevent recurrent effusion, surgical excision of a pericardial segment may be necessary. This provides a window through which the effusion drains, to be absorbed into the pleural and mediastinal lymphatics.

## Constrictive pericarditis

Constrictive pericarditis is no longer a common disease in the UK, largely due to the declining incidence of TB, which was responsible for most cases in the past.

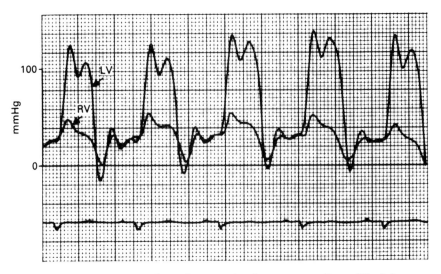

**Fig. 7.6** Constrictive pericarditis. These are simultaneous recordings of the left ventricular (LV) and right ventricular (RV) pressure signals. Note the dip-and-plateau configuration during diastole (cf. restrictive cardiomyopathy) with equalization of the diastolic pressures in both chambers. Equalization of left- and right-sided filling pressures also occurs in restrictive cardiomyopathy and cardiac tamponade.

## Aetiology

Pericarditis of any type may lead to constriction. Nevertheless, in the UK, most cases are idiopathic in origin.

## Pathophysiology

Constrictive physiology is very similar to that seen in restrictive cardio-myopathy and tamponade (see Fig. 4.2). Fibrosis and shrinkage of the pericardial sac impede diastolic relaxation of the ventricles and prevent adequate filling. Compensatory increments in filling pressures occur and, because constriction usually affects both ventricles equally, the filling pressures also equilibrate. Thus, atrial pressures and ventricular diastolic pressures on both sides of the heart are elevated and equal in constrictive pericarditis (Fig. 7.6). Systolic function is usually normal but may be impaired in some cases, due to myocardial involvement in the disease process.

## Clinical manifestations

Constrictive pericarditis is a chronic debilitating illness. Though symptoms and signs of low cardiac output are usually present, the consequences of elevated systemic venous pressure, together with salt and water retention, dominate the clinical picture. The appearances are

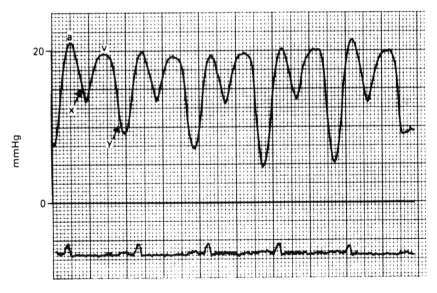

**Fig. 7.7** Constrictive pericarditis — right atrial pressure signal. Note right atrial pressure is considerably elevated, with prominence of the 'Y' descent.

those of severe right heart failure, with distension of the neck veins, hepatomegaly, ascites and peripheral oedema. Kussmaul's sign is invariably present, but a paradoxical pulse is seen less commonly. The waveform of the JVP is unusually dynamic, due to prominence of both the X and the Y descent; the former, however, may be less marked in cases with impaired systolic function (Fig. 7.7). Auscultation reveals an

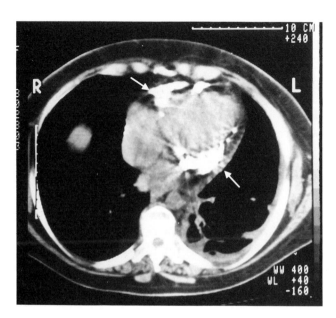

**Fig. 7.8** Constrictive pericarditis — computed tomography. This transverse thoracic tomogram at the level of the heart shows dense pericardial calcification (arrowed), particularly in the interventricular groove anteriorly and posteriorly. The calcified pericardium has a white appearance similar to that of bone.

early third heart sound (pericardial knock), due to rapid ventricular filling early in diastole.

## Diagnosis

The ECG usually shows diminished voltage deflexions with non-specific ST-segment and T-wave changes. The CXR may be normal; indeed, the combination of a normal heart size and signs of severe right-sided failure is suggestive of constriction. So is the presence of pericardial calcification (best seen on the lateral chest X-ray), although this is relatively uncommon in non-tuberculous constriction. The echocardiogram is rarely helpful. A better indication of pericardial thickening and calcification is provided by computed tomography (Fig. 7.8). Cardiac catheterization shows that the diastolic filling pressures in both ventricles are equal and elevated and have a characteristic dip-and-plateau configuration (see Fig. 7.6).

## Differential diagnosis

This includes other causes of right heart failure and cirrhosis of the liver. In most cases of right heart failure, the heart is enlarged and right ventricular dilatation can be demonstrated by echocardiography. Associated pulmonary vascular or left ventricular disease is often present. Cirrhosis produces ascites and debilitation, but does not show the cardiovascular manifestations of constrictive pericarditis. The differentiation of constrictive pericarditis from restrictive cardiomyopathy is difficult, because both produce almost identical physiological changes. If direct evidence of pericardial disease can be obtained by computed tomography, constriction is likely. Moreover, constriction nearly always shows exact equalization of right- and left-sided filling pressures. In restriction, on the other hand, the normal differential may be partially preserved, such that right-sided filling pressures are somewhat lower than on the left. Nevertheless, thoracotomy may sometimes be necessary for confirmation of the differential diagnosis.

## Treatment

Diuretics can be used to control salt and water overload, and in some cases no other treatment is necessary. However, it should be recognized that diuretics do nothing to correct the constriction and, by reducing ventricular filling, may exacerbate the fundamental haemodynamic derangement. Thus, if symptoms are severe, pericardiectomy is the treatment of choice. The procedure is technically difficult but, if excision of the diseased pericardium is successful, the results are excellent.

## Further reading

Cameron J., Westerle S.N., Baldwin J.C. and Hancock E.W. The etiologic spectrum of constrictive pericarditis. *Am. Heart J.* 1987, **113**, 354–9.

Hawkins J.W. and Vacek J.L. What constitutes definitive therapy of malignant pericardial effusion? Medical versus surgical treatment. *Am. Heart J.* 1989, **118**, 428–32.

Kralstein J. and Frishman W. Malignant pericardial diseases: diagnosis and treatment. *Am. Heart J.* 1987, **113**, 785–90.

Permanyer-Miralda G., Sagrista-Sauleda J. and Soler-Soler J. Primary acute pericardial disease: a prospective series of 231 consecutive patients. *Am. J. Cardiol.* 1985, **56**, 623–30.

# 8 Rheumatic Fever and Infective Endocarditis

## Summary

Rheumatic fever is an inflammatory condition, usually occurring between the ages of 5 and 15, that affects the heart, joints, skin and brain. It probably represents an autoimmune response to pharyngeal infection with group A haemolytic streptococcus. Once the commonest cause of valvular heart-disease in the UK, its incidence has now declined, due to complex environmental factors and changes in the streptococcus itself. It presents with fever and arthralgia; evidence of carditis (particularly murmurs of mitral or aortic regurgitation) is found in 50% of cases, although heart failure is rare. Polyarthritis, erythema marginatum and chorea may also occur. Diagnosis is by application of Jones' criteria in patients with serological evidence of recent streptococcal infection. Treatment is with aspirin and recovery can be expected in about 6 weeks. However, in patients with carditis, progressive scarring and shrinkage of the valve cusps may lead to chronic rheumatic heart-disease 15–20 years later.

Infective endocarditis usually involves the left-sided heart valves, although any other endocardial location may also be affected. High-risk groups include the elderly, patients with pre-existing heart defects, valve lesions or prostheses, intravenous (IV) drug abusers and immunosuppressed patients. *Streptococcus viridans* from the upper respiratory tract is the commonest infective agent, but a wide range of other bacterial and fungal organisms have also been implicated. Infective endocarditis is characterized pathologically by accumulations of blood products (vegetations) at the site of infection and by progressive destruction of the affected valve. It may present acutely with toxaemia and heart failure, particularly when caused by *Staphylococcus aureus*, but in the commoner *Streptococcus viridans* cases it is an insidious flu-like illness, associated with the heart murmur of mitral or aortic regurgitation. Major complications include embolization of vegetations, mycotic aneurysm and immune complex disease, with vasculitis, arthritis, glomerular nephritis and renal failure. The diagnosis is clinical and should be considered in every patient with fever and a heart murmur. Early treatment with bactericidal antibiotics for 4–6 weeks is potentially life-saving and in suspected cases should not be delayed beyond the time necessary to collect three blood cultures. Treatment should start with intravenous benzyl penicillin and gentamicin, on the assumption that *Streptococcus viridans* is the infective agent, but may need adjusting when the results of blood cultures are available. Severe valvular regurgitation causing heart failure requires surgical treatment. Antibiotic prophylaxis against endocarditis is essential in all patients with valvular heart disease or other endocardial defects, in order to prevent bacteraemia during dental surgery and other non-sterile invasive procedures.

## Rheumatic fever

Rheumatic fever is an inflammatory disease that follows pharyngeal infection by group A haemolytic streptococci. The major organs and tissues affected are the heart, joints, skin and central nervous system.

### *Aetiology*

One per cent of patients with group A haemolytic streptococcal pharyngitis develop rheumatic fever 2–3 weeks later. Evidence implicating the streptococcus in the aetiology of rheumatic fever is based upon:
1   Epidemiological studies.
2   Serological testing in acute rheumatic fever, which usually provides evidence of recent streptococcal infection.
3   The efficacy of penicillin prophylaxis in patients with streptococcal pharyngitis.

However, the precise pathogenic role of the streptococcus is unknown. A direct infective process is unlikely, because organisms are never present in the lesions of rheumatic fever; similarly there is no evidence of toxic tissue damage. A number of features suggest an autoimmune process, including: (i) the characteristic latency period between throat infection and the development of rheumatic fever; (ii) the demonstration of gamma-globulins in the myocardial sarcolemma of patients who have died during the illness; (iii) the immunological cross-reaction between streptococcal antigens and myocardial sarcolemma; and (iv) the demonstration of circulating heart-reactive antibodies in a relatively high proportion of patients with rheumatic carditis. It must be emphasized, however, that many of these features are as likely to be the consequence of cardiac damage as they are to be its primary cause. Thus, the role of autoimmunity in the pathogenesis of rheumatic fever remains unproven.

### *Epidemiology*

Rheumatic fever occurs most commonly between the ages of 5 and 15 years. Its incidence in developed countries has declined dramatically during the last 50 years, but elsewhere in the world it continues to be a major health problem.

Environmental, bacteriological and host factors affect susceptibility to rheumatic fever. Crowding and social deprivation encourage the spread of streptococci and are the principal environmental factors predisposing to the disease. The nature of the organism itself is important because, when rheumatic fever does occur in the UK, it is usually much less severe than in under-developed countries. This may also relate to host susceptibility. Thus, the tendency for rheumatic fever to be familial and the high incidence of recurrence following an initial attack indicate heightened susceptibility in certain individuals, possibly due to genetic predisposition.

The declining incidence in developed countries cannot be attributed to any single factor. Improvements in housing and welfare are important but do not provide the full explanation because the incidence has fallen in all social strata, including the socially deprived inner-city areas. Penicillin, highly effective against streptococci, became widely available only after the declining incidence of rheumatic fever was well established. The virulence of the organism itself may have changed, since rheumatic fever is now not only less common but also less severe.

## *Pathology*

Rheumatic fever may affect any of the cardiac tissues, including the myocardium, pericardium and endocardium. Myocardial involvement is characterized by the Aschoff body, a granulomatous lesion which persists long after the acute illness has subsided. Rheumatic pericarditis is usually transient, and may produce a fibrinous effusion, but tamponade and constriction are very rare.

Rheumatic endocarditis is the most important cardiac lesion. Inflammation and oedema of the valve cusps are associated with verrucous nodules, which develop along the lines of valve closure. Acutely, this may cause severe valve damage, but, more commonly, valve function remains little affected in this phase of the illness. During healing, however, progressive scarring of the valve apparatus may occur.

## *Non-cardiac disease*

Arthritis is characterized by an exudative synovitis, which does not produce long-term damage to the joints. Subcutaneous nodules are granulomatous and disappear following the acute illness. Patients with chorea rarely die, and characteristic brain pathology has not been identified.

## Clinical manifestations

Fever and arthralgia are often the only symptoms. These may be attributed to a trivial, influenza-like illness, which is soon forgotten by the patient.

## Carditis

Although carditis affects about half of all patients with a first attack of rheumatic fever, it rarely causes symptoms. Thus, many patients who present with valvular disease later are unaware that they had rheumatic carditis during childhood. Chest pain due to pericarditis is the most common symptom but, in fulminant cases, symptoms of heart failure also occur. The examination reveals tachycardia and a gallop rhythm, both of which are non-specific responses to fever in children. Heart murmurs are heard in the majority of cases, particularly the pansystolic apical murmur of mitral regurgitation. An apical mid-diastolic murmur (Carey Coombes) also indicates mitral involvement but does not always predict mitral stenosis in later life. The early diastolic murmur of aortic regurgitation is somewhat less common but, like the mitral murmurs, is strongly suggestive of rheumatic carditis. On the other hand, soft mid-systolic (ejection) murmurs usually reflect hyperkinetic flow caused by fever and do not necessarily indicate rheumatic carditis.

## Other major manifestations

Polyarthritis usually affects the large joints of the extremities. Joints are often affected in turn and, as one recovers, others become involved. Subcutaneous nodules are small and painless and often go unnoticed by the patient. They occur over the extensor tendons of the hands, feet, knees and elbows and also over the spinal column.

Erythema marginatum is an evanescent rash characteristic of rheumatic fever. The lesions vary in size and have a pink serpiginous margin, often with a clear centre, usually occurring on the trunk but never on the face.

Chorea (Sydenham's chorea, St Vitus' dance) is a late manifestation of rheumatic fever, which may occur several months after pharyngitis. Its severity is variable but, in mild cases, the involuntary movements and grimaces are often mistaken for insolence by parents or teachers. At its worst, however, violent jerky movements of the entire body demand specially padded beds to prevent serious injury.

## Diagnosis

Rheumatic fever tends to be over-diagnosed in children with fever, arthralgia and soft ejection murmurs, all of which are non-specific mani-

| Major criteria | Minor criteria |
|---|---|
| Carditis | Fever |
| Polyarthritis | Arthralgia |
| Erythema marginatum | Previous rheumatic fever |
| Chorea | Elevated ESR |
| Subcutaneous nodules | Prolonged PR interval |

**Table 8.1** Jones' criteria for the diagnosis of rheumatic fever

festations of viral illness. Nevertheless, if recent streptococcal infection can be confirmed, by demonstration of elevated serum antistreptolysin O-titre, then Jones' criteria may be used (Table 8.1). The presence of two major criteria, or one major and two minor, indicates a high diagnostic probability.

## Differential diagnosis

This includes other causes of childhood arthritis, bacterial endocarditis and viral pericarditis. Still's disease — the major cause of childhood arthritis — runs a chronic course and other criteria for rheumatic fever are not present. Bacterial endocarditis, although associated with fever and heart murmurs, causes relentless clinical deterioration and positive blood cultures and other stigmata of the condition should be sought. Simple viral pericarditis is never associated with valvular disease, unlike rheumatic pericarditis, in which valvular involvement and heart murmurs are always present.

An unusual but difficult diagnostic problem is the child with penicillin sensitivity following treatment of streptococcal pharyngitis. This often produces fever and arthritis similar to rheumatic fever. An urticarial or maculopapular rash, however, is strongly suggestive of drug sensitivity.

## Treatment

Rheumatic fever may be prevented by prompt treatment of streptococcal throat infections with penicillin. A single intramuscular injection of 0.6–1.2 mega-units of benzathine penicillin is effective.

In established rheumatic fever, no specific treatment cures or changes the course of the illness. Bed rest is necessary in the acute phase, particularly if there are signs of carditis; a course of penicillin should be given to eradicate residual streptococcal infection. Salicylates are highly effective for treatment of fever and arthritis: aspirin, starting at 100 mg/kg/day in children, is given in sufficient dosage to relieve symptoms without causing frank toxicity (tinnitus, headache, hyperventilation). In patients unable to tolerate salicylates, steroids are equally effective and are preferred by some physicians when active carditis is present. There is no evidence to suggest that steroids are more beneficial than salicylates, however, or that either treatment prevents chronic valvular damage. Steroid dosage is variable but an initial dose of prednisone 60–120 mg daily may be necessary to suppress symptoms; thereafter the dose can be gradually reduced.

Rheumatic chorea is unaffected by salicylates and steroids. Mental and physical rest in bed reduces the severity of choreiform attacks. Mild sedatives such as diazepam are often helpful.

Following rheumatic fever, long-term prophylactic penicillin therapy should be continued up to the age of 25 or for at least 5 years in patients over 20. Recommended regimens are a monthly intramuscular injection of benzathine penicillin (1.2 mega-units) or oral penicillin V (125 mg twice daily). Oral sulphadiazine (1 g daily) may be used in penicillin-sensitive individuals.

## Course and prognosis

Acute rheumatic fever usually subsides within 6 weeks. Occasionally, however, the illness lasts 6 months or longer, particularly in patients with intractable carditis or chorea. Carditis probably affects the majority of young children with rheumatic fever but is less common in older patients: recurrent attacks occur frequently and, in patients with carditis, these exacerbate cardiac damage and increase susceptibility to heart failure and death. In most cases, however, heart failure is delayed until the development of chronic rheumatic heart-disease several years later. Chorea and arthritis rarely produce chronic sequelae.

## Chronic rheumatic heart-disease

Following an attack (or recurrent attacks) of rheumatic fever, cardiac function usually returns to normal. During healing of the inflamed valves, however, progressive scarring may lead to chronic rheumatic heart-disease, although this does not usually present until 15–20 years later. Adhesion of the valve commissures and shrinkage of the cusps and the subvalvular apparatus produce variable stenosis and regurgitation, exacerbated by valvular calcification. By the age of 30, many patients have had their first attack of congestive heart failure, which is often precipitated by the onset of atrial fibrillation (AF) or the stress of pregnancy. The mitral valve is most commonly affected, and is often associated with disease of the aortic valve. Functional impairment of the tricuspid valve is unusual and rheumatic pulmonary valve disease is almost never seen.

**Table 8.2**  Organisms causing endocarditis. The pathogens most commonly implicated are shown in bold

|  | Typical source of infection | First-choice antibiotics (pending sensitivity studies) |
|---|---|---|
| SUBACUTE DISEASE |  |  |
| **Streptococcus viridans** | Upper respiratory tract | Penicillin, gentamicin |
| **Streptococcus faecalis** | Bowel and urogenital tract | Ampicillin, gentamicin |
| **Anaerobic streptococci** | Bowel | Ampicillin, gentamicin |
| **Staphylococcus epidermidis** | Skin | Flucloxacillin, gentamicin |
| Fungi—*Candida*, histoplasmosis | Skin and mucous membranes | Amphotericin B*, 5-fluorocytosine* |
| *Coxiella burnetti* | Complication of Q fever | Chloramphenicol*, tetracycline |
| *Chlamydia psittacosi* | Contact with infected birds | Tetracycline* and erythromycin |
| ACUTE DISEASE |  |  |
| **Staphylococcus aureus** | Skin | Flucloxacillin, gentamicin |
| **Streptococcus pneumoniae** | Complication of pneumonia | Penicillin, gentamicin |
| *Neisseria gonorrhoeae* | Venereal | Penicillin, gentamicin |

* These drugs are not cidal and valve replacement is nearly always necessary to eradicate infection.

## Infective endocarditis

Infective endocarditis usually involves the heart valves (native or prosthetic) but may also occur in association with congenital or acquired defects; occasionally, infection develops around the endocardial insertion of pacemaker electrodes. Infection of the endothelial lining of arterial aneurysms or arteriovenous fistulae is rare but produces a similar illness.

## *Aetiology*

Endocarditis is now seen increasingly in the elderly, unlike 50 years ago when it was more common in young adults. Organisms implicated in the aetiology of endocarditis are shown in Table 8.2. The most common of these is *Streptococcus viridans*, a normal commensal of the upper respiratory tract. This is a relatively indolent organism, which produces a chronic, subacute, illness. Other more virulent organisms, notably *Staphylococcus aureus*, produce an acute, rapidly progressive, illness. Regardless of the organism, however, the outcome is invariably fatal if endocarditis is not treated.

Endocarditis may affect healthy patients with entirely normal hearts. Nevertheless, patients at greater risk are those with pre-existing valvular disease or congenital or acquired cardiac defects. Other high-risk groups are shown in Table 8.3. High-velocity flow favours the endothelial deposition of organisms in bacteraemic patients. Thus, aortic and mitral valve disease, ventricular septal defect and patent ductus arteriosus are the conditions most commonly associated with infective endocarditis.

**Table 8.3** Groups at increased risk of endocarditis

1  The elderly (>60 years)
2  Patients with intrinsic cardiovascular disease. High risk lesions are:
    ventricular septal defect
    aortic regurgitation
    mitral regurgitation
    aortic stenosis
    patent ductus arteriosus
    coarctation of the aorta
3  Patients with valve prostheses, tissue grafts and other intracardiac foreign material
4  Mainlining drug addicts — right-sided valvular endocarditis occurs relatively commonly in this group
5  Immunosuppressed patients

Right-sided endocarditis is rare, usually affecting mainlining drug addicts.

The source of infection cannot usually be identified. *Streptococcus viridans* bacteraemia is almost invariable during dental surgery (drilling, scaling, extractions), but less than 15% of patients with endocarditis give a history of this. Instrumentation of the genitourinary (GU) or gastrointestinal (GI) tracts also causes bacteraemia but is not often implicated. Drug addicts commonly use dirty needles and expose themselves to a variety of organisms which may infect the left- or right-sided heart valves, and infected intravenous cannulae are a potential cause of staphylococcal endocarditis in hospitalized patients.

## *Pathology*

Endocarditis leads to accumulation of fibrin, platelets and other blood products at the site of infection. This produces a vegetation, which is relatively avascular and tends to isolate the infective organism from host defences and antimicrobial agents. Valve destruction produces worsening regurgitation and commonly leads to heart failure. In staphylococcal endocarditis, valve destruction is rapid, but in less aggressive infections (e.g. *Streptococcus viridans*) the progression of disease is slower and large craggy vegetations develop. Embolization to any of the major organs or the extremities is common and may cause metastatic abscesses, particularly in the spleen or brain. Pulmonary embolism, from right-sided cardiac lesions, also occurs. Extension of infection into the adjacent myocardial or arterial walls produces conduction defects, valve ring abscesses or mycotic aneurysms. The chronic infection that characterizes endocarditis may lead to immune complex disease, with vasculitic involvement of the kidneys, joints or skin.

## Clinical manifestations

In acute bacterial endocarditis caused by *Staphylococcus aureus*, the onset is often dramatic, with severe prostration leading rapidly to heart failure and septicaemic shock. In subacute disease, the onset is insidious, with influenza-like symptoms, including fever, night sweats, arthralgia and fatigue. Petechial haemorrhages in the skin and under the nails (splinter haemorrhages) are a common but non-specific finding. Valvular endocarditis produces regurgitant murmurs (typically aortic or mitral), due to destruction of the valve leaflets. Other classical manifestations of endocarditis, including Osler's nodes (tender erythematous nodules in the pulps of the fingers), Janeway lesions (painless erythematous lesions on the palms), clubbing of the fingers and splenomegaly, are now rarely seen.

## Complications

Heart failure is the major complication of endocarditis and the usual cause of death. Vegetations may embolize peripherally, threatening limbs or major organs, and metastatic abscesses may occur, particularly in the spleen or brain. Embolization in the vasa vasorum causes mycotic aneurysm, which may be infected or sterile. These often develop locally in the sinuses of Valsalva, but may also occur in the peripheral circulation. Rupture can occur during the acute phase of the illness or at any time following. Local abscess formation in the aortic valve ring may produce heart block by damaging the conducting tissue in the inter-ventricular septum. Right-sided endocarditis is commonly associated with pneumonia caused by infected embolization to the lungs.

Immune complex disease complicating infective endocarditis is a cause of vasculitic rash and arthritis. More important, however, is glomerulonephritis, which may progress to renal failure.

## Diagnosis

Endocarditis is predominantly a clinical diagnosis and should be considered in every patient with fever and a heart murmur. Laboratory findings include leucocytosis, usually with neutrophilia, and normo-chromic normocytic anaemia is almost invariable. Urinalysis commonly reveals haematuria due to glomerulonephritis. Blood cultures are positive in the majority of cases and should always be obtained before antibiotic treatment is started. Aerobic, anaerobic and fungal cultures should be performed. Occasionally, bone marrow cultures are helpful for detection of candida and brucella endocarditis. Coxiella and chlamydia can never be cultured from the blood and must be diagnosed by serological tests.

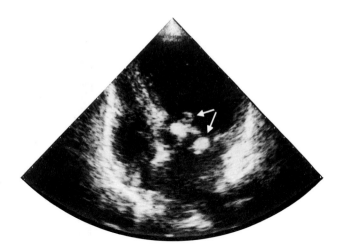

**Fig. 8.1** Infective endocarditis. This two-dimensional echocardiogram (apical four-chamber view) shows dense vegetations adherent to both leaflets of the mitral valve (arrowed).

Failure to detect bacteraemia may be due to:

**1** Pretreatment with antibiotics.

**2** Inadequate sampling — up to six blood samples should be taken over 24 hours.

**3** Infection with unusual micro-organisms.

The echocardiogram identifies underlying valvular disease, and vegetations may also be seen if these are large enough (Fig. 8.1). It is often impossible to visualize vegetations on prosthetic valves. The trans-oesophageal technique is helpful in difficult cases and Doppler studies identify regurgitant jets through the damaged valves. It should be emphasized, however, that failure to image vegetations by echocardiography does not rule out the diagnosis of endocarditis.

## Differential diagnosis

Infective endocarditis must be differentiated from other causes of fever and heart murmurs. Rheumatic fever is no longer common in the UK but, in children, may be difficult to distinguish from endocarditis. Fever of any cause may be associated with soft ejection systolic murmurs due to hyperkinetic circulation. Nevertheless, if murmurs of valvular regurgitation do not develop, the diagnosis of valvular endocarditis is unlikely.

## Treatment

Initial diagnosis is made on clinical grounds and treatment must not be delayed beyond the time necessary to obtain three or four blood samples for culture. Bactericidal antibiotic therapy should then be started and the course should continue for at least 4 weeks, or up to 6 weeks in complicated cases of prosthetic valve infection. It is recommended that, for the first 2 weeks, combination therapy is given, with two antibiotics injected intravenously, using a central line. During this time, serially diluted blood samples should be back-titrated against the cultured organism in the bacteriology laboratory to ensure adequate bactericidal activity. After 2 weeks of intravenous treatment, the course may be completed with oral drugs, using a single antibiotic.

Streptococcal infection accounts for over 70% of cases. Thus, while awaiting the results of blood culture, initial treatment should be with benzylpenicillin — 12 mega-units daily — and low-dose gentamicin, which enhances penicillin activity. The dose of gentamicin must be titrated against blood concentrations, in order to achieve peak and trough values of 3–5 mg/litre and <1 mg/litre, respectively. When the results of blood culture become available, alternative antibiotics may be necessary. In culture-negative cases treatment with penicillin and gentamicin should continue while a search for unusual organisms such as fungi, coxiella and chlamydia is undertaken.

Pyrexia usually settles within a few days of starting treatment but persistent elevation of the erythrocyte sedimentation rate (ESR) for up to 4 weeks is common. Recurrence of pyrexia is often the result of antibiotic sensitivity but it may also indicate superinfection with a new organism. Fungi are particularly troublesome and difficult to treat. For this reason a weekly injection of amphotericin is often recommended during the course of treatment. Any sign of infection around an intravenous site demands removal of the catheter; the tip should be sent for culture and a new line inserted under full aseptic conditions.

The valve damage caused by endocarditis may require surgical treatment, which, if possible, should be delayed until antibiotic therapy has cleared the infection, although the development of heart failure demands more urgent valve replacement. Conduction defects, recurrent embolism and resistant infection, particularly in prosthetic valve endocarditis, are other relative indications for early surgery. Fungal endocarditis usually requires surgical treatment because all the available antifungal drugs are fungistatic (not fungicidal). Eradication of fungal infection by medical treatment is therefore very difficult.

### Prophylaxis

Antibiotic prophylaxis against endocarditis is required for all patients with valvular heart disease, or other endocardial defects caused by acquired or congenital disease. Patients with mitral valve prolapse only need prophylaxis when there is an associated systolic murmur of mitral regurgitation. A permanent pacemaker in patients with conducting tissue disease is not an indication for prophylaxis.

The purpose of prophylaxis is to prevent bacteraemia during dental surgery and other non-sterile invasive procedures. A single oral dose of amoxycillin 3 g should be given 1 hour before dental work (scaling, filling, extraction) to protect against *Streptococcus viridans* infection. In patients allergic to penicillin, single oral doses of either erythromycin 1.5 g (with a further 500 mg 6 hours after the procedure) or clindamycin 600 mg should be substituted. For patients undergoing instrumentation or surgery of the upper respiratory tract (e.g. bronchoscopy), prophylaxis requirements are the same as for dental procedures. Instrumentation or surgery of the GI and GU tracts does not require prophylaxis unless the patient has a prosthetic heart valve or gives a history of previous endocarditis, when amoxycillin combined with intramuscular gentamicin 120 mg is recommended. During childbirth antibiotic prophylaxis is unnecessary for normal vaginal deliveries but is recommended for instrumented deliveries and for all mothers with prosthetic valves or a history of previous endocarditis.

## *Prognosis*

When penicillin therapy was introduced, mortality in endocarditis fell from 100% to about 30%. Since that time, mortality has shown little tendency to decline further, despite the increasing availability of powerful antibiotics. This is probably the result of multiple factors, including the emergence of antibiotic-resistant organisms, the introduction of prosthetic heart valves, the widespread use of immunosuppressive therapy, the worsening problems of intravenous drug abuse and the older, more debilitated age-group that is now at risk. Probably the major impediment to effective treatment in endocarditis is delay in diagnosis. The insidious onset of the illness often causes the correct diagnosis to be overlooked until it is too late. Thus, endocarditis must be considered in all patients with a feverish illness and a heart murmur, particularly those patients known to be at high risk.

## Further reading

Bayliss R., Clark C., Oakley C.M. *et al.* Incidence, mortality and prevention of infective endocarditis. *J. R. Coll. Physicians Lond.* 1986, **20**, 15–24.

Bisno A.L. Acute rheumatic fever: forgotten but not gone. *N. Engl. J. Med.* 1987, **316**, 476–8.

Bisno A.L. Group A streptococcal infections and acute rheumatic fever. *N. Engl. J. Med.* 1991, **325**, 783–93.

Gray I.R. Infective endocarditis 1937–1987. *Br. Heart J.* 1987, **57**, 211–13.

Rapaport E. The changing role of surgery in the management of infective endocarditis. *Circulation* 1978, **58**, 598–601.

Robbins M.J., Soeiro R., Frishman W.H. and Strom J.A. Right-sided valvular endocarditis: etiology, diagnosis and an approach to therapy. *Am. Heart J.* 1986, **111**, 128–35.

Working Party of the British Society for Antimicrobial Therapy. Antibiotic prophylaxis of infective endocarditis. *Lancet* 1990, **335**, 88–9.

# 9 Valvular Heart-disease

## Summary

Valvular heart-disease adversely affects ventricular loading and tends to diminish cardiac output. Compensatory mechanisms will often preserve haemodynamic stability but, if the lesion is severe, heart failure eventually supervenes. Diagnosis can usually be made clinically, but echocardiography and Doppler technology permit more precise assessment of lesion severity without the need for cardiac catheterization. Surgery has revolutionized the management of valvular heart-disease and, if timed before ventricular dysfunction or pulmonary hypertension have become irreversible, can produce complete haemodynamic correction.

*Mitral stenosis* is always rheumatic and is associated with progressive increments in left atrial pressure, which establish a pressure gradient across the valve to maintain left ventricular (LV) filling. As pressure rises, dyspnoea gets worse, deteriorating abruptly with the onset of atrial fibrillation (AF). Auscultation reveals a loud first heart sound (S1) and an opening snap in early diastole, followed by a low-pitched mid-diastolic murmur. Treatment is with diuretics, but, if dyspnoea remains troublesome, valve surgery is necessary. Patients in AF require digoxin to slow the ventricular rate and anticoagulants to protect against systemic embolization.

*Mitral regurgitation* may be caused by valvular, subvalvular or dilating LV disease. The regurgitant jet causes left atrial pressure to rise and volume-loads the left ventricle, which dilates. Atrial fibrillation is common and presentation is with dyspnoea and an apical pansystolic murmur, often associated with a third heart sound. Treatment is initially medical, as for mitral stenosis, with surgery in reserve for severe symptoms.

*Aortic stenosis* is usually caused by degenerative calcific disease affecting the elderly. The LV hypertrophies to generate a pressure gradient across the aortic valve sufficient to preserve forward flow. In end-stage disease the LV dilates and fails, and a paradoxical reduction in the pressure gradient may then occur. Presentation is with dyspnoea, angina and, in severe cases, syncope and left ventricular failure (LVF). The carotid pulse has a slow upstroke and auscultation reveals a mid-systolic murmur and a fourth heart sound. The development of symptoms heralds a poor prognosis and is an indication for surgery.

*Aortic regurgitation* may be caused by valve leaflet or aortic root disease. The regurgitant jet volume-loads the left ventricle, which dilates and, in severe cases, eventually fails. It is commonly an incidental finding, but, when severe, causes dyspnoea and angina. The carotid pulse has a sharp upstroke with a wide pulse pressure, and auscultation reveals a high-pitched, early diastolic murmur at the aortic area, associated with a mid-systolic flow murmur. Treatment with vasodilators and diuretics is helpful, but progressive LV dilatation demands valve replacement.

*Tricuspid stenosis* is nearly always rheumatic but is rare, unlike *tricuspid regurgitation*, which is common and usually a functional consequence of right ventricular failure (RVF). The jugular venous pulse (JVP) is elevated, with giant 'v' waves, and auscultation reveals a pansystolic murmur at the left sternal edge. Treatment is with diuretics, and surgery is rarely required.

*Pulmonary stenosis* is one of the commoner congenital heart defects and, if severe, may require treatment by balloon valvuloplasty. *Pulmonary regurgitation* is usually a result of severe pulmonary hypertension and requires no specific treatment, being of negligible haemodynamic significance.

## Introduction

The heart valves open and close in response to cyclical changes in intracardiac and arterial pressures. This directs the cardiac output forwards into the pulmonary and systemic circulations without impeding flow. Valvular dysfunction is the result of incompetence or stenosis, which produces backward flow (regurgitation) or impeded flow, respectively. Regurgitant valve lesions volume-load the heart, whilst stenotic lesions of the ventricular outflow valves (aortic, pulmonary) pressure-load the ventricles. Stenosis of the ventricular inflow valves (mitral, tricuspid) impede filling and reduce preload. The abnormal loading which results from valve dysfunction commonly leads to heart failure, although this may be delayed by the effects of compensatory mechanisms (see p. 79). Nevertheless, because full development of these compensatory mechanisms takes time, chronic valve lesions are better tolerated than acute.

The important role of echocardiography in the diagnosis of valvular heart disease has already been emphasized. Used in conjunction with Doppler studies, the severity of valvular stenosis and regurgitation can be evaluated. These non-invasive investigations make cardiac catheterization unnecessary for diagnostic purposes, but it is recommended in patients who require valve replacement — particularly the older age-group (men over 35, women over 45), who are at risk of coronary heart disease. This not only adds precision to the diagnosis of the valve lesion, but also permits coronary arteriography, so that, when necessary, bypass grafting can be performed at the same time as valve replacement.

Surgery has revolutionized the management of valvular heart-disease and can produce complete haemodynamic correction. The timing of valve surgery is important. If it is delayed until ventricular dysfunction or pulmonary hypertension has become irreversible, the risks are greater and the results less satisfactory. In mitral stenosis, dilatation of the valve (valvotomy) is effective if the valve is competent and not calcified. Regurgitation through the atrioventricular valves can sometimes be corrected by repair procedures. In most cases of valvular heart-disease, however, surgical correction requires replacement of the valve with a tissue graft or a prosthesis. Porcine xenografts are widely used because, unlike prostheses, they are not thrombogenic and do not expose the patient to the inconvenience and risk of long-term anticoagulation. Nevertheless, tissue grafts usually calcify and fail within 7–10 years. For this reason, prostheses are often preferred — usually ball-and-cage or tilting-disc mechanisms. Both types are reliable but tilting-disc valves present less obstruction to flow (Fig. 9.1). Long-term anticoagulation is essential following insertion of a prosthetic valve.

It is convenient to consider each of the important valve lesions separately. It must be recognized, however, that an individual valve may be both incompetent and stenosed. Moreover, disease involving more than one valve is not uncommon, particularly in rheumatic disease and endocarditis. Multivalvular disease increases the haemodynamic burden on the heart and produces heart failure earlier.

## Mitral stenosis (MS)

### Aetiology

Mitral stenosis is nearly always rheumatic in origin, rarely occurring as a congenital defect.

### Pathophysiology

In adults the normal mitral valve orifice is $4–6\,cm^2$. However, flow across the valve remains unimpeded until the valve area is about half this. As stenosis worsens, adequate left ventricular filling demands a progressive increase in left atrial pressure, which establishes a diastolic pressure gradient across the mitral valve (Fig. 9.2). Left ventricular contraction

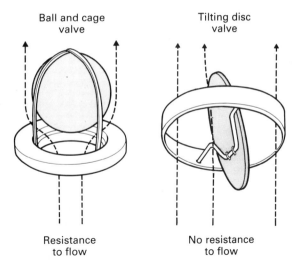

Ball and cage
valve

Tilting disc
valve

Resistance
to flow

No resistance
to flow

**Fig. 9.1** Prosthetic heart valves. The ball-and-cage prosthesis causes greater resistance to flow than the tilting-disc prosthesis.

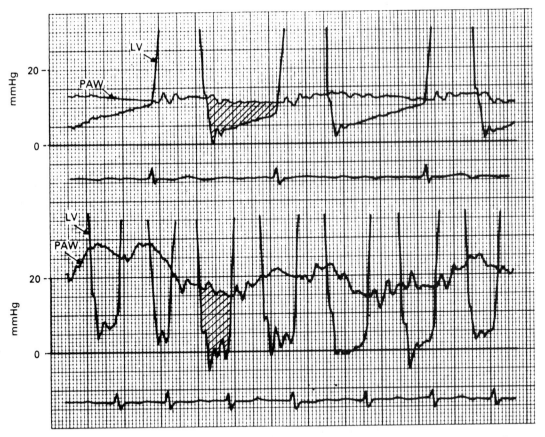

**Fig. 9.2** Mitral stenosis. These are simultaneous recordings of the left ventricular (LV) and pulmonary artery wedge (PAW) pressure signals. Recordings at rest are shown above and recordings during exercise below. Note that the diastolic pressure gradient across the mitral valve (shaded area) increases considerably during exercise due to the sharp rise in pulmonary artery wedge pressure. This accounts for the exercise-related dyspnoea that occurs in mitral stenosis.

is unaffected but, because filling is impeded, adequate cardiac output cannot always be maintained, particularly during exercise.

As pressure rises in the left atrium, it dilates and is prone to fibrillate. This compromises left ventricular filling still further, due partly to the loss of atrial systole and partly to the rapid heart rate, which reduces diastolic filling time. Thus, the onset of atrial fibrillation (AF) often produces abrupt clinical deterioration.

MS, therefore, is associated with a chronically elevated and labile left atrial pressure, causing pulmonary congestion and pulmonary hypertension, which lead to right ventricular failure. In advanced MS, obliterative disease in the pulmonary arterioles increases pulmonary vascular resistance and exacerbates pulmonary hypertension and right ventricular failure. Following the development of obliterative pulmonary vascular disease, pulmonary hypertension is irreversible and remains unaffected by mitral valve surgery.

## Clinical manifestations

MS produces orthopnoea, exertional fatigue and dyspnoea, in the same way as other causes of left heart failure (p. 3). In advanced disease, life-threatening attacks of acute pulmonary oedema occur. Chronic bronchial congestion produces cough and haemoptysis and predisposes towards winter bronchitis. The onset of AF is often associated with abrupt clinical deterioration, which may also occur during the third trimester of pregnancy, due to the increase in circulatory volume.

Cyanotic discoloration of the cheeks produces the typical mitral facies. The pulse is commonly irregular, due to AF. Auscultation at the cardiac apex reveals a loud first heart sound and an opening snap in early diastole, followed by a low-pitched mid-diastolic murmur; presystolic accentuation of the murmur occurs only in patients who are in sinus rhythm. In advanced MS, the loud first sound and the opening snap become less prominent as the mobility of the thickened valve leaflets becomes progressively restricted; the opening snap also tends to move closer to the second heart sound, as rising left atrial pressure forces open the mitral valve progressively earlier in diastole.

The development of right ventricular failure produces peripheral oedema and elevation of the jugular venous pulse. The dilated right ventricle displaces the apical impulse towards the left axilla and causes a left parasternal systolic thrust. Prominence of the pulmonary component of the second heart sound reflects pulmonary hypertension.

## Complications

AF is almost invariable in long-standing disease. Haemostasis in the dilated left atrium leads to thrombosis and commonly results in thrombo-

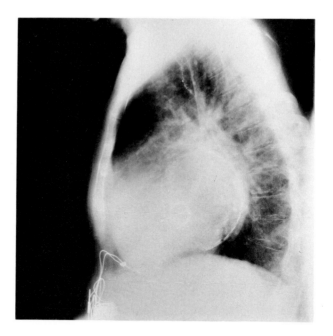

**Fig. 9.3** Mitral valve disease — lateral chest X-ray. The patient has a mitral valve prosthesis and also an epicardial pacemaker (see Chapter 10). There is dense calcification in the wall of the left atrium, which lies posterior to the prosthetic valve. The left atrium is dilated and there is also right ventricular dilatation with partial obliteration of the retrosternal space.

embolism. Pulmonary hypertension predisposes to chest infections (a common cause of death in MS), and may also lead to right ventricular failure. Although endocarditis is rare in pure MS, antibiotic prophylaxis should always be given prior to dental surgery and other non-sterile invasive procedures.

## *Diagnosis*

Left atrial enlargement produces a broad bifid P wave on the electro-cardiogram (ECG) before the onset of AF. Evidence of right ventricular hypertrophy occurs if pulmonary hypertension is severe (p. 37).

The chest X-ray (CXR) shows signs of left atrial enlargement (p. 48), often with a normal heart size. The heart size may increase with the development of right ventricular failure (RVF). Prominence of the upper lobe veins is almost invariable and, in advanced cases, pulmonary congestion or frank pulmonary oedema may be present. Calcification of the mitral valve or the left atrial wall is occasionally evident on penetrated or lateral films (Fig. 9.3).

The echocardiogram is diagnostic: thickening and variable rigidity of the valve leaflets are associated with dilatation of the left atrium. The two-dimensional image may show dilatation of the right-sided cardiac chambers but the left ventricle is normal (Fig. 9.4). The transoesophageal technique is particularly useful for identifying thrombus in the left atrial appendage. Doppler studies provide quantitative assessment of the pressure gradient across the mitral valve.

Cardiac catheterization permits measurement of the mitral valve

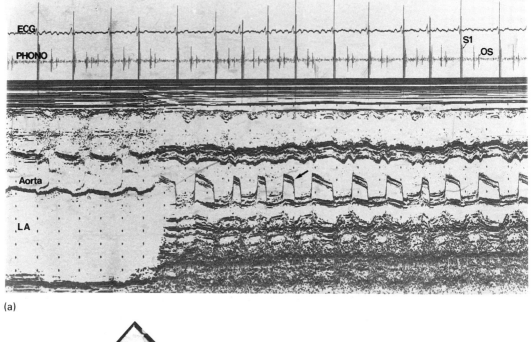

(a)

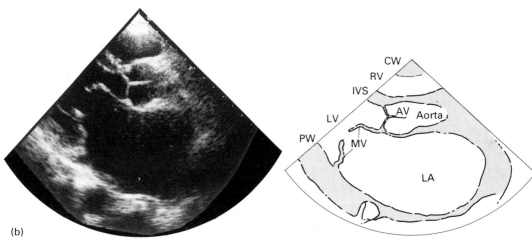

(b)

**Fig. 9.4**   Mitral stenosis — echocardiogram. The M-mode recording (a) shows thickening of the mitral valve (arrowed) with a normal-sized left ventricle. The left atrium lying behind the aorta is considerably dilated. The two-dimensional recording (b) confirms these findings and shows typical doming of the mitral valve leaflets during diastole. The ECG shows atrial fibrillation and the phonocardiogram shows a very loud first heart sound (S1) with an opening snap (OS) following shortly after the second heart sound.

pressure gradient at rest and during exercise (Fig. 9.2). In patients with severe pulmonary hypertension, the effects of inhaling 100% oxygen should be assessed; this usually produces a prompt reduction in pulmonary artery pressure, as oxygen is a potent pulmonary vasodilator, but this does not occur in patients with irreversible pulmonary vascular disease.

## Differential diagnosis

Mitral stenosis must be distinguished from left ventricular failure (LVF), which produces almost identical symptoms. Although a mid-diastolic murmur is not present, the third heart sound may cause confusion. Conditions normally associated with a mid-diastolic murmur (e.g. tricuspid stenosis, atrial septal defect) may also cause confusion. However, in all these conditions other auscultatory signs of mitral stenosis are not found and the echocardiogram shows a normal mitral valve.

## Treatment

This consists of diuretics to control pulmonary and systemic congestion, digitalis to control the ventricular rate in AF and anticoagulants to protect against thromboembolism. Anticoagulation with warfarin is mandatory in all patients with mitral stenosis following the onset of AF, to protect against thromboembolism. Antibiotic prophylaxis should be given prior to dental procedures.

The major indications for surgery are dyspnoea, unresponsiveness to medical treatment and RVF. Any patient who has a mitral valve gradient greater than 10 mmHg during exercise is likely to need surgery, which is either valvotomy, in which the valve cusps are separated along the commissures, or valve replacement. Closed valvotomy without direct visualization of the valve does not require cardiopulmonary bypass, but, if the surgeon wishes to inspect the valve, an open operation with full cardiopulmonary bypass is necessary. Valvotomy is the procedure of choice when the valve cusps are pliant and mobile, but valvular calcification or incompetence demands valve replacement. In uncomplicated cases, the mortality risk of mitral valve surgery is less than 2% but pulmonary hypertension or heart failure increases the risk to 10% or more.

The recent development of mitral balloon valvuloplasty avoids the need for surgery in some patients with non-calcified competent valves. The balloon catheter is advanced from the femoral vein into the right atrium and thence into the left atrium by trans-septal puncture. The balloon is then positioned across the stenosed mitral valve and inflated. This dilates the valve and can produce sustained benefit, unlike aortic balloon valvuloplasty, in which any improvement is nearly always temporary.

## *Prognosis*

Following rheumatic carditis, the development of symptomatic mitral stenosis may take up to 20 years, although pregnancy or the early development of atrial fibrillation often prompts an earlier presentation. Once symptoms are established, progressive deterioration leads to death within 5–10 years, unless the stenosis is relieved by surgery. Thus, without surgery, death usually occurs in middle age and may be caused by pulmonary oedema, chest infection, endocarditis or thromboembolism.

## Mitral regurgitation (MR)

### *Aetiology*

Mitral regurgitation is caused by valve-leaflet disease, subvalvular disease or dilatation of the left ventricle (Table 9.1).

### *Mitral valve prolapse*

This is a common and usually asymptomatic condition, in which one or both of the mitral valve leaflets bulge backwards into the left atrium during systole, producing mitral regurgitation in some cases. Mitral valve prolapse affects about 5% of the population and is particularly common in young women; the cause is unknown but it may be associated with a variety of cardiac and systemic disorders. Most cases are idiopathic, however, and are characterized by myxomatous degeneration of the voluminous (redundant) valve-leaflet tissue. Although patients are usually asymptomatic, some complain of non-specific chest pain, the cause of which is not clear. Others complain of palpitations, which are sometimes related to ventricular premature beats or paroxysmal supraventricular tachycardias, although a clear association between mitral valve prolapse

**Table 9.1**   Causes of mitral regurgitation

| | |
|---|---|
| *Valve-leaflet disease* | Mitral valve prolapse |
| | Rheumatic disease |
| | Infective endocarditis* |
| *Subvalvular disease* | Chordal rupture* |
| | Papillary muscle dysfunction |
| | Papillary muscle rupture* |
| *Dilating left ventricular disease* | 'Functional' mitral regurgitation |

* These disorders produce acute regurgitation.
Note that the subclassification into valve-leaflet and subvalvular disease is to some extent artificial because all the causes of valve-leaflet disease are usually associated with subvalvular dysfunction.

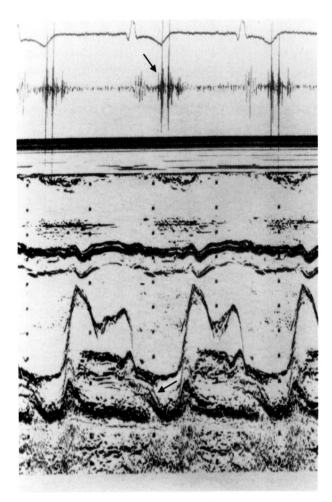

**Fig. 9.5**  Mitral valve prolapse. The M-mode recording shows typical backward displacement of the posterior leaflet of the mitral valve (arrowed) during systole. The simultaneous phonocardiogram shows a click in mid-systole (arrowed), which is followed by two much louder clicks and a systolic murmur.

and cardiac arrhythmias has yet to be established. The auscultatory signs may vary from day to day, but typically there is a mid-systolic click followed by a murmur. Occasionally, the murmur is pansystolic, while in other cases only a mid-systolic click is present. The echocardiogram is usually diagnostic, showing posterior displacement of the mitral valve leaflet(s) immediately following the click (Fig. 9.5). For most cases, no treatment is necessary but, in severe MR, valve replacement is occasionally required. Antibiotic prophylaxis, prior to dental surgery and other non-sterile invasive procedures, is recommended only when mitral valve prolapse is associated with a murmur indicating MR.

## Chordal rupture

This is usually idiopathic, affecting patients over 50, but may be related to endocarditis or rheumatic fever. It produces acute MR, the severity of which relates to the extent of chordal rupture.

## Papillary muscle disease

Myocardial ischaemia can lead to dysfunction or rupture of the papillary muscles. Papillary muscle dysfunction is usually well tolerated but, when myocardial infarction (MI) is complicated by papillary muscle rupture, the mitral valve is completely unsupported. Torrential MR and pulmonary oedema then occur, and urgent valve replacement is essential to prevent death.

## Pathophysiology

MR volume-loads the left ventricle, due to increased filling from the left atrium. In chronic disease, this causes compensatory dilatation and hypertrophy. The lesion is usually well tolerated because the systolic leak of regurgitant blood into the left atrium reduces left ventricular wall tension considerably. The reduction in afterload permits diversion of energy to myocardial shortening, such that forward output is maintained. Moreover, progressive dilatation of the left atrium increases its distensibility (compliance) and prevents marked elevation of atrial pressure during ventricular systole. This protects against pulmonary oedema and the development of pulmonary hypertension. AF commonly supervenes.

## Clinical manifestations

MR remains asymptomatic until the left ventricle begins to fail. In acute MR, this often occurs abruptly, but in chronic disease it may take several years. Symptoms include orthopnoea, exercise-related fatigue and dyspnoea. Because pulmonary hypertension is unusual in MR, signs of RVF are rarely prominent.

The pulse is commonly irregular, due to AF, but there is no reduction in pulse volume until LVF is advanced. Auscultation reveals an apical pansystolic murmur, which radiates into the left axilla. In mitral valve prolapse, the murmur usually occurs later in systole and is preceded by a click (see above). A third heart sound is often present, due to rapid filling from the volume-loaded left atrium.

## Complications

Patients with MR are prone to thromboembolism from the dilated left atrium, particularly after the onset of AF when anticoagulation is mandatory. There is also a considerable risk of endocarditis, and antibiotic prophylaxis prior to dental surgery and other non-sterile invasive procedures is essential. Although MR is generally well tolerated, in severe cases the chronic volume overload leads inexorably to LVF and irreversible contractile dysfunction. Pulmonary hypertension and right ventricular failure, however, are less common than in MS.

## Diagnosis

The ECG shows P mitrale before the onset of AF. The CXR shows signs of left atrial dilatation and the heart size is usually increased due to left ventricular enlargement. In rheumatic disease, calcification of the mitral valve may be evident. The lung fields remain normal until the development of LVF.

The echocardiogram confirms left atrial and left ventricular dilatation, although left ventricular contractile function remains well preserved until the development of failure. Diagnostic abnormalities of the valve itself occur in mitral valve prolapse and rheumatic disease, and vegetations can usually be imaged in endocarditis (see Fig. 8.1). Dynamic abnormalities of the valve (e.g. flail leaflet) may be present in chordal or papillary muscle rupture but, in many cases of subvalvular mitral regurgitation, the valve appears normal. Nevertheless, Doppler echocardiography identifies the regurgitant jet in the left atrium and permits assessment of the severity of the lesion. At cardiac catheterization, left ventricular angiography confirms the diagnosis and defines left ventricular contractile function (see Fig. 3.15). In acute MR, the regurgitant jet produces a prominent 'v' wave in the pulmonary artery wedge pressure signal (Fig. 9.6). This occurs less commonly in chronic MR because the dilated left atrium is compliant and the regurgitant jet does not produce such an abrupt rise in pressure.

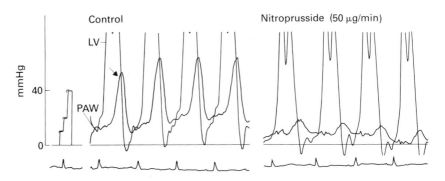

**Fig. 9.6**  Acute mitral regurgitation. Simultaneous recordings of the left ventricular (LV) and pulmonary artery wedge (PAW) pressure signals are shown before and after nitroprusside infusion. Note that before nitroprusside there is considerable elevation of the left ventricular diastolic and pulmonary artery wedge pressures. A giant 'v' wave is clearly visible (arrowed). Vasodilator therapy with nitroprusside reduces the ventricular filling pressures and also reduces regurgitant flow with disappearance of the 'v' wave.

## Differential diagnosis

MR must be distinguished from other conditions causing systolic murmurs. The pansystolic murmur of tricuspid regurgitation is augmented by inspiration and is located at the lower left sternal edge without radiation into the left axilla. The pansystolic murmur of ventricular septal defect is also best heard at the lower left sternal edge. Nevertheless, following MI, acute ventricular septal defect may be difficult to distinguish from MR caused by papillary muscle rupture (see Table 5.8). The murmur of aortic stenosis is often clearly audible at the cardiac apex but can be identified by its mid-systolic timing and its association with a slow-rising carotid pulse. In all these situations, echocardiography and Doppler studies are usually diagnostic.

## Treatment

Diuretics are often sufficient to control dyspnoea. The development of AF requires digitalis, to prevent a rapid ventricular response, and anticoagulants, to protect against thromboembolism from the dilated left atrium. Antibiotic prophylaxis against endocarditis is essential.

Vasodilators, such as prazosin or ACE inhibitors, play an important role. By lowering aortic pressure, forward flow into the aorta increases and regurgitation is reduced. Vasodilators are particularly useful in acute MR, and a nitroprusside infusion often produces dramatic haemodynamic improvement and relief from pulmonary oedema in patients with papillary muscle rupture complicating MI (Fig. 9.6). Treatment of this type can be used to stabilize the circulation pending emergency valve replacement. Troublesome symptoms which cannot be controlled medically and any evidence of left ventricular contractile dysfunction are indications for valve replacement in chronic MR.

## Prognosis

Chronic MR is only slowly progressive and is compatible with a normal lifespan. However, if the volume-loaded left ventricle develops contractile failure, the prognosis is considerably worse and death usually occurs within 5–10 years. Prognosis is also influenced by aetiology and the outlook in ischaemic disease (papillary muscle dysfunction), for example, is less favourable than in rheumatic disease.

## Aortic stenosis (AS)

## Aetiology

With the decline in rheumatic fever in the UK, calcific disease has become the commonest cause of AS. Indeed, calcific AS is now the most common of all valve lesions, with the possible exception of mitral valve prolapse. It is a degenerative process, affecting the elderly, in which calcification of a previously normal valve causes progressive obstruction to flow. Congenital bicuspid aortic valve is the second most common cause of AS but does not present until middle age, when calcification of the valve leaflets usually occurs (see p. 314). Rheumatic AS is now relatively unusual and rarely occurs without associated mitral disease. All the important causes of AS are also causes of aortic regurgitation, and a combination of both defects commonly occurs in the same patient.

## Pathophysiology

Aortic stenosis obstructs left ventricular outflow and produces a pressure gradient across the valve during systole (see Fig. 3.18). The LV hypertrophies, enabling it to generate sufficient pressure to maintain normal flow through the diseased valve. Not until the aortic, valve area is less than $1 cm^2$ (about one-quarter its normal value) is AS regarded as critical. Stenosis of this severity requires a peak systolic pressure gradient of more than 50 mmHg to maintain normal flow.

Hypertrophy diminishes left ventricular compliance, such that adequate filling depends upon a high end-diastolic pressure. Vigorous left atrial systole (reflected by a prominent 'a' wave) contributes importantly by boosting ventricular filling and, for this reason, AF is poorly tolerated.

As aortic stenosis worsens, deterioration in left ventricular contractile function eventually occurs. The pressure gradient across the aortic valve can no longer be sustained and forward flow declines. The heart dilates and frank congestive failure develops.

## Clinical manifestations

Dyspnoea, angina and syncope are the principal symptoms but they rarely occur before the valve area is critically reduced.

Elevation of the left atrial pressure causes exertional dyspnoea, which is particularly severe following the development of frank LVF. This is a late event in the natural history of AS and, in addition to dyspnoea, produces orthopnoea and exercise-related fatigue.

Angina is caused by the exaggerated oxygen demands of the hypertrophied LV. Although the coronary arteries are often normal, they are unable to deliver sufficient oxygen, particularly when demand is heightened during exertion. Coincidental coronary artery disease makes symptoms worse.

Syncope usually occurs during exertion, because flow through the stenosed aortic valve cannot increase sufficiently to maintain blood-pressure as skeletal muscle vasodilates. Vasodilator drugs can produce

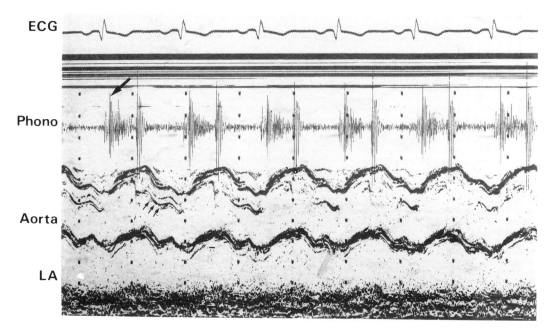

**Fig. 9.7**   Aortic stenosis — bicuspid aortic valve. In this M-mode echocardiogram the diastolic closure line of the aortic valve (small arrows) lies eccentrically within the aortic root, suggesting a bicuspid valve. The valve is normal in other respects. The ejection click (arrowed) and murmur typical of this condition are recorded on the phonocardiogram.

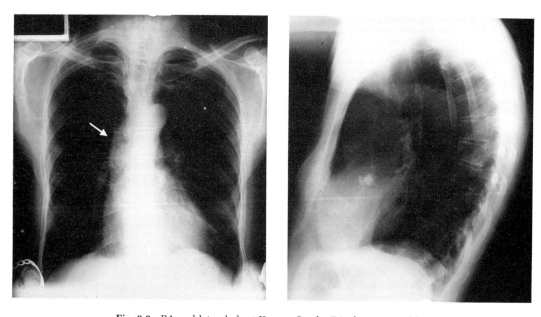

**Fig. 9.8**   PA and lateral chest X-rays. On the PA chest X-ray dilatation of the aortic root is clearly visible (arrowed) and the calcified valve leaflets can be identified. Note that the heart size is not enlarged because aortic stenosis produces left ventricular hypertrophy without dilatation. On the lateral chest X-ray the calcified valve is more clearly visible.

hypotension and syncope by the same mechanism and must be used with caution in AS. Syncope may also result from paroxysmal ventricular arrhythmias (Stokes–Adams attacks) or, rarely, from the development of complete heart block (see below).

Examination of the carotid pulse reveals a slow upstroke and plateau, associated with reduced volume. The apex beat is not usually displaced unless there is associated aortic regurgitation. It is thrusting and may have a double impulse, due to vigorous atrial contraction immediately before ventricular systole. Systolic thrills are often palpable over the aortic area and the carotid arteries. Auscultation reveals a medium-pitched mid-systolic murmur, which may be heard all over the left precordium but is usually loudest at the base of the heart, radiating into the neck. It is occasionally preceded by an ejection click if the valve cusps are pliant and not heavily calcified (Fig. 9.7). Other auscultatory findings include a fourth heart sound, reflecting vigorous atrial systole, and reversed splitting of the second heart sound, which may be single — especially when the valve is heavily calcified (see Fig. 1.9).

## Complications

Endocarditis is an ever-present risk. Antibiotic prophylaxis prior to dental surgery and other non-sterile invasive procedures is essential. Cardiac arrhythmias are common. AF may produce abrupt clinical deterioration but more important are ventricular arrhythmias, which are a cause of syncope and sudden death. Heart block, requiring pacemaker therapy, is an occasional complication of calcific AS and is caused by calcific destruction of the conducting tissue in the adjacent part of the interventricular septum. In advanced AS, the chronic pressure load eventually leads to LVF, with irreversible contractile impairment.

## Diagnosis

The ECG shows exaggerated voltage deflexions, reflecting left ventricular hypertrophy. This may be associated with T-wave inversion in the lateral leads (strain pattern) in advanced cases and, occasionally, left bundle branch block occurs. The CXR shows a normal heart size, unless there is associated aortic regurgitation. Post-stenotic dilatation of the ascending aorta is usually evident and the penetrated film may reveal valvular calcification (Fig. 9.8).

The echocardiogram is diagnostic in most cases. The aortic valve is thickened and rigid. Symmetrical left ventricular hypertrophy is almost invariable (Fig. 9.9). Doppler studies provide a quantitative assessment of the pressure gradient across the valve and may also demonstrate asso-ciated aortic regurgitation (AR). The majority of patients with AS are

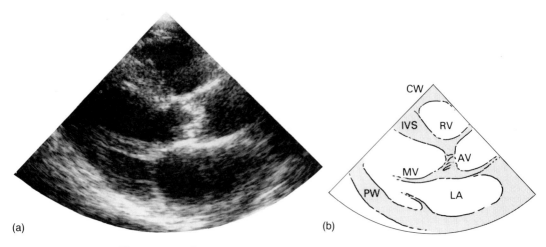

(a)

(b)

**Fig. 9.9**  Two-dimensional echocardiogram (long-axis view). The aortic valve is grossly thickened and highly echogenic, suggestive of calcification. Concentric left ventricular hypertrophy is clearly visible.

middle-aged or elderly and many of them have angina. Coronary arteriography is therefore an essential part of the preoperative evaluation in order that diseased vessels, if present, may be bypassed at the same time as valve replacement. During cardiac catheterization, the pressure gradient across the aortic valve should be measured (see Fig. 3.18). Aortic root angiography permits assessment of associated AR (see Fig. 3.14).

## Differential diagnosis

The differential diagnosis of AS includes hypertrophic cardiomyopathy and hypertension. Both conditions may be associated with angina, a mid-systolic ejection murmur and ECG changes similar to AS, but in neither condition is the carotid pulse slow-rising, nor does the echocardiogram show a thickened aortic valve.

Innocent systolic murmurs (see p. 23) should not be confused with AS. They are usually soft and never produce a slow-rising carotid pulse.

## Treatment

Subcritical AS requires no specific treatment while it remains asymptomatic, although vigorous exertion should be discouraged because of the risk of ventricular arrhythmias. Antibiotic prophylaxis against infective endocarditis is essential.

Surgical treatment is usually by valve replacement. Valvotomy is effective in infants with congenital bicuspid valves but is impossible in adults with calcific disease which prohibits effective division of the

**Table 9.2** Causes of aortic regurgitation (AR)

| | |
|---|---|
| *Valve-leaflet disease* | Congenital bicuspid valve |
| | Calcific disease |
| | Rheumatic disease |
| | Infective endocarditis* |
| *Aortic root dilating disease* | Marfan's syndrome |
| | Ankylosing spondylitis |
| | Syphilis |
| | Hypertension |
| | Aortic dissection* |
| | Aortic root aneurysm |
| | Deceleration injury* |

* These disorders produce acute AR. In the remainder the course is chronic.

commissures. Percutaneous aortic balloon valvuloplasty, now the procedure of choice in infants (see p. 315), is unhelpful in adults for the same reason. Indications for valve surgery in AS are:

**1** Any symptoms attributable to AS.

**2** LVF. Regular monitoring of ventricular function by echocardiography or nuclear ventriculography is essential.

**3** Critical AS (i.e. peak systolic pressure gradient > 50 mmHg). This is usually regarded as an indication for valve replacement even in the asymptomatic patient with well-preserved ventricular function.

## Prognosis

AS is well tolerated and most patients are over 60 before they die, but, following the development of symptoms, death usually occurs within 3 years. The outlook is worse in patients with LVF. Valve replacement improves the prognosis of these symptomatic patients considerably.

## Aortic regurgitation (AR)

### Aetiology

AR is caused either by disease of the valve cusps or aortic root disease (Table 9.2). In calcific disease AR is usually trivial but in bicuspid valvular disease and rheumatic disease it may be the dominant lesion. Infective endocarditis is an important cause of acute AR, as are deceleration injuries, which cause acute aortic regurgitation by traumatic rupture of the valve.

Aortic root disease causes AR by dilatation of the valve annulus. This may occur acutely in aortic dissection but usually it is a chronic process, seen in cystic medial necrosis of the aorta (with or without other manifestations of Marfan's syndrome), ankylosing spondylitis and other connective tissue and rheumatological disorders. The majority of cases, however, are idiopathic. Syphilis is no longer a common cause of aortic root disease.

## Pathophysiology

Regurgitant flow in AR is greatest immediately following valve closure and declines in mid-diastole as pressure in the aortic root falls. Increments in heart rate reduce the regurgitant volume by shortening diastole.

AR volume-loads the LV. When this occurs acutely, the Starling reserve of the ventricle is often exceeded, resulting in pulmonary oedema and low-output failure. In chronic AR, however, left ventricular dilatation and hypertrophy effectively compensate for the volume load. The increase in diastolic filling increases stroke volume (Starling mechanism), such that forward cardiac output is maintained despite the regurgitant flow. Left ventricular dilatation is relatively more pronounced than hypertrophy and compliance remains normal or increases. Thus, the volume-loaded left ventricle does not always exhibit significant elevation of end-diastolic pressure. The Starling mechanism and the compliance properties of the ventricle ensure that chronic AR is well tolerated, without producing low cardiac output or pulmonary oedema. Nevertheless, the compensatory potential of left ventricular dilatation and hypertrophy is limited (see p. 81) and, in advanced disease, contractile function deteriorates, leading to heart failure.

## Clinical manifestations

Acute aortic regurgitation may present dramatically with pulmonary oedema and low-output failure. Chronic AR, however, usually remains asymptomatic for several years before the development of exertional fatigue and dyspnoea marks the onset of LVF. Angina affects 50% of cases and is caused by the increased oxygen requirements of the dilated, hypertrophied ventricle (cf. aortic stenosis).

The carotid pulse is readily visible in the neck — Corrigan's pulse. It has a rapid upstroke and collapses in early diastole as blood regurgitates into the left ventricle. The pulse pressure is widened, with exaggeration of the systolic peak and the diastolic nadir. During blood-pressure measurement, the Korotkoff sounds often persist to zero so that phase V cannot be identified (see p. 14), and phase IV must be used for the diastolic measurement.

The apex beat is displaced towards the left axilla and has a prominent impulse, due to left ventricular enlargement. Auscultation at the aortic area reveals a high-pitched early diastolic murmur, which radiates down to the left sternal edge; a mid-systolic murmur, due to turbulent forward flow through the aortic valve, is usually also present. It relates to increased stroke volume and does not necessarily indicate aortic stenosis. In severe disease, the regurgitant jet causes preclosure of the anterior leaflet of the mitral valve during diastole. This produces an apical mid-diastolic murmur (Austin Flint murmur).

## Complications

Infective endocarditis is a major complication. In advanced disease, progressive left ventricular dilatation and irreversible contractile dysfunction results in heart failure (Fig. 9.10).

## Diagnosis

The ECG shows evidence of left ventricular hypertrophy. The CXR shows an enlarged heart and dilatation of the ascending aorta. Penetrated films may reveal calcification of the aortic valve.

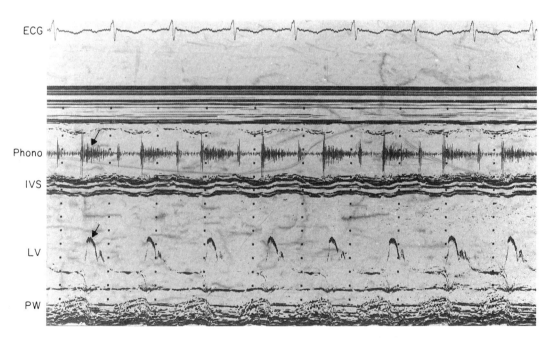

**Fig. 9.10** Aortic regurgitation — end-stage disease. This M-mode echocardiogram shows severe left ventricular dilatation with global contractile impairment. Note the fine vibrations on the anterior leaflet of the mitral valve (arrowed) caused by the regurgitant jet. The early diastolic decrescendo murmur has been recorded immediately following the second heart sound (arrowed). The prognosis in this case is very poor, but might have been better if aortic valve replacement earlier in the natural history of the disease had prevented deterioration in left ventricular contractile function.

The echocardiogram may show an abnormally thickened aortic valve. In aortic root disease, however, the valve itself appears normal although the aorta is dilated. The regurgitant jet may produce fine vibrations on the anterior leaflet of the mitral valve and, less commonly, on the inter-ventricular septum. The left ventricle shows variable dilatation and vigorous contractile function until this deteriorates in end-stage disease (Fig. 9.10). Doppler studies identify the regurgitant jet and permit assessment of its severity.

Cardiac catheterization is usually necessary before aortic valve surgery, in order to examine the coronary anatomy. Left ventricular and aortic root angiography define contractile function and the severity of AR, respectively (see Fig. 3.14). In patients with associated AS, the valve gradient can be measured.

## Differential diagnosis

AR must be distinguished from other conditions associated with an early diastolic murmur. Pulmonary regurgitation is relatively unusual and is nearly always associated with evidence of severe pulmonary hypertension. In patent ductus arteriosus and ruptured sinus of Valsalva aneurysm, the murmurs are continuous but are loudest at end-systole/early diastole. Moreover, these conditions are associated with a wide pulse pressure. Confusion with AR is therefore easy. Echo–Doppler studies, however, can usually confirm the differential diagnosis.

## Treatment

In acute AR associated with LVF, valve replacement should not be delayed. In chronic AR, symptoms are rarely obtrusive until the onset of LVF. Mild dyspnoea may respond to diuretic therapy, but vasodilators are often more useful because reductions in peripheral resistance and reflex tachycardia increase forward flow and reduce the regurgitant fraction. Antibiotic prophylaxis against infective endocarditis is essential.

When AR becomes symptomatic, valve replacement is usually indicated, particularly when symptoms are associated with echocardiographic or radionuclide evidence of LV contractile deterioration. If surgery is delayed until left ventricular dysfunction has become irreversible, the results are less satisfactory.

## Prognosis

The prognosis is determined principally by the severity of left ventricular dysfunction. Thus, mild AR with normal ventricular function is compatible with a normal lifespan but, in more severe cases, LVF often develops in middle age. Thereafter, prognosis is poor and similar to that of other causes of LVF (see p. 95). Timely valve replacement improves prognosis considerably.

## Tricuspid stenosis (TS)

### *Aetiology*

This is almost invariably rheumatic in origin and is usually associated with mitral valve disease. It is uncommon, not only because rheumatic disease tends to spare the right side of the heart but also because the tricuspid valve is very large and can tolerate substantial commissural fusion and leaflet fibrosis before obstruction to flow becomes significant.

### *Pathophysiology*

Obstruction to tricuspid flow causes elevation of the right atrial pressure and establishes a pressure gradient across the valve, increased by inspiration. Vigorous atrial contraction contributes importantly to right ventricular filling and produces a giant 'a' wave in the JVP. As tricuspid stenosis deteriorates, pulmonary flow decreases. This may produce a paradoxical symptomatic improvement in patients with associated MS by reducing pulmonary artery and pulmonary capillary pressures. Nevertheless, this improvement is at the expense of worsening cardiac output and right heart failure.

### *Clinical manifestations*

TS is usually associated with rheumatic mitral valve disease, which tends to dominate the clinical presentation causing dyspnoea. As TS becomes more severe, however, dyspnoea may improve (see above), to be replaced by symptoms of right heart failure, including oedema and abdominal discomfort caused by hepatomegaly and ascites. Muscular fatigue, caused by low cardiac output, is also common.

The examination reveals an elevated JVP with a giant 'a' wave. The 'a' wave disappears with the onset of AF. A low-pitched mid-diastolic murmur, augmented during inspiration, is present at the lower left sternal edge, with presystolic accentuation in sinus rhythm.

### *Diagnosis*

In isolated TS the ECG may show tall peaked P waves indicating right atrial enlargement, but the CXR is usually normal. The two-dimensional echocardiogram confirms thickening and rigidity of the tricuspid valve and right atrial enlargement. Doppler studies permit quantification of the pressure gradient.

## Differential diagnosis

TS must be differentiated from other causes of a mid-diastolic murmur and right heart failure, particularly MS and atrial septal defect.

## Treatment

In most cases the lesion is mild and haemodynamically unimportant; severe right heart failure, however, requires valve surgery. Valvotomy is rarely satisfactory and valve replacement is the procedure of choice.

## Tricuspid regurgitation (TR)

This is usually functional and secondary to right ventricular dilatation in advanced RVF, when it exacerbates the existing haemodynamic derangement. Other causes of TR, including rheumatic disease, infective endocarditis, Ebstein's anomaly and carcinoid disease, are rare.

Tricuspid regurgitation volume-loads the right ventricle and leads to (or, more commonly, exacerbates) symptoms and signs of right heart failure. A pansystolic murmur is audible at the left sternal edge and may be associated with a mid-diastolic tricuspid flow murmur. The regurgitant jet produces pulsatile systolic waves in the jugular veins, called giant 'v' waves (Fig. 9.11). Sometimes pulsatile expansion of the enlarged liver

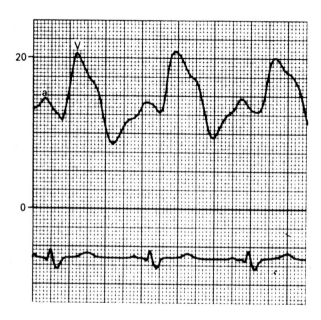

**Fig. 9.11** Tricuspid regurgitation. The right atrial pressure recording shows a typical giant 'v' wave caused by the regurgitant jet.

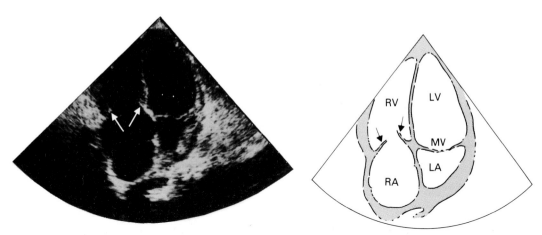

**Fig. 9.12**  Tricuspid regurgitation — carcinoid. The two-dimensional echocardiogram is a systolic frame (note that the mitral valve is closed), but the damaged tricuspid valve leaflets (arrowed) are tethered and remain widely separated, allowing tricuspid regurgitation. Thus, the right atrium is severely dilated.

can be detected. In functional TR, signs of pulmonary hypertension are usually present, including a loud pulmonary component to the second heart sound.

TR is essentially a clinical diagnosis, based on the pansystolic murmur at the lower left sternal edge and giant 'v' waves in the JVP. Doppler studies identify the regurgitant jet. The echocardiogram may show a normal tricuspid valve if regurgitation is functional, but there is always dilatation of the right-sided cardiac chambers (Fig. 9.12).

TR is usually well tolerated, even when it occurs acutely in endo-carditis. Treatment with diuretics controls systemic congestion and reduces right ventricular volume, which improves functional regurgita-tion. Tricuspid valve surgery is only rarely necessary.

## Pulmonary valve disease

Rheumatic disease of the pulmonary valve is rare. Endocarditis occurs occasionally (usually in intravenous drug abusers), but the most common pulmonary valve defects are congenital valvular stenosis and valvular regurgitation due to pulmonary hypertension. Congenital pulmonary stenosis is discussed in Chapter 15. Pulmonary regurgitation produces an early diastolic murmur at the upper left sternal edge (Graham Steell murmur), which is almost identical to that of AR. Nevertheless, in pul-monary regurgitation signs of pulmonary hypertension are usually prominent and the carotid pulse is normal, so differentiation between pulmonary and aortic regurgitation should not be difficult. Pulmonary regurgitation is well tolerated, producing negligible haemodynamic embarrassment, and prognosis is determined by the associated pulmonary hypertension.

## Further reading

Anonymous. Mitral valve prolapse. *Lancet* 1989, **i**, 1173–5.

Chesler E. and Gornick C.C. Maladies attributed to myxomatous mitral valve. *Circulation* 1991, **83**, 328–38.

Collins J.J. The evolution of artificial heart valves. *N. Engl. J. Med.* 1991, **324**, 624–6.

Frankl W.S. Valvular heart disease: the technologic dilemma. *J. Am. Coll. Cardiol.* 1991, **17**, 1037–8.

Hall R. Aortic stenosis, aortic regurgitation, rheumatic mitral valve disease, non-rheumatic mitral valve disease. In Julian D.G., Camm A.J., Fox K.M., Hall R.J.C. and Poole-Wilson P.A. (eds), *Diseases of the Heart.* London, Baillière Tindall, 1989, pp. 705–827.

Hancock E.W. Timing of valve replacement for aortic stenosis. *Circulation* 1990, **82**, 310–12.

Levine M.J. and McKay R.G. Percutaneous balloon valve dilatation. *Br. Med. J.* 1989, **298**, 620–1.

Rahimtoola S.H. Vasodilator therapy in chronic severe aortic regurgitation. *J. Am. Coll. Cardiol.* 1990, **16**, 430–2.

Selzer A. Changing aspects of the natural history of valvular aortic stenosis. *N. Engl. J. Med.* 1987, **317**, 91–8.

Strauss B. and Marquis J.F. Percutaneous valvuloplasty as a treatment for aortic and mitral valve disease. *Am. Heart J.* 1990, **119**, 1184–92.

Taggart D.P. and Wheatley D.J. Mitral valve surgery: to repair or replace? *Br. Heart J.* 1990, **64**, 234–5.

# 10 Conduction Tissue Disease and Pacemakers

## Summary

Idiopathic fibrosis, a condition affecting the elderly, is the most common cause of conduction tissue disease; ischaemic disease and cardiomyopathy are also important. Although the conduction tissue is often diffusely involved, sinoatrial (SA) and atrioventricular (AV) disease are conveniently considered separately.

*SA disease* The commonest manifestation is sinus bradycardia, which, if the rate fails to increase normally with exercise (chronotropic incompetence), may cause fatigue and dyspnoea. Prolonged sinus pauses lead to dizzy attacks and syncope; in the bradycardia–tachycardia syndrome, paroxysmal tachyarrhythmias (usually atrial fibrillation) cause palpitations and, occasionally, thromboembolism. Because symptoms are typically intermittent, diagnosis may require ambulatory Holter monitoring to document the electrocardiogram (ECG) abnormality. Treatment of bradycardias and sinus pauses is by atrial pacing (dual-chamber pacing for patients with associated AV disease) but is only necessary in patients experiencing symptoms. Associated tachyarrhythmias may require treatment with antiarrhythmic drugs but, if these exacerbate SA dysfunction, a pacemaker may be necessary to protect against severe bradycardia. Atrial fibrillation (AF) increases the risk of thromboembolism, and prophylactic anti-coagulation (warfarin) or aspirin is usually recommended.

*AV-disease* may involve the AV node or the bundle branches. First-degree AV block causes delayed conduction but is asymptomatic because heart rate is unaffected. The ECG shows a prolonged PR interval and no treatment is necessary. In second-degree AV block, failure of conduction is intermittent, but symptoms (fatigue, dizziness) occur only if insufficient sinus impulses are conducted to maintain an adequate ventricular rate. Second-degree block may be within the AV node (Wenckebach), when the PR interval is prolonged and increases progressively, culminating in a dropped beat; the process may then repeat itself. Symptoms are unusual and pacemaker therapy, therefore, is rarely necessary. When second-degree block affects the bundle branches (Mobitz type II), the ECG usually shows a normal PR interval with bundle branch block, intermittent block in the other bundle branch resulting in dropped beats. Pacing is mandatory because of the risk of prolonged asystole. Third-degree (complete) AV block is characterized by complete AV dissociation, with regular P waves (unless the atrium is fibrillating) and regular but slower QRS complexes occurring independently of one another. Block may be at the AV node (congenital block, inferior myocardial infarction), when a reliable junctional escape rhythm usually prevents symptoms, making pacing unnecessary. More often it occurs further down the conduction system in the bundle branches, where escape rhythms are slow and unreliable and pacing is mandatory because of the risk of prolonged asystole.

*Pacemakers* Ventricular pacing (VVI) is usually only indicated in complete AV block associated with atrial fibrillation, when, ideally, a rate-responsive unit (VVIR) should be used. Other patients with complete AV block should be offered a dual-chamber (DDD) unit because this reestablishes AV synchrony and allows the sinus node to control heart rate, which increases normally with exercise. In SA disease, atrial pacing (AAI) may be the method of choice, although patients with chronotropic incompetence require a rate-responsive unit (AAIR); DDD pacing is required in patients with associated atrioventricular block.

## Introduction

Disease of the cardiac conduction tissues can occur at any level from the sinus node, through the sinoatrial junction, the atrioventricular (AV) node, the bundle of His to the bundle branches and Purkinje system (Fig. 10.1).

## Sinoatrial (SA) disease

### Aetiology

Causes of SA disease are shown in Table 10.1. The most common is idiopathic fibrosis, which affects the conduction tissue at any level and occurs particularly in the elderly.

### Pathology

The sinus node, the conduction tissue with the highest intrinsic firing rate, is the pacemaker of the normal heart. The spontaneous discharge of the sinus node is influenced by a variety of neurohumoral factors, particularly vagal and sympathetic stimulation, which, respectively, slow and speed the sinus rate. The normal sinus rate varies with activity and with age. A rate of 40 beats/min is often normal during sleep and rates up to 200 beats/min may be achieved during exertion. Sinus arrhythmia (in

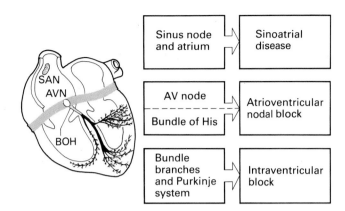

**Fig. 10.1** Classification of conduction tissue disease. SAN — sinoatrial node; AVN — atrioventricular node; BOH — bundle of His.

**Table 10.1** Causes of sinoatrial disease

Idiopathic fibrosis
Ischaemic heart-disease
Amyloidosis
Collagen vascular diseases
Infective causes (diphtheria, rheumatic fever and viral myocarditis)
Pericardial disease
'Antiarrhythmic' drugs
Radiotherapy
Post cardiac surgery
Trauma and hypothermia

which the rate increases during inspiration and decreases during expiration) is common in the young but tends to disappear with advancing age. Progressive slowing of the sinus rate occurs after the age of 55–60.

Sinus node discharge can be recorded endocardially, using special electrodes. It is not, however, visible on the surface ECG, although the atrial depolarization it initiates produces the P wave. Sinus node discharge may be suppressed by drugs or disease, or it may be blocked and fail to activate the atrium. Under these circumstances, pacemaker function can be assumed by escape foci in atrial tissue, the AV node, His–Purkinje tissue or the ventricular myocardium. The intrinsic rates of all these escape pacemakers are slower than the normal sinus rate and usually decrease progressively down the conduction system (Fig. 10.2).

## Clinical manifestations

SA disease is often asymptomatic. Presentation is usually with episodes of dizziness or syncope caused by severe bradycardia or prolonged sinus pauses without an effective escape rhythm. Pauses longer than 3 or 4 seconds are usually necessary to produce symptoms, although the elderly may be more susceptible. Additional complaints may include

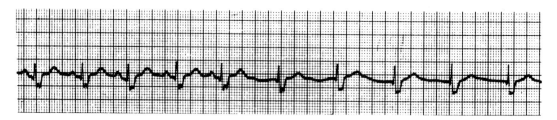

**Fig. 10.2** Junctional escape rhythm. Sinus rhythm ceases abruptly after the fifth beat and a junctional (AV node/bundle of His) focus takes over. Because ventricular depolarization proceeds by normal pathways, the QRS complexes of the escape rhythm are identical to the sinus complexes. However, P waves are not seen and the rate is slower.

exertional fatigue and dyspnoea, due to the failure of a physiological increase in heart rate (chronotropic incompetence). Patients may complain of palpitations, due to associated tachycardias, and thromboembolic events may also occur.

## Complications

Paroxysmal tachycardias, which may be atrial or junctional, often occur in association with bradyarrhythmias. This is known as the bradycardia–tachycardia syndrome (see below). More important is thromboembolism, which is particularly common in patients with paroxysmal tachycardias.

## Diagnosis

### Arrhythmia detection (see p. 39)

ECG documentation is essential for accurate diagnosis but the resting recording is rarely helpful in SA disease. Ambulatory ECG monitoring is usually required, but symptoms are often infrequent and documentation of the arrhythmia may be impossible without repeated Holter recordings. Although patient-activated recorders are preferable, symptoms are often transitory, and a device with a loop facility should be chosen, which, when triggered manually by the patient, provides a record of the ECG in the seconds leading up to the episode. Electrophysiological studies are rarely helpful because measurements of SA function are very insensitive, often yielding false-negative results in patients with SA disease.

### Electrocardiographic diagnosis

#### Sinus bradycardia

This may be defined as a resting sinus rate below 50 beats per minute. Like other bradycardias, it may be associated with atrial, junctional or

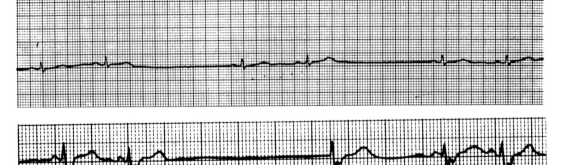

**Fig. 10.3** Sinus pauses. The upper panel shows intermittent *sinoatrial block* (after the second and fourth complexes), which has prevented sinus impulses from depolarizing the atrium. No P waves are seen but, because the sinus discharge continues uninterrupted, the pauses are each a precise multiple of the preceding PP interval. The lower panel shows *sinus arrest* with junctional escape. This occurs after the second complex, when there is a long pause terminated by the junctional escape beat (no P wave). Thereafter, sinus rhythm becomes re-established.

ventricular escape rhythms. Sinus bradycardia is physiological during sleep and in trained athletes, but in other circumstances may reflect SA disease, particularly when associated with chronotropic incompetence (see p. 210).

**Sinus pauses**

Sinus pauses may be caused by SA block or sinus arrest. In SA block, a normal sinus impulse occurs but its exit to the atria is blocked and the P wave is absent. In sinus arrest, the pause is caused by intermittent failure of sinus node discharge. SA block can sometimes be distinguished from sinus arrest if the pause is a precise multiple of preceding PP intervals. However, this is not reliable, and in practical and prognostic terms there is little point in attempting to distinguish between the different causes of sinus pauses (Fig. 10.3).

**Bradycardia–tachycardia syndrome**

Paroxysmal atrial or junctional tachyarrhythmias often occur in patients with SA disease. The tachycardias may be escape rhythms after pauses or may occur during periods of normal SA function. Atrial fibrillation (Fig. 10.4) is one of the more common arrhythmias and the main cause of thromboembolic events associated with this condition.

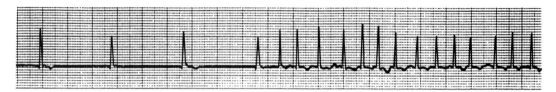

**Fig. 10.4** Bradycardia–tachycardia syndrome. A very slow junctional rhythm gives way to rapid atrial fibrillation.

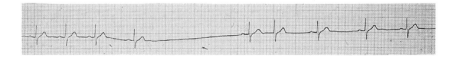

**Fig. 10.5** Carotid sinus hypersensitivity. The beginning of the trace shows normal sinus rhythm. Carotid sinus massage produces a long sinus pause, which continues until massage is stopped.

## Differential diagnosis

SA disease must be distinguished from other cardiac and non-cardiac causes of dizzy attacks and syncope (see p. 5).

*Carotid sinus syndrome* is caused by carotid sinus hypersensitivity. Pressure over the carotid sinus may cause sinus bradycardia, sinus arrest or AV block, as well as vasodilatation (Fig. 10.5). Patients may complain of syncope caused by shaving or a tight shirt collar. Carotid sinus massage is usually diagnostic (see p. 43). Pacing corrects bradycardias in the carotid sinus syndrome. The vasodilator component, however, may be difficult to treat and is often exacerbated if VVI rather than dual-chamber pacing is used (see below).

*Malignant vasovagal syndrome* also has bradycardic and vasodilator elements, caused usually by exaggerated vagal responses to emotional or painful stimuli. Diagnosis is by tilt testing (see p. 42). Repeated syncopal attacks may become very disabling and require dual-chamber pacing.

### Treatment

Most asymptomatic patients with sinus bradycardia or sinus pauses require no specific treatment. Drugs such as beta-blockers, which suppress the sinus node, should be avoided. Patients who have symptomatic bradycardias or pauses require pacemaker therapy to maintain the heart rate and prevent syncope. Atrial pacing is preferred because, unlike ventricular pacing, it reduces the risk of thromboembolism. It also maintains normal cardiac activation and heart rate, improves exercise tolerance and often prevents associated tachyarrhythmias. If abnormalities of AV conduction are manifest or suspected, additional ventricular pacing is required, using a dual-chamber pacemaker (see below).

Associated tachyarrhythmias may require treatment with anti-arrhythmic agents, but most drugs of this type will exacerbate SA dys-function, when a pacemaker is necessary to protect against severe bradycardia. Atrial fibrillation increases the risk of thromboembolism, and anticoagulation with warfarin is usually recommended. In patients under 50, however, the risk is lower, particularly if the left atrium is not dilated, and aspirin is a reasonable alternative.

## Prognosis

The prognosis of SA disease depends mainly on the underlying cause and on the thromboembolic risk. Death is rarely a direct consequence of sinus bradyarrhythmias.

## Atrioventricular (AV) block

### Aetiology (Table 10.2)

The commonest cause of AV block in the Western world is idiopathic fibrosis of the bundle branches, particularly in the elderly. Ischaemic heart-disease and cardiomyopathy are also important. Chagas' disease is the most common cause in Central and South America.

**Table 10.2** Causes of AV block

Idiopathic fibrosis (Lenegre's disease/Lev's disease)
Ischaemic heart-disease
Calcific aortic stenosis
Congenital AV block (isolated or associated with other congenital malformations)
Cardiomyopathy (including Chagas' disease)
Infection (tuberculosis, diphtheria, syphilis)
Sarcoidosis
Myeloma and other tumours (including Hodgkin's disease)
Connective tissue disease (ankylosing spondylitis, rheumatoid disease)
Myxoedema
Muscular dystrophies
'Antiarrhythmic' drugs
Radiotherapy
Cardiac surgery
Trauma
Hypothermia

## Pathophysiology

AV block can occur either in the AV node or in the His–Purkinje system. When conduction is merely delayed (e.g. first-degree AV block, bundle branch block), the heart rate is unaffected. When conduction is completely interrupted, however, the rate may slow and cause symptoms. In second-degree AV block, failure of conduction is intermittent and, if sufficient sinus impulses are conducted to maintain an adequate ventricular rate, symptoms do not occur. In third-degree AV block, there is complete failure of conduction and continuing ventricular activity depends on the emergence of an escape rhythm; the higher the level in the conduction system at which block occurs, the faster the escape rhythm. If block is within the AV node, the escape rhythm is often, though not always, fast enough to prevent major syncope. If both bundle branches are blocked, the ventricular escape rhythm may be very slow and unreliable and lead to syncope and death.

## Clinical manifestations

First-degree AV block is asymptomatic and can only be diagnosed from the ECG. In second-degree AV block, symptoms depend on the number of conducted impulses and, although patients are often asymptomatic, fatigue and dyspnoea commonly occur. The development of higher degrees of block may cause syncope.

In third-degree (complete) AV block, the symptoms depend on the level in the conduction system at which block occurs. In congenital AV

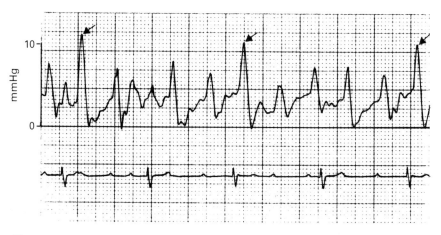

**Fig. 10.6**  Cannon 'a' waves in congenital complete heart block. The ECG shows complete dissociation of atrial and ventricular activity. The random coincidence of atrial and ventricular systole (occurring shortly after the QRS complex) produces intermittent cannon 'a' waves (arrowed) on the right atrial pressure recording.

block and acute inferior myocardial infarction, block is usually at the level of the AV node and a reliable junctional escape rhythm is common. However, in most other cases, block occurs further down the conduction system in the bundle branches, where escape rhythms are slow and unreliable. Exertional fatigue and dyspnoea are common and frank heart failure may occur, particularly in patients with associated valvular or myocardial disease. Very slow rates and prolonged pauses cause dizziness and syncope (Stokes–Adams attacks).

Examination in third-degree AV block reveals a slow regular pulse, usually less than 50 beats/min. The atrial and ventricular rhythms are dissociated and, if the sinus node is functioning normally, intermittent cannon 'a' waves in the jugular venous pulse (Fig. 10.6) and beat-to-beat variation in the intensity of the first heart sound are present. If the atrium is fibrillating, however, these signs are absent.

## Diagnosis

### Detection of AV block

All forms of AV block may be persistent or intermittent. If persistent, they are easily diagnosed from the resting ECG. If intermittent, ambulatory monitoring is usually required (see p. 40). Abnormalities on the resting ECG (e.g. prolonged PR interval or bundle branch block with axis deviation) pointing to underlying conduction abnormalities must be interpreted cautiously because, in the absence of symptoms, they are often clinically unimportant and, even in patients with syncope, paroxysmal ventricular tachycardia is as likely to be responsible as intermittent complete heart block.

Electrophysiological study (see p. 41) is more useful for diagnosing intermittent complete AV block than SA disease, but the predictive accuracy remains low and ambulatory monitoring techniques are preferred.

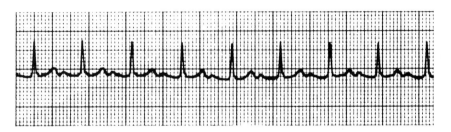

**Fig. 10.7** First-degree AV block. Note the prolongation of the PR interval (0.28 sec).

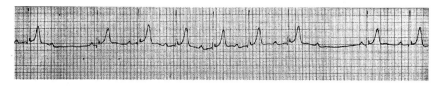

**Fig. 10.8**  Second-degree AV block — Wenckebach type. The PR interval shows progressive prolongation until failure of AV conduction occurs and a beat is dropped.

### First-degree AV block (Fig. 10.7)

Delayed AV conduction causes a prolonged PR interval (more than 0.20-sec) on the ECG. Ventricular depolarization, however, usually occurs rapidly, using normal His–Purkinje pathways. Thus, the QRS complexes are narrow and of normal duration unless there is associated bundle branch block.

### Second-degree AV block — Wenckebach type (Fig. 10.8)

This is also called Mobitz type I block and occurs within the AV node. Successive sinus beats find the AV node increasingly refractory, until failure of conduction occurs. The delay permits recovery of nodal function and the process may then repeat itself. The ECG often shows a prolonged PR interval, which increases progressively, culminating in a dropped beat. The QRS complexes are usually narrow and of normal duration.

### Second-degree AV block — Mobitz type II (Fig. 10.9)

This usually indicates advanced conduction tissue disease affecting the bundle branches. There is usually persistent block in one bundle branch, and intermittent block in the other branch resulting in complete failure of AV conduction and dropped beats. The PR interval in conducted beats is constant and often normal.

Patients with 2:1 AV block may have Wenckebach or Mobitz type II

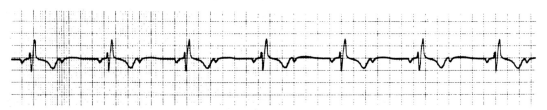

**Fig. 10.9**  Second-degree AV block — Mobitz type II. The ECG shows 2:1 AV block, in which every second sinus discharge fails to penetrate the ventricle. Note that, in those beats which are conducted, the QRS complex shows a bundle branch block pattern and the PR interval is normal — both typical features of Mobitz type II AV block.

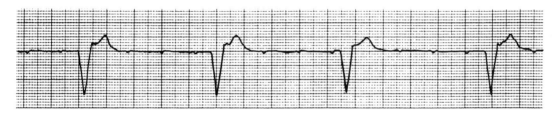

**Fig. 10.10** Third-degree AV block below the bundle of His. There is complete dissociation of atrial and ventricular activity. The ventricular escape rhythm arises distally in the ventricular conducting system and has a broad QRS complex. Compare with Figs 5.21 and 10.6, in which block is at the level of the AV junction.

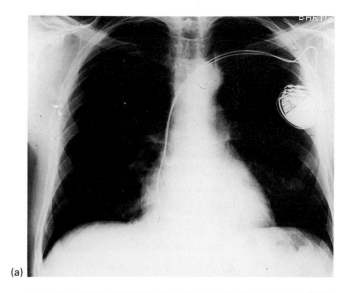

(a)

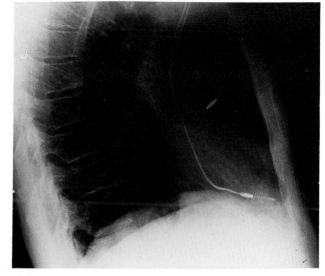

**Fig. 10.11** Permanent dual-chamber pacemaker. The PA and lateral chest X-rays (panels a and b, respectively) show a modern dual-chamber pacemaker in the left prepectoral position attached to right atrial and ventricular pacing electrodes.

(b)

block. The precise level of the block can be difficult to determine in these cases, but generally, if there is a prolonged PR interval in the conducted beat and normal QRS complexes, then the block is more likely to be of the Wenckebach type, with AV nodal disease. If the conducted PR interval is normal but there is bundle branch block, it is more likely to be Mobitz type II block, with His–Purkinje disease.

### *Third-degree — complete — AV block* (Fig. 10.10)

Complete failure of AV conduction produces dissociated atrial and ventricular rhythms. The ECG shows regular P waves (unless the atria are fibrillating) and regular but slower QRS complexes, occurring independently of one another. When block is within the AV node, a junctional escape rhythm often occurs, with a narrow QRS complex and a reliable rate of 40–60 beats/min. When block is within the bundle branches, the ventricular escape rhythm is generally slow and unreliable, with broad QRS complexes. Complete AV block may be misdiagnosed as 2:1 AV block when the atrial rate is approximately twice the ventricular rate and only a short rhythm strip is examined.

### *Right bundle branch block* (see Fig. 2.11)

This may be a congenital defect, occurring as an isolated phenomenon. However, it is more commonly the result of organic conduction tissue disease, which may be idiopathic or associated with other cardiac disorders, notably coronary disease. Right ventricular depolarization is delayed and this results in a broad QRS complex, with an rSR pattern in lead V1 and a prominent S wave in leads I and V6.

### *Left bundle branch block* (see Fig. 2.11)

Although this may occur as an isolated finding it usually indicates organic conduction tissue disease, which, like right bundle branch block, may be idiopathic or associated with other cardiac disorders. Left ventricular depolarization is delayed and there is a broad QRS complex, with a large slurred or notched R wave in leads I and V6. Block may be confined to the anterior or posterior divisions of the left bundle (hemiblock), when it is associated with left or right axis deviation, respectively, on the ECG.

### **Treatment**

All patients with complete AV block require a permanent pacemaker unless block is likely to be temporary (acute myocardial infarction, drug effect). A pacemaker is also required if the risk of developing complete AV block is high, e.g. in Mobitz type II block, and selected patients with trifascicular block (prolonged PR interval, right bundle branch block and left axis deviation), in whom AV conduction is dependent on the remaining division of the left bundle branch. Pacing relieves symptoms and, importantly, prevents prolonged asystole and sudden death. Only in congenital AV block are the indications for pacemaker therapy less well defined. These patients often remain asymptomatic for prolonged periods and the usual recommendation has been for pacing only in the event of symptoms. However, elective early pacing is favoured by some cardiologists because it may prevent the later development of irreversible cardiomegaly.

## Temporary pacemakers

Temporary pacemakers are used predominantly for the treatment of bradycardias (very occasionally for tachycardias), when the conduction disturbance is temporary and reversible or when pacing is required as a 'bridge' to a permanent device. Transvenous, endocardial pacing catheters are used most commonly. The catheter is inserted through either a central (usually subclavian or internal jugular) or peripheral vein and positioned within the right ventricle; temporary right atrial pacing can also be performed. Temporary epicardial pacing is reserved for patients who have undergone heart surgery: epicardial wires, placed peroperatively, are used to protect against bradycardia during the recovery period.

Endocardial temporary pacing catheters are usually bipolar, with the two electrodes mounted at the distal end (cathode at the tip, anode about 1 cm more proximally). The electrodes are connected to an external pulse generator, which consists of electronic circuitry and a battery power source. Complications, uncommon in experienced hands, include haemorrhage due to venous puncture, pneumothorax if the subclavian approach is used, infection and cardiac perforation.

## Permanent pacemakers

A permanent pacemaker consists of a hermetically sealed pulse generator driven by a lithium/lithium iodide cell. It is inserted under local anaesthetic into a subcutaneous 'pocket' (usually in the left prepectoral position) and attached to one, or often two, pacing catheters, using a special connector block. The pacing catheters are introduced transvenously, either through the cephalic vein or, failing this, by direct subclavian puncture, and are positioned in the right side of the heart (Fig. 10.11). Modern pacemaker pulse generators weigh between 25 and 35 g, are about 6 mm thick and last approximately 7 years before the battery

expires. Most are programmable, using an external radiofrequency programmer, which allows performance to be optimized by controlling the
pacing rate, voltage output, sensitivity and a variety of other more
sophisticated variables. In general, the lowest output compatible with
reliable pacing should be selected in order to prolong battery life. The
choice of rate depends on the indication for pacing. Modern pacemakers
are usually bipolar, with the anode and cathode mounted at the distal end
of the pacing catheter, closely applied to the endocardium; some older
pacemakers are unipolar, with the cathode at the distal end of the pacing
catheter and the anode provided by the metal casing of the pulse
generator.

Pacing catheters are usually coaxially wound, insulated coils connected to the pulse generator and terminating within the heart in a pair of
platinum or carbon electrodes. The distal cathodal electrode is specially
treated to reduce electrical resistance. This in turn reduces the pacing
'threshold' and permits the voltage output to be programmed to a low
level. A fixation device at the catheter tip, usually fine tines or a retract-
able screw, helps anchor it within the heart and prevent catheter displacement. Atrial pacing catheters usually have a J-shaped tip to facilitate
positioning within the right atrial appendage.

An international five-letter code describes the various methods of
pacing (Table 10.3). For practical purposes, however, only the first three
letters are usually used, describing the chamber paced, the chamber
sensed and the mode of response to sensing. The fourth letter R is applied
when the unit is rate-responsive, permitting a physiological increase in
heart rate with exercise; the fifth letter is rarely used. The most widely
used pacing methods are AAI, VVI, DDD and DDI. Any of these may be
rate-responsive, when R is added.

### VVI pacing (Fig. 10.12)

This is still the most commonly used method of pacing, even though it is
no longer the method of choice for the majority of cases. The right
ventricle is paced at a preselected rate, programmed into the pulse

**Table 10.3** Methods of pacing: five-letter code

| Chamber paced | Chamber sensed | Response to sensing | Programming and rate-responsiveness | Antitachycardia capability |
|---|---|---|---|---|
| O = None | O = None | O = None | O = None | O = None |
| A = Atrium | A = Atrium | T = Triggered | P = Simple | P = Pacing |
| V = Ventricle | V = Ventricle | I = Inhibited | M = Multiprogrammable | S = Shock |
| D = Dual (A + V) | D = Dual (A + V) | D = Dual (T + I) | C = Communicating | P = Dual (P + S) |
|  |  |  | R = Rate-responsive |  |

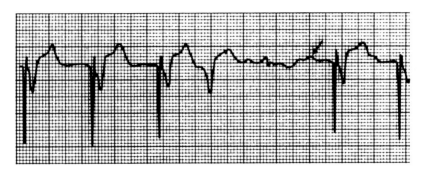

**Fig. 10.12** VVI pacing. The first three complexes are paced and are preceded by a pacing artefact. A spontaneous ventricular premature beat then inhibits the pacemaker and is followed by a sinus beat conducted with delay (prolonged PR interval). The next sinus impulse (arrowed) is not conducted and the ventricular pacemaker takes over again.

generator, which depends on the indication for pacing. Spontaneous ventricular beats, whether normally conducted or ectopic, are sensed and inhibit the pulse generator. This prevents competitive 'fixed-rate' pacing (VOO), in which delivery of electrical pulses during the vulnerable period of the cardiac cycle may initiate potentially lethal tachyarrhythmias (see Fig. 5.19). Thus, the pacemaker is only activated when the spontaneous ventricular rate falls below the preselected pacing rate. If the pacemaker is prophylactic against occasional sinus pauses, a slow rate (perhaps 50/min) is sufficient to guard against syncopal attacks, but in complete AV block, in which the escape rhythm is slow and unreliable, a faster pacing rate is necessary. A function called 'hysteresis' can also be selected, which allows the sensed rate at which the pacemaker is activated to be lower than the pacing rate. Hysteresis is useful for intermittent conduction disturbances because it ensures that the pacemaker is not activated unnecessarily often.

VVI pacing is simple, no doubt accounting for its continued widespread use. However, it is not the optimal pacing method for either SA disease or AV block. AV dissociation is an inevitable consequence of VVI pacing, because it fails to maintain the normal physiological conduction sequence of atrial followed by ventricular activation. This may cause 'pacemaker syndrome', where atrial and ventricular depolarizations occur simultaneously, with adverse haemodynamic effects. Moreover, because this is a ventricular pacing method, normal atrial contraction is lost and in patients with SA disease this can increase the risk of thromboembolism. In addition, VVI pacing does not permit a physiological increase in heart rate with exercise, unless a rate-responsive (VVIR) unit is chosen. Perhaps the only major indication for VVI pacing is AV block associated with atrial fibrillation, in which synchronous atrial activation can never be

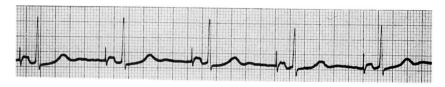

**Fig. 10.13** AAI pacing. The atrial pacing artefacts are seen, followed by a P wave and then a normally conducted QRS complex.

restored. A VVIR unit should usually be selected in these cases (see below).

### AAI pacing (Fig. 10.13)

This is an atrial pacing method, in which the pacing electrode is positioned in the right atrial appendage. The atrium is sensed and spontaneous contractions inhibit the pulse generator. Thus, pacing only occurs during atrial standstill to prevent prolonged asystolic pauses. Clearly, AAI pacing cannot be used in patients with AV block. However, it is the method of choice in patients with isolated SA disease, in whom AV conduction is normal. In patients with chronotropic incompetence, the rate-responsive variant (AAIR) ensures a normal heart rate response to exercise.

### DDD pacing (Fig. 10.14)

This is a dual-chamber pacing method, using two bipolar pacing catheters, one positioned in the right atrium and the other in the right ventricle (see

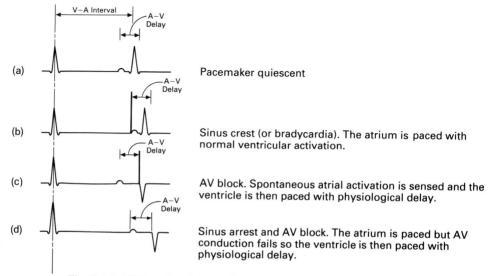

**Fig. 10.14** DDD pacing. See text for details.

Fig. 10.11). If SA and AV function is normal and the patient is in stable sinus rhythm at a satisfactory rate, the pacemaker remains quiescent (Fig. 10.14a). Reductions in atrial rate caused by sinus arrest or bradycardia are sensed by the atrial pacer, which is then activated to maintain the rate above a preselected level (Fig. 10.14b). AV delay is monitored and, so long as the atrial beats (spontaneous or paced) are conducted promptly to the ventricle, initiating depolarization, the ventricular pacer remains inhibited; ectopic beats also inhibit the ventricular pacer. However, if ventricular depolarization fails to occur, the ventricle is paced (Fig. 10.14c), and if neither atrial nor ventricular depolarizations occur spontaneously, both chambers are paced (Fig. 10.14d). Thus, neither, either or both chambers of the heart may be paced with this form of pacemaker. If AV block is present, but the sinus node is functioning normally with a physiological response to exercise, the ventricular rate will follow the atrial rate during exercise in a synchronized manner. This mode therefore re-establishes AV synchrony and allows the sinus node to control the heart rate. It can be combined with the rate-responsive mode (DDDR) if there is chronotropic incompetence.

DDD pacing comes closest to restoring normal physiology in patients with AV block, with or without associated SA disease, and is the method of choice in this group. However, it depends upon an intact atrial rhythm and cannot be used in AF, although reprogramming to other pacing modes is possible should AF develop after the system has been implanted. The major complication of DDD pacing is endless-loop tachycardia. It occurs in the minority of patients who retain normal ventriculoatrial conduction, despite anterograde AV block. In these patients, ventricular pacing, following either a spontaneous or a paced P wave, can cause retrograde and premature activation of the atrium, which in turn triggers ventricular pacing (after the appropriate AV delay), completing the circuit and providing the substrate for endless-loop tachycardia. Modern pacemakers have certain safeguards which protect against endless-loop tachycardia but, if they are not effective, DDI pacing provides an alternative method.

### DDI pacing

This is a dual-chamber pacing method similar to DDD. Both the atria and the ventricles are sensed and both can be paced. However, an increase in atrial rate above a preselected level does not trigger an increase in ventricular rate. This prevents endless-loop tachycardia and is useful when conduction disturbance is only intermittent, particularly in patients with malignant vasovagal and carotid sinus syndromes (see pp. 5 and 42).

The disadvantage of DDI pacing is that an exertional increase in the atrial rate will not trigger a similar increase in the ventricular rate, but this can be overcome by incorporation of rate responsiveness (DDIR).

### Rate-responsive pacing

DDD pacemakers are rate-responsive if the atrial rhythm is intact and increases normally with exercise. However, they cannot be used in patients with AF or other atrial arrhythmias. Rate-responsive pacemakers are now available which sense a specific physiological response to exertion and then trigger an appropriate increase in either atrial or ventricular rate (or both), depending on the type of unit. The most widely used device senses physical activity from vibration and muscle noise. Others sense minute ventilation, body acceleration, temperature or adrenergic activity, as reflected by the QT interval.

Rate-responsive pacing improves exercise tolerance and patient well-being. The DDD pacemaker comes closest to normal physiology and for most patients with AV block is the rate-responsive device of choice. However, patients with isolated SA disease benefit from AAIR units and patients with AV block in whom the atrium is fibrillating benefit from VVIR units (see above).

## Complications of pacemakers

### Infection

This may be localized to the pacemaker pocket or be more generalized, and is often difficult to eradicate without removing the pacing system; endocarditis is rare. Erosion through the skin of the pulse generator or its connecting electrodes is less common than in the past, when devices were much larger.

### Battery failure

This is the usual, and ultimately inevitable, cause of pacemaker failure. In older pacemakers, impending failure was signalled by incremental reductions in the pacing rate, which occurred in a predictable fashion. In modern pacemakers, the rate remains constant and battery depletion is monitored by measurement of battery impedance, using telemetry. Premature battery failure is usually caused by a component failure within the pacemaker that results in an internal short circuit. This is now uncommon, however, because quality control has reduced the rate of premature failure to less than 1:5000 devices.

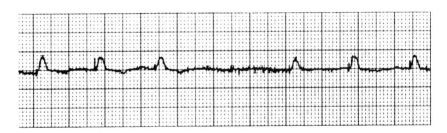

**Fig. 10.15**  Myopotential inhibition. After the third paced complex, random myopotentials caused by increased muscular activity inhibit the pacemaker, producing a prolonged pause on the ECG. As the myopotentials decrease, normal pacemaker function becomes re-established.

### Pacing electrode

Problems with the sensing device are seen occasionally. Undersensing, in which the pacemaker fails to sense spontaneous cardiac activity, leads to inappropriate pacing. The competition between spontaneous and paced beats causes uncomfortable palpitations and may be dangerous if ventricular arrhythmias are triggered (see Fig. 5.19). Oversensing, when electrical noise is sensed and pacing is inappropriately inhibited, can cause syncopal attacks. A special form of oversensing may occur during vigorous exertion in patients with unipolar systems (see p. 220), when pectoral muscle myopotentials inhibit the pacemaker (Fig. 10.15). Similarly, inappropriate stimulation of the pectoral muscles may cause troublesome twitching. However, these problems have largely disappeared with the use of bipolar pacemakers, in which the electrical circuit is confined to the terminal portion of the pacing wire, far removed from the pectoral muscles.

Displacement of the pacing electrode can occur early after implantation, but this is now rare because active fixation electrodes secure the tip of the wire against the endocardium. Myocardial perforation has also become a rare complication since the introduction of modern flexible electrodes. Fracture of the pacing catheter is an occasional cause of premature pacemaker failure.

### Exit block

The pacing threshold (voltage output necessary to initiate depolarization) normally shows a small rise early after implantation, but in some patients the rise is exaggerated, leading to loss of capture. This is called exit block and is the result of fibrous infiltration into the tip of the electrode, a problem that has become less common with improvements in materials used in tip manufacture.

**Other complications**

Thrombosis affecting the subclavian vein or superior vena cava is occasionally troublesome, although thromboembolism is unusual. Other complications, such as pacemaker syndrome and endless-loop tachycardia, have been described above.

## Pacemaker follow-up

Pacemaker patients should be seen every 6 months for clinical assessment. Careful analysis of the ECG and manipulation of settings, using the programmer, permit accurate diagnosis and correction of most pacemaker problems and malfunctions. At each visit, the pacing threshold should be checked and the voltage output programmed down to the lowest level compatible with safe pacing, in order to prolong battery life. The extent of battery depletion should be monitored by battery impedance measurement (see above); prophylactic replacement of the pulse generator is recommended when 1 year's life remains. Patients require hospital admission (often as a day case) for the replacement procedure, at which the old generator is removed and the new one attached to the existing pacing electrodes.

## Prognosis

First-degree block poses no direct threat to the patient and prognosis relates to the aetiology of the underlying conduction tissue disorder. Nevertheless, the ECG and 24-hour Holter recordings should be monitored at regular intervals because progression to higher degrees of AV block is not uncommon. Isolated bundle branch block also poses no threat, although when right bundle branch block is associated with left axis deviation and prolongation of the PR interval (trifascicular block) the risk of progression to complete AV block is particularly high and prophylactic pacing is often recommended. Wenckebach AV block is benign in most cases, occurring in some normal individuals, and pacing is not usually necessary. In Mobitz type II and third-degree AV block, the risk of prolonged asystole and sudden death demands pacing, even if block is transient, unless the conduction disturbance is clearly a temporary response to drug therapy or acute myocardial infarction. Following pacemaker insertion, the risk of asystole and sudden death is removed and prognosis relates to the aetiology of the underlying conduction tissue disorder. In idiopathic fibrosis of the conduction system, for example, prognosis is excellent but in ischaemic heart-disease it is much worse.

## Further reading

Furman S. Rate-modulated pacing. *Circulation* 1990, **82**, 1081–94.

Nathan A.W. and Davies D.W. Is VVI pacing outmoded? *Br. Heart J.* 1992, **67**, 205–8.

Working Party of the British Pacing and Electrophysiology Group. Recommendations for pacemaker prescription for symptomatic bradycardia. *Br. Heart J.* 1991, **66**, 185–91.

# 11 Cardiac Arrhythmias

## Summary

Cardiac arrhythmias (atrial, junctional or ventricular) are usually caused by a re-entry mechanism, less commonly by enhanced automaticity. Symptoms (palpitations, angina, dyspnoea and syncope) are determined less by the origin of the arrhythmia, more by the ventricular rate and the presence and severity of underlying heart-disease. Atrial arrhythmias and most junctional arrhythmias are conducted by the atrioventricular (AV) node, producing a narrow, morphologically normal, QRS complex. Occasionally, rate-related (or pre-existing) bundle branch block produces a broad-complex tachycardia, difficult to distinguish from ventricular tachycardia (VT). Nevertheless, differential diagnosis is nearly always possible from scrutiny of the electrocardiogram (ECG).

*Atrial arrhythmias* Atrial premature beats have an early bizarre P wave, usually followed by a normal QRS complex. In atrial fibrillation (AF), P waves are replaced by irregular fibrillatory waves (rate 400–600/min), only a proportion of which are conducted, to produce an irregular ventricular rate of 130–200 beats/min. Atrial flutter produces sawtooth flutter waves (rate 300 beats/min), which are usually conducted with 2:1 block, to give a ventricular rate of 150 beats/min.

*Junctional arrhythmias* These re-entrant arrhythmias are caused either by an abnormal atrionodal pathway or an accessory AV pathway. Atrionodal pathways are the substrate for AV junctional re-entrant tachycardias (AVJRT, rate 140–250 beats/min). The accessory AV pathway in the Wolff–Parkinson–White (WPW) syndrome pre-excites the ventricles during sinus rhythm, producing a short PR interval and slurring of the initial QRS deflexion (delta wave). It provides the substrate for re-entrant tachycardias, which are usually orthodromic (conduction anterogradely by the AV node, retrogradely by the accessory pathway) with a narrow QRS complex. Occasionally, the re-entrant circuit is in the opposite direction (antidromic), causing pre-excitation with a broad-complex tachycardia. AF may be dangerous if the accessory pathway permits rapid conduction of the fibrillatory impulses, resulting in an uncontrolled ventricular response (over 300 beats/min), which may degenerate into ventricular fibrillation (VF).

*Ventricular arrhythmias* Ventricular premature beats produce an early, broad QRS complex and are usually benign in themselves, requiring no treatment. VT, on the other hand, often indicates important heart-disease and requires urgent treatment. In the differential diagnosis of broad-complex tachycardias, ECG findings suggesting VT include a very broad QRS (>140 ms), extreme axis deviation, evidence of AV dissociation (P waves 'marching through' the tachycardia), capture or fusion beats, concordant QRS deflexions in V1–V6, and an RSr' complex in V1 or a QS complex in V6. VF, characterized by irregular fibrillatory waves with no discernible QRS complexes, demands immediate direct-current (DC) cardioversion or death is inevitable.

*Treatment* Primary aims are termination of sustained arrhythmias and prevention of paroxysmal arrhythmias; in refractory atrial arrhythmias, treatment is often aimed at controlling the ventricular rate. An empirical approach is satisfactory for benign atrial or junctional arrhythmias: AV nodal blockers (digoxin, beta-blockers, verapamil) for rate control in AF, intravenous (IV) verapamil or adenosine for terminating AVJRT or orthodromic tachycardia in WPW syndrome, and drugs from Vaughan Williams classes IA (disopyramide), IC (flecainide) or III (amiodarone) for termination and prevention of most other supraventricular arrhythmias. For ventricular arrhythmias, class IB drugs (lignocaine, mexiletine) are also effective, but in VT (or the dangerous variant of WPW syndrome) there is no role for empirical measures, and the efficacy of treatment must be confirmed by provocative testing. Non-pharmacological antiarrhythmic therapy is playing an increasing role. Antitachycardia pacing terminates most re-entrant arrhythmias acutely, but catheter ablation of accessory AV or atrionodal pathways and arrhythmogenic foci in the atria or ventricles provides a better long-term solution. Where this fails, surgical treatment is often successful. DC shock remains treatment of choice for terminating life-threatening arrhythmias; implantable defibrillators are now available for patients with refractory VT or VF not amenable to catheter ablation or arrhythmia surgery.

## Introduction

Cardiac arrhythmias may originate anywhere in the atrial, junctional or ventricular conduction tissue, requiring only a pathological substrate and a trigger mechanism. Cardiac causes include congenital abnormalities, such as accessory AV pathways in patients with junctional arrhythmias, and organic disease, particularly ischaemia and cardiomyopathy. Arrhythmias may also be caused by a variety of non-cardiac disorders, including metabolic disorders, electrolyte imbalance and drug toxicity.

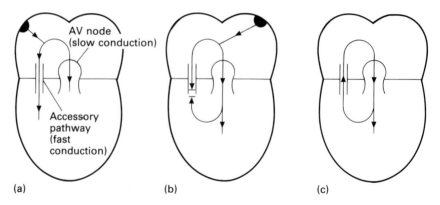

Fig. 11.1 A re-entrant circuit. See text for discussion.

## Pathophysiology

Major mechanisms responsible for most tachyarrhythmias are re-entry and enhanced automaticity.

### Re-entry (Fig. 11.1)

Re-entry may occur within the atria or the ventricles, or may involve the AV junction via an accessory pathway. The substrate is provided by two or more non-homogeneous conduction pathways with different electrical characteristics. The trigger is usually provided by a premature beat, which causes transient unidirectional block in one of the pathways. A typical re-entry circuit is seen in the Wolff–Parkinson–White (WPW) syndrome, involving the AV node (slow conductor) and an accessory AV pathway (fast conductor). The sinus impulse is conducted slowly through the AV node but more rapidly through the accessory pathway, pre-exciting the ventricles (Fig. 11.1a). An atrial premature beat, however, may find the accessory pathway refractory, particularly if it occurs very early after the previous sinus beat (Fig. 11.1b). Thus the premature beat is conducted slowly by the AV node into the His–Purkinje system, depolarizing the ventricles without pre-excitation. By this time, the accessory pathway has recovered and can conduct the impulse retrogradely into the atria, thereby completing the circuit and initiating self-sustaining re-entry arrhythmia (Fig. 11.1c). The anatomical distribution of the re-entry circuit is large in the WPW syndrome, but when re-entry occurs in the atria or ventricles it is much smaller, often consisting of only a few myocardial cells, which together constitute a microcircuit with slow and fast conducting limbs.

### Enhanced automaticity

Automaticity (or spontaneous depolarization) is a property common to all the specialized conducting tissues. The automatic discharge of the sinus node normally proceeds at a faster rate than the remainder of the conducting tissues, which remain suppressed. Nevertheless, a variety of stimuli, including ischaemia, drug toxicity and trauma, can enhance the automaticity of an ectopic focus within the atria or ventricles, allowing it to depolarize more rapidly than the sinus node. This produces a premature beat. Repeated automatic discharge at a rate in excess of the sinus node results in sustained atrial or ventricular tachyarrhythmias.

## Clinical manifestations

Tachyarrhythmias may be entirely asymptomatic. Symptoms, when they do occur, are determined by the ventricular rate and also by the presence and severity of underlying heart-disease.

Palpitations are the most common symptom caused by tachyarrhythmias. They are usually regular and, in patients with paroxysmal attacks, start and terminate abruptly. Irregular palpitations occur in atrial fibrillation and also in patients with ectopic beats, due to the compensatory pauses or the forceful beats that follow.

Angina may occur if the rapid ventricular rate causes oxygen demand to exceed supply and, although troublesome in patients with coronary artery disease, may also occur in the presence of normal coronary arteries.

Dyspnoea, due to heart failure, commonly occurs in patients with rapid tachyarrhythmias, particularly when there is associated left ventricular or valvular disease. Arrhythmias are an important treatable cause of heart failure.

Syncopal episodes (Stokes–Adams attacks) occur when paroxysmal tachyarrhythmias produce abrupt reductions in cardiac output, associated with cerebral hypoperfusion. Paroxysmal ventricular arrhythmias are usually responsible and, if sustained, may be fatal. Sudden death is an inevitable consequence of sustained ventricular fibrillation (VF).

## Complications

Myocardial ischaemia, heart failure and death are the major complications. Thromboembolism may occur, particularly in patients with atrial fibrillation who are not anticoagulated with aspirin or warfarin.

## Arrhythmia detection (see p. 39)

ECG documentation of the arrhythmia is essential for accurate diagnosis. This may require ambulatory ECG monitoring for paroxysmal arrhythmias, but, in patients presenting with a sustained arrhythmia, a full 12-lead ECG should always be obtained. This is particularly important for patients with broad-complex tachycardias, because it helps determine whether the arrhythmia is atrial or ventricular in origin. Availability of a 12-lead ECG also helps interpret the clinical significance of arrhythmias induced during provocative testing. Simple provocative tests, such as exercise testing, have a role in patients with exertional symptoms, but electrophysiological study (EPS) is usually more helpful, particularly for diagnosing junctional and ventricular arrhythmias and assessing responses to therapy. During EPS, premature stimuli are delivered to the atria or ventricles with the aim of stimulating re-entry arrhythmias (AV junctional re-entrant tachycardia, ventricular tachycardia). In the normal heart, sustained arrhythmias of this type cannot usually be provoked. Arrhythmia provocation during programmed stimulation is often diagnostic, particularly when the arrhythmia reproduces symptoms or is morphologically identical to the spontaneous arrhythmia recorded previously. The test can be repeated after administration of antiarrhythmic drugs to assess the efficacy of treatment.

## Atrial arrhythmias

Atrial arrhythmias commonly occur without overt heart-disease. However, they may be associated with a variety of cardiac disorders, including pericardial, rheumatic, coronary and cardiomyopathic disease. Non-cardiac disorders associated with atrial arrhythmias are pulmonary disease, thyrotoxicosis, phaeochromocytoma, hypothermia, hypoxia, acidosis, electrolyte imbalance (notably hypokalaemia and hypomagnesaemia) and toxic stimuli, such as caffeine, alcohol, anaesthetic agents, digoxin and other antiarrhythmic drugs. Patients recovering from major surgery, particularly cardiac procedures, are also susceptible to atrial arrhythmias.

Atrial arrhythmias are conducted by the AV node, and ventricular depolarization, therefore, is by normal His–Purkinje pathways. This usually results in a narrow (morphologically normal) QRS complex. However, rate-related (or pre-existing) bundle branch block produces a broad complex (more than 0.12 sec), which may be difficult to distinguish from ventricular tachycardia (see below). Atrial arrhythmias in the WPW syndrome may also be associated with a broad QRS complex if rapid AV conduction through the accessory pathway pre-excites the ventricles.

Atrial arrhythmias are often asymptomatic and are not usually dangerous. Nevertheless, they may predispose to thromboembolism and, like any arrhythmia, may precipitate heart failure or ischaemia if the rate is very rapid or if there is underlying valvular, myocardial or coronary disease.

## *Atrial premature beats (APBs)* (Fig. 11.2)

These are caused by the premature discharge of an ectopic atrial focus. This produces an early P wave, morphologically distinct from the normal sinus P waves, which is essential for the diagnosis. The premature impulse

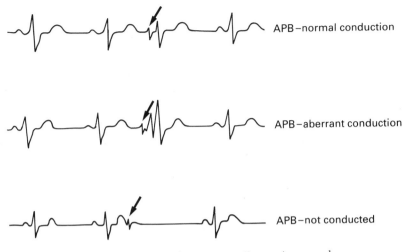

Fig. 11.2  Atrial premature beats. The premature P wave is arrowed.

usually enters and depolarizes the sinus node, such that a partially compensatory pause occurs before the next sinus beat. Because the atrial discharge is premature, the AV node is often partially refractory and conduction is slow, resulting in a prolonged PR interval. If one or other of the bundle branches is also refractory, a broad QRS complex may occur. Very premature beats sometimes find the AV node completely refractory and are blocked, producing a pause on the ECG; this may be misdiagnosed as a sinus pause if the premature P wave is not identified. Atrial premature beats do not usually require treatment unless they cause troublesome palpitations or are responsible for initiating other arrhythmias.

*Prevention*: disopyramide, flecainide, amiodarone.

### *Atrial tachycardia* (Fig. 11.3)

This is a relatively uncommon arrhythmia, although in the past the term 'paroxysmal atrial tachycardia (PAT)' has often been misused to describe AV junctional (nodal) re-entrant tachycardias (see below). Most cases are re-entrant, but it may also be caused by enhanced automaticity, particularly in digoxin toxicity. The atrial rate varies between 120 and 240 beats/min, and with rapid rates there is often variable AV block.

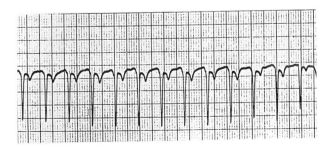

Fig. 11.3  Atrial tachycardia with 1:1 AV conduction.

(a)

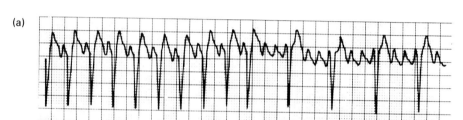

(b)

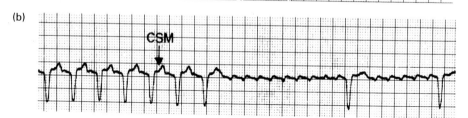

**Fig. 11.4**   Atrial flutter. (a) This shows typical sawtooth flutter waves, initially with 2:1 AV conduction. Later block increases abruptly and conduction becomes 4:1. The flutter rate is a little faster than 300/min. (b) The ventricular rate of this tachycardia is 150, which is highly suggestive of atrial flutter with 2:1 block. Not until AV block is increased by carotid sinus massage (CSM) do the flutter waves become apparent. In this example the flutter rate is just below 300/min.

*Termination*: disopyramide, flecainide, amiodarone; direct-current (DC) cardioversion, antitachycardia pacing.

*Rate control*: digoxin, verapamil or diltiazem, beta-blockers.

*Prevention*: disopyramide, flecainide, amiodarone.

### *Atrial flutter* (Fig. 11.4)

This is a re-entrant arrhythmia with an atrial rate of approximately 300 beats/min. There is usually 2:1 AV block, giving a ventricular rate of 150 beats/min. Higher degrees of block may occur, and some patients show variable block, due to Wenckebach periodicity within the AV node. The ECG characteristically shows a sawtooth flutter wave, which may not be evident in all leads but should be looked for whenever a narrow-complex tachycardia is associated with a ventricular rate of 150. Sometimes block can be increased transiently by vagal manoeuvres (e.g. carotid sinus massage), allowing the flutter waves to become apparent. Atrial flutter may degenerate into atrial fibrillation or develop from it. Anticoagulation to prevent thromboembolic complications is usually recommended but treatment of the arrhythmia is often difficult.

*Termination*: flecainide, disopyramide plus verapamil, amiodarone; DC cardioversion, antitachycardia pacing.

*Rate control*: digoxin, verapamil or diltiazem, beta-blockers; catheter ablation to block AV nodal conduction has a role (see below).

*Prevention*: flecainide, disopyramide, amiodarone, beta-blockers.

### *Atrial fibrillation (AF)* (see Figs 1.4 and 9.4)

In AF, atrial activity is chaotic and mechanically ineffective. P waves are therefore absent and are replaced by irregular fibrillatory waves (rate 400 to 600/min). Only a proportion of the atrial impulses are conducted through the slowly conducting AV node, to produce an irregular ventricular rate of 130–200 beats/min. In the presence of a rapidly conducting accessory pathway in the WPW syndrome, ventricular rates of more than 300 beats/min may occur. Anticoagulation is indicated in most patients with AF, whether chronic or paroxysmal, to prevent embolic complications. Aspirin is a reasonable alternative, especially in the younger patient without organic heart-disease.

*Termination*: flecainide, disopyramide plus verapamil, amiodarone; DC cardioversion.

*Rate control*: digoxin, verapamil or diltiazem, beta-blockers; catheter ablation to block AV nodal conduction in refractory cases.

*Prevention*: flecainide, disopyramide, amiodarone, beta-blockers.

### *Multifocal atrial tachycardia* (Fig. 11.5)

This is not uncommon in the elderly, and can be caused by chest infection or digitalis toxicity. Competing atrial–ectopic foci result in a rapid and somewhat irregular rhythm, with multiform P waves, usually associated with narrow QRS complexes. Correction of the arrhythmia is often difficult, and treatment should be directed at the underlying cause.

### Junctional arrhythmias

These are the commonest supraventricular tachycardias (SVTs) and are usually paroxysmal, without obvious cardiac or extrinsic causes. They are re-entrant arrhythmias, caused either by an abnormal pathway between the atrium and the AV node (atrionodal pathway) or by an accessory AV pathway (bundle of Kent), as seen in WPW syndrome.

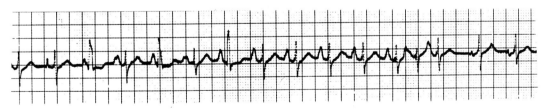

**Fig. 11.5** Multifocal atrial tachycardia. The arrhythmia is somewhat irregular, but each QRS complex is preceded by a P wave. P wave morphology, however, is very variable and a least four different configurations are apparent in this example.

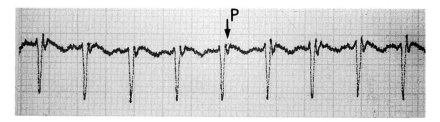

**Fig. 11.6**  AV junctional re-entrant tachycardia (AVJRT). Note the very early retrograde P wave (arrowed).

## AV junctional (nodal) re-entrant tachycardia (AVJRT)
(Fig. 11.6)

The substrate for this arrhythmia is a slow atrionodal pathway, not dual AV nodal pathways as previously thought. This abnormal pathway provides the basis for a small re-entrant circuit (see p. 230). In sinus rhythm, the ECG is usually normal, although occasionally there is a short PR interval, which, in association with AVJRT, is called the Lown–Ganong–Levine (LGL) syndrome. During tachycardia, the heart rate is 140 to 250 beats/min. P waves are usually very early after the QRS complexes in 1:1 ratio but are not always visible; rarely AV or VA block alters the ratio. Because AV conduction is by normal His–Purkinje pathways, QRS morphology is typically normal, though, like atrial arrhythmias, rate-related (or pre-existing) bundle branch block produces a broad complex, which may be difficult to distinguish from ventricular tachycardia (see below).

*Termination*: vagal manoeuvres, verapamil or adenosine (by rapid IV injection); antitachycardia pacing, DC cardioversion.

*Prevention*: flecainide, disopyramide, verapamil, beta-blockers, amiodarone; catheter ablation or surgery to destroy the slow atrionodal pathway.

## Wolff–Parkinson–White (WPW) syndrome

WPW syndrome is common, affecting approximately 0.12% of the population. It is a congenital disorder in which there is an accessory pathway (bundle of Kent) between the atria and ventricles (Fig. 11.7). During sinus rhythm, atrial impulses conduct more rapidly through the accessory pathway than the AV node. Thus, the initial phase of ventricular depolarization occurs early through the accessory pathway (pre-excitation) and spreads slowly through the myocardium (Fig. 11.8). The PR interval is therefore short and the initial deflection of the QRS complex is slurred, producing a 'delta wave'. The remainder of ventricular depolarization, however, is rapid, because the delayed arrival of the impulse conducted through the AV node completes ventricular depolarization by normal His–Purkinje

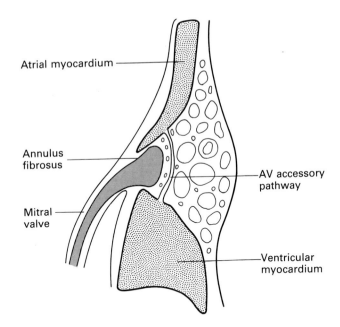

**Fig. 11.7**  Wolff–Parkinson–White syndrome — the AV accessory pathway (in longitudinal section) connecting the atrium and ventricle.

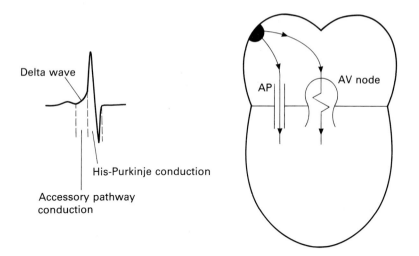

**Fig. 11.8**  Wolff–Parkinson–White syndrome — ECG abnormalities caused by pre-excitation. AP — accessory pathway.

pathways. The vector of the delta wave on the 12-lead ECG (Fig. 11.9) indicates the approximate location of the accessory pathway within the heart, but this is of practical importance only for the surgeon or cardiologist who is operating upon or ablating the pathway.

Cardiac tachyarrhythmias affect about 60% of patients with WPW syndrome and are usually re-entrant (rate 140–250 beats/min), triggered by a premature beat. In most patients, the re-entrant tachycardias are

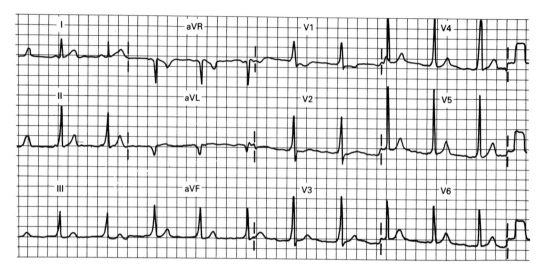

**Fig. 11.9**   Wolff–Parkinson–White syndrome — 12-lead ECG. Note the short PR interval. A positive delta wave is clearly visible, particularly in the inferior leads (II, III and aVF). The patient has Wolff–Parkinson–White syndrome type A with a left lateral accessory pathway.

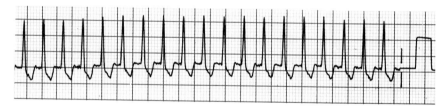

**Fig. 11.10**   Wolff–Parkinson–White syndrome — AV orthodromic re-entrant tachycardia. This is morphologically indistinguishable from AVJRT (see Fig. 11.6).

orthodromic, with anterograde conduction through the AV node and retrograde conduction through the accessory pathway. Because anterograde conduction is through the AV node, the QRS complexes are narrow, without pre-excitation, unless there is rate-related (or pre-existing) bundle branch block (Fig. 11.10). Occasionally the re-entrant circuit is in the opposite direction (antidromic), causing a very broad, pre-excited, tachycardia.

*Termination*: Vagal manoeuvres, verapamil or adenosine (by rapid IV injection); antitachycardia pacing, DC cardioversion.

*Prevention*: flecainide, disopyramide, verapamil, amiodarone, beta-blockers; catheter ablation or surgery to destroy the accessory pathway.

### Atrial fibrillation in WPW syndrome

Patients with the WPW syndrome are more prone to AF than the general population. This is of little consequence if the accessory pathway is

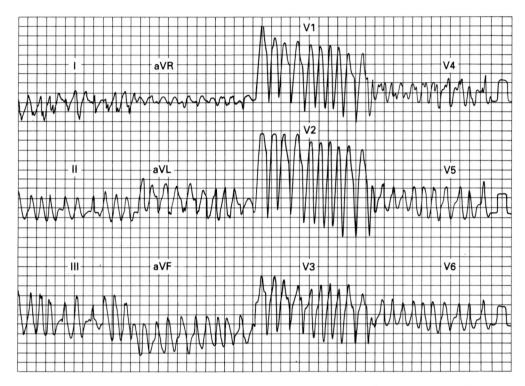

**Fig. 11.11** Wolff–Parkinson–White syndrome — 12-lead ECG showing rapid pre-excited AF. This patient is at risk of sudden death if not adequately treated.

incapable of rapid conduction. In a minority of patients, however, the fibrillatory impulses are conducted very rapidly through the accessory pathway, producing an uncontrolled ventricular response, with a rate of more than 300 beats/min (Fig. 11.11). This may degenerate into VF, resulting in sudden death.

*Termination*: IV flecainide, disopyramide, amiodarone; DC cardioversion.

*Prevention*: flecainide, disopyramide, amiodarone, beta-blockers; catheter ablation of accessory pathway (digoxin is contraindicated because it enhances conduction in the accessory pathway).

## *Concealed accessory pathways*

In some patients with accessory pathways, anterograde conduction through the pathway cannot occur. Thus, in sinus rhythm, impulses are conducted normally by the AV node, resulting in a narrow QRS complex without pre-excitation. The ECG, therefore, is normal and the accessory pathway concealed. However, the pathway can conduct retrogradely, providing the substrate for orthodromic re-entrant tachycardia. Clearly, AF poses no threat to the patient because the pathway will not conduct anterogradely. Treatment is the same as in the WPW syndrome.

**Table 11.1**  Substrates for ventricular arrhythmias

Myocardial infarction (acute or chronic)
Dilated cardiomyopathies
Hypertrophic cardiomyopathy
Other cardiomyopathies
Valvular heart-disease (especially mitral prolapse and aortic stenosis)
Hypertensive heart-disease
Congenital heart-disease
Long QT syndrome
Cardiac tumours
Various metabolic disorders
Anitarrhythmic drugs

## Ventricular arrhythmias

Ventricular arrhythmias, particularly ectopic beats, may be benign and occur without overt heart-disease. They are commonly triggered by toxic stimuli, such as caffeine or sympathomimetic drugs. Nevertheless, ventricular arrhythmias may also reflect important underlying heart-disease (Table 11.1) and are an important cause of sudden death.

Because of their origin in the ventricular myocardium, depolarization is by abnormal pathways, producing a broad QRS complex, usually more than 0.12 sec in duration. Retrograde VA conduction may result in a P wave early after the QRS complex, but penetration of the sinus node is unusual and for this reason ventricular ectopic beats are usually followed by a fully compensatory pause before the next sinus beat. In ventricular tachycardia, however, retrograde VA conduction does not usually occur, and this results in dissociated atrial and ventricular rhythms, in which the atrial rhythm continues uninterrupted, though at a slower rate than the ventricular tachycardia, producing cannon 'a' waves in the jugular venous pulse (JVP) (see p. 16).

### *Ventricular premature beats (VPBs)* (see Fig. 6.4)

These are caused by the premature discharge of a ventricular ectopic focus, which produces an early, broad QRS complex. There is usually a fully compensatory pause before the next sinus beat. Treatment is not indicated on prognostic grounds, and indeed may unpredictably produce more serious arrhythmias. If symptoms are intolerable (which is rare), class I or III antiarrhythmic drugs can be used, cautiously.

### *Accelerated ventricular rhythm* (see Fig. 5.17)

This usually occurs as a complication of myocardial infarction (MI) and is discussed in Chapter 5.

## *Ventricular tachycardia (VT)*

This is defined as three or more consecutive ventricular beats at a rate above 100/min. It usually reflects important underlying heart-disease but may occur in an apparently normal heart. VT is usually regular and monomorphic (constant QRS morphology), except when it complicates acute MI, when it is commonly irregular and polymorphic (variable QRS morphology). The tachycardia originates from a single ventricular site and depolarization of the ventricular myocardium is by slow, muscle-to-muscle conduction, resulting in a broad-complex tachycardia. This distinguishes it from most supraventricular tachycardias, in which the QRS complexes are narrow. However, differential diagnosis may be more difficult for supraventricular tachycardia with a broad complex due to rate-related (or pre-existing) bundle branch block. Symptoms are unhelpful because they depend on heart rate and underlying ventricular function, not the origin of the tachycardia. Clinical circumstance may provide a guide: early after myocardial infarction, for example, broad-complex tachycardia is more likely to be ventricular in origin. In most cases, however, the differential diagnosis of broad-complex tachycardias depends on careful scrutiny of the ECG (Fig. 11.12). Findings that support a diagnosis of VT include:

**1**  Very broad QRS complex (more than 140 ms).

**2**  Extreme left or right axis deviation.

**3**  AV dissociation evidenced by P waves, at a slower rate than the QRS complexes, 'marching through' the tachycardia (Fig. 11.13).

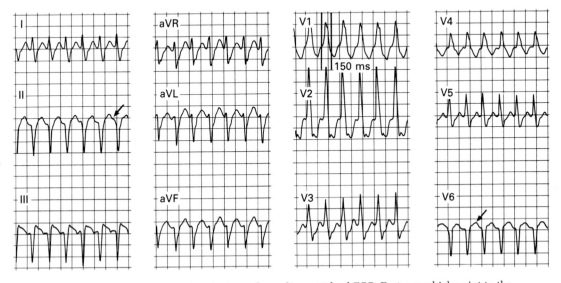

**Fig. 11.12**  Ventricular tachycardia — 12-lead ECG. Features which point to the ventricular origin of this tachycardia include the very broad QRS complex (150 ms) with an indeterminate axis, dissociated P waves (arrowed), an RSr′ complex in V1 and a QS complex in V6.

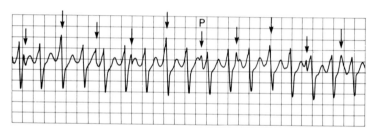

**Fig. 11.13**  Ventricular tachycardia — AV dissociation. The independent P waves are arrowed marching through the tachycardia.

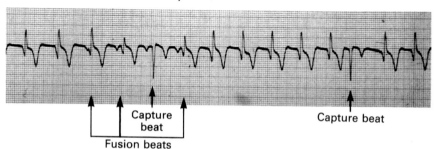

**Fig. 11.14**  Ventricular tachycardia — capture and fusion beats. The panel on the left shows the patient in sinus rhythm. The panel on the right shows VT: after the first two complexes, two fusion beats followed by a capture beat (normal QRS morphology) are seen. Another capture beat is seen towards the end of the strip.

**4**  Ventricular capture and/or fusion beats, in which the dissociated atrial rhythm penetrates the ventricle by conduction through the AV node and interrupts the tachycardia, producing either a normal ventricular complex (capture) or a broad hybrid complex (fusion) that is part sinus and part ventricular in origin (Fig. 11.4).

**5**  Concordance of the QRS deflexions in V1 to V6, either all positive or all negative.

**6**  Configurational features of the QRS complex, including an RSr' complex in V1 ('left rabbit ear') and a QS complex in V6 (Fig. 11.12). Comparison with the ECG during sinus rhythm may be helpful.

VT nearly always needs urgent treatment, either with intravenous antiarrhythmic drugs, antitachycardia pacing or, most effectively, DC shock. Prognosis is often poor and, in patients with recurrent attacks, the efficacy of preventive therapy should be confirmed by exercise testing and Holter monitoring. Serial electrophysiological studies may be needed to find an effective drug. Patients refractory to antiarrhythmic drugs should

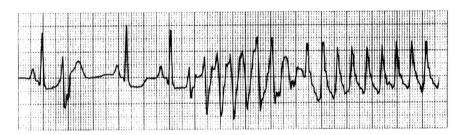

**Fig. 11.15** Long QT syndrome with *torsades de pointes*. The second complex is an early ventricular premature beat interrupting sinus rhythm (note the long QT interval). A second ventricular premature beat triggers a broad complex tachycardia with changing wavefronts (first negative, later positive), confirming the ventricular origin of the tachycardia.

be considered for an implantable cardioverter defibrillator (ICD) or anti-arrhythmic surgery.

*Termination*: IV lignocaine, disopyramide, flecainide, amiodarone; anti-tachycardia pacing, DC cardioversion (external or ICD).

*Prevention*: mexiletine, disopyramide, flecainide, amiodarone; anti-arrhythmic surgery.

### *Long QT syndrome and* torsades de pointes

Abnormalities of ventricular repolarization may produce the long QT syndrome, characterized by an abnormally long QT interval on the ECG. This is inherited as an autosomal dominant trait in the Romano–Ward syndrome and as an autosomal recessive trait in the Lange–Nielsen syndrome (when it is associated with congenital deafness). It may also be caused by drugs (e.g. disopyramide, phenothiazines) and hypokalaemia. Patients with the syndrome are at risk of sudden death due to complex ventricular arrhythmias, particularly *torsades de pointes*, so called because of its changing wavefronts (Fig. 11.15). In the idiopathic forms of long QT syndrome, treatment is aimed at preventing life-threatening arrhythmias with beta-blockers (with or without atrial pacing), or left stellate ganglionectomy in refractory cases. Drug-induced *torsades de pointes* should be treated by drug withdrawal, electrolyte correction, if necessary, and atrial pacing.

### *Ventricular fibrillation (VF)* (Fig. 11.16)

This may be a primary arrhythmia or may degenerate from VT. It is characterized by irregular fibrillatory waves with no discernible QRS complexes. There is no cardiac output and death is inevitable unless resuscitation is instituted rapidly. VF in the first 24–48 hours after acute

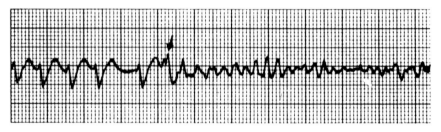

**Fig. 11.16** Ventricular fibrillation. The first five complexes are atrial fibrillation, but a very early ventricular premature beat (arrowed) triggers ventricular fibrillation.

MI does not usually warrant long-term prophylactic therapy after resuscitation, but in all other circumstances the risk of recurrence is high and therapy should be instituted as for VT.

*Termination*: DC cardioversion (external or ICD).

*Prevention*: mexiletine, disopyramide, flecainide, amiodarone; antiarrhythmic surgery.

## Treatment

The aims of treatment are to correct symptoms and also to improve prognosis in those patients at risk of major morbidity or sudden death. These aims are usually met by preventing paroxysmal arrhythmias and terminating sustained arrhythmias, although, in patients with refractory atrial arrhythmias (particularly AF), treatment must be directed at controlling the rate of the ventricular response and reducing the risk of thromboembolism. ECG documentation of the arrhythmia is essential before starting treatment. In the patient with a relatively benign atrial or junctional arrhythmia, treatment is usually chosen empirically, with more sophisticated testing reserved for cases refractory to this approach. However, in the patient with a dangerous WPW syndrome or VT, there is no role for empirical measures, and treatment must be guided by appropriate tests to confirm its efficacy. This will usually involve provocative testing to ensure effective suppression of the arrhythmia. In all cases, other cardiac or non-cardiac disorders must be treated, particularly myocardial ischaemia, heart failure, metabolic and electrolyte disturbance and drug intoxication.

## *Antiarrhythmic drugs*

Table 11.2 shows the Vaughan Williams classification of antiarrhythmic drugs. All these drugs, however, may themselves exacerbate cardiac arrhythmias, due to pro-arrhythmic side-effects. Thus, a cautious and rational approach to treatment should be adopted. ECG documentation of the

**Table 11.2**  The Vaughan Williams classification of antiarrhythmic drugs

| Vaughan Williams classification | IV bolus dose | Chronic oral therapy — daily dose (mg) | Therapeutic plasma level (mg/litre) |
|---|---|---|---|
| *Class IA* | | | |
| Disopyramide | 2 mg/kg | 400–600 | 2–5 |
| Procainamide | Up to 1000 mg | 3000–4500 | 4–8 |
| Quinidine | N/A | 500–1000 | 3–6 |
| *Class IB* | | | |
| Lignocaine | 2 mg/kg | N/A | 2–5 |
| Mexiletine | 2 mg/kg | 400–720 | 0.6–2 |
| *Class IC* | | | |
| Flecainide | 2 mg/kg | 200 | 0.2–0.8 |
| Propafenone | N/A | 450–900 | — |
| *Class II* | | | |
| Metoprolol | 5 mg | 50–200 | |
| Propranolol | 1–10 mg | 40–320 | 0.05–0.1 |
| *Class III* | | | |
| Amiodarone | 300 mg | 100–400 | 1–2 |
| Sotalol | 0.4–1 mg/kg | 80–480 | — |
| *Class IV* | | | |
| Diltiazem | N/A | 180–360 | — |
| Verapamil | 0.15 mg/kg | 120–360 | 0.1–0.2 |

arrhythmia is essential before starting treatment. Because the therapeutic range for most drugs is very narrow, regular measurements of plasma concentrations should, if possible, be obtained, particularly during early treatment, and, if the arrhythmia persists despite therapeutic levels, an alternative drug from a different class should be substituted. A partial response might justify the addition of a second agent, but combination regimens of this type should, if possible, be avoided because of the risk of drug interactions and exaggerated side-effects. Class III and class IA drugs, for example, both prolong the QT interval and their combination can induce the long QT syndrome, which is associated with severe ventricular arrhythmias. Class II and class IV agents both slow conduction through the AV node. The combination is generally safe if the drugs are given orally but intravenous use of one with concomitant use of the other must be avoided, because of the risk of complete heart block and asystole.

## Class I drugs

These are the local anaesthetic or sodium-blocking drugs and they slow phase 0 of the action potential (see p. 27). Effects on repolarization are variable and provide the basis for a subclassification into groups A, B and

C, which prolong, shorten and have little effect on the QT interval, respectively.

Class IA drugs are effective against atrial and ventricular arrhythmias. Quinidine is the prototype but is not often used because of well-documented pro-arrhythmic and gastrointestinal side-effects. Disopyramide is effective against atrial and ventricular arrhythmias but is moderately pro-arrhythmic and has marked negative inotropic properties, demanding caution in patients with heart failure. Anticholinergic side-effects include blurred vision, dry mouth and urinary retention. Procainamide is less negatively inotropic but is also pro-arrhythmic and can cause the lupus syndrome with long-term use.

Lignocaine and mexiletine are the most widely used class IB drugs, mainly useful against ventricular arrhythmias. Lignocaine has its major role in the treatment of ventricular arrhythmias complicating acute myocardial infarction, but is not very effective in other circumstances. Intravenous administration is always necessary because of first-pass metabolism in the liver. Major side-effects include bradycardia, hypotension, drowsiness and convulsions, particularly if the drug is administered too rapidly. Negative inotropic effects are minimal. Mexiletine is in all respects similar but can be given orally. Gastrointestinal side-effects, especially nausea, may be troublesome.

Flecainide and propafenone are potent class IC agents, useful for atrial, junctional and ventricular arrhythmias. Both are moderately negatively inotropic but are well tolerated, although therapeutic margins are narrow. Pro-arrhythmic effects are well documented.

## Class II drugs

These are the beta-blockers, which protect the heart against excessive adrenergic stimulation. They are useful in combination with digoxin for controlling the ventricular rate in AF, but their antiarrhythmic effects are generally weak except in thyrotoxicosis. They are occasionally useful in junctional arrhythmias, although large doses are necessary, which are often not tolerated. They also have a special role for long-term therapy after myocardial infarction, when they increase the fibrillation threshold and reduce the incidence of arrhythmic death. Propranolol is usually chosen for intravenous use, but for long-term oral use there is little to choose between beta-blockers in terms of their antiarrhythmic efficacy.

## Class III drugs

Amiodarone is the most important drug in this class, although sotalol, a beta-blocker, also has class III activity. Amiodarone prolongs the action potential, increasing the effective refractory period throughout the conduction system. It has unusual pharmacokinetics, with a plasma half-life of 7 to 8 weeks, and it may take several months to achieve steady state. Amiodarone is effective against a wide range of arrhythmias and may be used intravenously, although it is toxic to vascular endothelium and should be given into a central vein. It may be pro-arrhythmic, though not as frequently as class IA or IC drugs, and has only minor negative inotropic effects. Chronic therapy is associated with a variety of side-effects, including photosensitivity rash, skin discoloration, corneal infiltrates, thyrotoxicosis or hypothyroidism, pulmonary infiltrates, hepatic dysfunction, neuropathies, myopathies and encephalitis. For this reason, amiodarone should rarely be used as a first-line agent.

## Class IV drugs

These drugs are calcium antagonists. Verapamil has been the most important drug in this class, although diltiazem is also useful. Selective blockade of the slow calcium channel decreases depolarization and slows conduction through the AV node. Thus class IV drugs have an important role for controlling the ventricular rate in AF, particularly in combination with digoxin. Given intravenously they are useful for terminating junctional arrhythmias, and they can also be used prophylactically, although in WPW they shorten the refractory period of the accessory pathway, increasing the ventricular rate in AF. Verapamil and diltiazem are negatively inotropic and should be used with caution in heart failure.

## Digitalis

Digoxin, the most commonly used cardiac glycoside, defies classification by Vaughan Williams criteria. In addition to its mild positive inotropic properties, the drug slows conduction through the AV node by a direct effect on depolarization and by its vagotonic action. In AF it is the drug of choice for slowing the ventricular rate except in WPW syndrome when it is contraindicated; it is only rarely useful for prophylaxis against paroxysmal attacks. It has almost no other role for the treatment of arrhythmias. Digoxin can be given by slow intravenous infusion for loading purposes, but is most commonly used orally. The therapeutic range is narrow and dose increases may need to be titrated against plasma concentrations. It is excreted by the kidneys, and in patients with renal failure the dose must be reduced. Other factors which increase the risk of digoxin toxicity include old age, hypokalaemia and hypomagnesaemia. Important side-effects are loss of appetite, nausea, vomiting, visual disturbances and bradyarrhythmias. Digoxin may also cause a variety of tachyarrhythmias, by enhancing automaticity. Digoxin therapy produces important ECG changes, including prolongation of the PR interval and sagging of the ST segment, with T-wave inversion. These abnormalities do not necessarily indicate toxicity.

## Adenosine

Adenosine is a newly available drug which, like digoxin, defies classification by Vaughan Williams criteria. Its short half-life of less than 10 sec requires it to be given by very rapid intravenous injection, followed by a large bolus of saline flush. It is a potent AV nodal blocker and a dose of 0.1 or 0.2 mg/kg will nearly always terminate junctional arrhythmias; even if complete AV block occurs, its short half-life ensures almost immediate recovery. Other side-effects (flushing, nausea, hypotension) are similarly evanescent. Thus, adenosine is safe and is particularly useful in the critically ill, haemodynamically compromised patient, although in other situations IV verapamil remains the drug of first choice for terminating junctional arrhythmias.

## Non-pharmacological treatment

### Autonomic manoeuvres

The reflex vagotonic response to carotid sinus massage and the Valsalva manoeuvre slow AV conduction and may terminate junctional re-entrant arrhythmias. These manoeuvres also facilitate the diagnosis of atrial arrhythmias (see Fig. 11.4).

### Antitachycardia pacing

Re-entrant arrhythmias can always be terminated by antitachycardia pacing, using either a temporary pacing catheter or a permanent antitachycardia pacemaker. Carefully timed single or double premature stimuli (Fig. 11.17) or a longer burst of overdrive pacing is usually effective. Occasionally, however, this causes unpredictable and potentially danger-

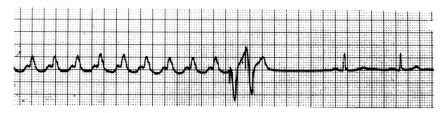

**Fig. 11.17**  Antitachycardia pacing — the broad-complex tachycardia is terminated by two intracardiac stimuli, which break the re-entrant circuit and allow sinus rhythm to become re-established.

ous acceleration of the tachycardia — in the atrium to AF and in the ventricle to rapid VT or VF. Although pacing continues to be used as a temporary measure for termination of re-entrant tachycardias, permanent antitachycardia pacemakers have become virtually redundant in the current era of catheter ablation. They are now rarely used for atrial or junctional arrhythmias but continue to have a role in the treatment of paroxysmal VT, although the risk of VF demands that they are incorporated into an implantable cardioverter defibrillator (see below).

## Catheter ablation

Electrode catheters attached to an energy source may be placed strategically within the heart and used to cause selective damage to the conduction system. DC electrical energy, from a defibrillator, or radiofrequency energy (similar to surgical diathermy) is used most commonly. The technique was used originally for ablation of the AV node in patients with troublesome atrial arrhythmias (particularly paroxysmal or sustained AF) resistant to conventional drug therapy (Fig. 11.18). It results in complete AV block, which prevents conduction of the arrhythmia to the ventricles, thereby abolishing palpitations and other consequences of a rapid ventricular response (see p. 231). Following the procedure, permanent ventricular pacing is required, ideally with a rate-responsive unit (VVIR).

The role of catheter ablation has been extended, however, and it now finds its major application in the management of junctional arrhythmias (Fig. 11.19). Skilled operators, using radiofrequency energy, are able to ablate accessory pathways in virtually any part of the heart. The technique is new but results are excellent and produce complete correction of re-

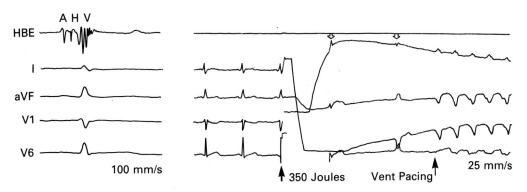

**Fig. 11.18**  Catheter ablation of AV node. The patient, with troublesome paroxysmal AF, was in sinus rhythm at the time of the ablation procedure. The His bundle electrogram is seen in the His bundle channel (HBE). The His bundle electrode is disconnected and attached to a defibrillator. Following the shock, successful ablation is achieved, resulting in complete AV heart block with ventricular pacing.

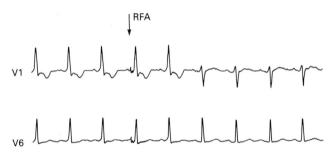

Fig. 11.19  Catheter ablation of accessory pathway in Wolff–Parkinson–White syndrome. The patient, with obvious pre-excitation (note the delta wave), undergoes radiofrequency ablation of the pathway after the third beat (RFA). After a further two beats the accessory pathway is successfully destroyed and pre-excitation is lost, never to return.

entrant tachycardias in patients with atrial–nodal pathways and WPW syndrome.

## Arrhythmia surgery

This was once restricted to the induction of complete AV block in patients with intractable atrial arrhythmias, but catheter ablation has now rendered the procedure obsolete. Current indications for arrhythmia surgery are the WPW syndrome and life-threatening, drug-refractory, ventricular arrhythmias. Surgery in WPW syndrome is reserved for patients in whom catheter ablation has failed. It involves close collaboration between the cardiologist, who maps the position of the accessory pathway, and the cardiac surgeon, who either resects it or destroys it with a cryoprobe. Surgery for ventricular arrhythmias also requires peroperative mapping of the arrhythmogenic focus prior to its resection. Most ventricular arrhythmias originate from the endocardial surface, and limited endocardial resection, leaving the rest of the muscle intact, preserves LV function and prevents further arrhythmias. The operative mortality is approximately 10–15% and is higher in those with very poor LV function or recent myocardial infarction.

## External direct-current countershock (Fig. 11.20)

Electrode paddles placed against the chest wall permit the delivery of a high-energy DC shock across the heart. Anaesthesia is necessary if the patient is conscious. This technique corrects the majority of acute-onset

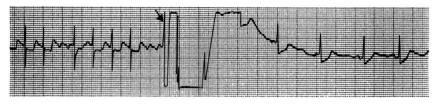

Fig. 11.20  External DC countershock. Atrial flutter is terminated by a DC shock (arrowed), allowing sinus rhythm to become re-established.

atrial, junctional and ventricular arrhythmias by completely depolarizing the heart and allowing the sinus node to re-establish itself. The rapid, almost instantaneous, response makes DC shock the treatment of choice in emergency cases. The shock is always synchronized with the QRS complex (except in VF), to reduce pro-arrhythmic effects. A low-energy shock (50 joules) will usually terminate atrial tachycardia, flutter, junctional arrhythmias and monomorphic VT. However, higher energy (up to 360 joules) is required for AF, polymorphic or very rapid VT and VF. In patients undergoing elective cardioversion of chronic AF, anticoagulation reduces the risk of thromboembolism. Digoxin does not contraindicate DC shock, but it should not be used in digoxin toxicity (except in emergency) because it may induce asystole or severe ventricular arrhythmias.

### Implantable cardioverter defibrillator (ICD)

This device can detect and treat most sustained ventricular arrhythmias. It is indicated in refractory VT or VF, when ablation or arrhythmia surgery is inappropriate or unsuccessful. Until recently, implantation required a thoracotomy to sew the defibrillator patches directly on to the heart, but defibrillator coil electrodes are now available for transvenous insertion. The defibrillator itself (about the size of a pack of cards) is implanted in the abdomen beneath the rectus muscle. The ICD monitors heart rate and automatically delivers a DC shock when an abrupt rate increase indicates VT or VF (Fig. 11.21). The number of shocks that can be delivered is limited by the battery life of the defibrillator. However, most ICDs now have antitachycardia pacing capability and only use shocks if this fails to terminate VT or if VF occurs.

The ICD is palliative and does not prevent arrhythmias from occurring.

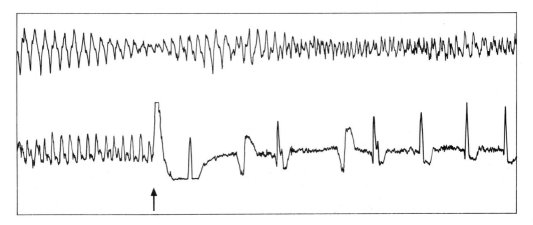

**Fig. 11.21** Implantable cardioverter defibrillator. Ventricular fibrillation is terminated by a DC shock (arrowed) from an ICD.

Nevertheless, it has been shown to improve survival considerably in this high-risk group of patients.

## *Cardiac transplantation*

Some patients with severe ventricular arrhythmias and very poor LV function are best treated by cardiac transplantation.

## Prognosis

Prognosis in patients with cardiac arrhythmias depends on the nature of the arrhythmia and the underlying cause. Atrial arrhythmias are commonly associated with a normal life expectancy, although when caused by ischaemia, mitral valve disease or heart failure the prognosis is less good. Most patients with junctional arrhythmias have a normal prognosis, with the important exception of the Wolff–Parkinson–White syndrome associated with a rapidly conducting accessory pathway, when the risk of sudden death is high unless the patient is adequately treated. Ventricular arrhythmias are more sinister and, although premature beats may occur in normal individuals, more complex arrhythmias are usually associated with severe underlying heart-disease, when the prognosis is poor.

## Cardiac arrest

### *Aetiology*

Cardiac arrest is usually caused by VF or asystole but may also be caused by rapid VT. These arrhythmias are usually the result of severe myocardial ischaemia or infarction but may also complicate hypoxia, electrolyte imbalance and a variety of drug interventions. Autonomic reflexes in response to endotracheal intubation or urethral catheterization occasionally cause cardiac arrest.

### *Clinical manifestations*

In cardiac arrest, there is no effective cardiac output. The diagnosis is made clinically by loss of the arterial pulse followed rapidly by unconsciousness, apnoea and dilatation of the pupils. Irreversible brain damage usually occurs if the circulation is not re-established within 3–4 min, though factors such as hypothermia may prolong this time.

### *Treatment*

A firm thump over the sternum occasionally converts ventricular tachycardia or fibrillation to sinus rhythm; if this fails, full cardiopulmonary resuscitation should be instituted. The patient is placed supine on a firm surface with the neck extended. The airway must be cleared, and positive-pressure ventilation and external cardiac massage can then be started. These should be continued uninterrupted until adequate spontaneous circulatory and respiratory function are restored. All drugs during resuscitation should be given into a central vein, but if this is impossible double doses of adrenaline, lignocaine and atropine can be given by the endotracheal tube. Acidosis commonly develops in a prolonged resuscitation and may be corrected by IV sodium bicarbonate (50 ml of an 8.4% solution), though ideally requirements should be titrated against arterial gas analysis.

## Positive-pressure ventilation

The lungs should be inflated about 12 times/min. Adequate oxygenation of the blood can usually be achieved by hand ventilation, using a face mask, or by mouth-to-mouth techniques. Endotracheal intubation, however, should not be delayed, because this not only improves alveolar ventilation but also protects the airway against regurgitated gastric contents.

## External cardiac massage

This is applied by sharp compression of the lower end of the sternum about 60 times/min. As soon as possible, the patient should be attached to an ECG monitor in order to determine the cardiac rhythm. Further management is directed at restoring an effective spontaneous cardiac output.

## Ventricular fibrillation

This is treated with DC shock, using 200 joules first, which, if unsuccessful, may be repeated once before higher energy (360 joules) is resorted to. Patients resistant to cardioversion should be given adrenaline (1 mg) before trying again, with repeat injections every 5 min as necessary. This produces a coarser fibrillatory pattern, which is often more susceptible to cardioversion. Antiarrhythmic drugs, such as lignocaine (100 mg given slowly intravenously), may make resistant VF more responsive to DC cardioversion.

## Asystole

Successful treatment is difficult. First choice is adrenaline (1 mg), repeated every 5 min as necessary. Patients unresponsive to the first dose of adrenaline should be given atropine 2 mg. If asystole persists, it is always worth trying DC shock. When available, external or transoesophageal pacing may help, or a pacemaker catheter can be introduced into the right ventricle. A paced rhythm can usually be established by these means, but electromechanical dissociation often prevents restoration of effective cardiac output. Calcium chloride (10 ml in 10% solution) should only be used if the patient is hyperkalaemic, hypocalcaemic or known to be on calcium antagonists.

If these measures succeed in restoring spontaneous circulatory function, further management is directed towards the maintenance of a stable cardiac rhythm and oxygenation of the blood. Prophylactic antiarrhythmic drugs are often necessary and many patients require mechanical ventilation.

## *Prognosis*

Following resuscitation, prognosis depends upon the cause of arrest and the resultant ischaemic cerebral damage. Prompt resuscitation prevents neurological sequelae and, in those cases caused by drugs and other toxic insults, life expectancy may be normal. In the majority of cases, however, cardiac arrest reflects severe underlying heart-disease and the prognosis is usually poor. An important exception is primary VF in acute MI, when the prognosis following resuscitation is only a little worse than for other survivors.

## Further reading

Akhtar M. Clinical spectrum of ventricular tachycardia. *Circulation* 1990, **82**, 1561–73.

Cairns J.A. and Connolly S.J. Nonrheumatic atrial fibrillation: risk of stroke and role of antithrombotic therapy. *Circulation* 1991, **84**, 469–81.

Camm A.J. and Garratt C.J. Drug therapy: adenosine and supraventricular tachycardia. *N. Engl. J. Med.* 1991, **325**, 1621–9.

Castellanos A. and Myerburg R.J. Changing perspectives in the preexcitation syndrome. *N. Engl. J. Med.* 1987, **317**, 109–11.

Chesebro J.H., Fuster V. and Halperin J.L. Atrial fibrillation — risk marker for stroke. *N. Engl. J. Med.* 1990, **323**, 1556–8.

Cunningham D. and Rowland E. Endocavitary ablation of atrioventricular conduction. *Br. Heart J.* 1990, **64**, 231–3.

Garratt C., Ward D.E. and Camm A.J. Lessons from the cardiac arrhythmia suppression trial. *Br. Med. J.* 1989, **299**, 805–6.

Horowitz L.N. Proarrhythmia: taking the bad with the good. *N. Engl. J. Med.* 1988, **319**, 304–5.

Kastor J.A. Multifocal atrial tachycardia. *N. Engl. J. Med.* 1990, **322**, 1713–17.

Kim S.G. Management of survivors of cardiac arrest: is electrophysiologic testing obsolete in the era of the implantable defibrillator? *J. Am. Coll. Cardiol.* 1990, **16**, 756–62.

Klein L.S., Miles W.M. and Zipes D. Antitachycardia devices: realities and promises. *J. Am. Coll. Cardiol.* 1991, **18**, 1349–62.

Mason J.W. Drug therapy: amiodarone. *N. Engl. J. Med.* 1987, **316**, 455–65.

Plum F. Vulnerability of the brain and heart after cardiac arrest. *N. Engl. J. Med.* 1991, **324**, 1278–80.

Resuscitation Council (UK). Guidelines for cardiopulmonary resuscitation. *Br. Med. J.* 1989, **299**, 442–7.

Rosenthal M.E. and Josephson M.E. Current status of antitachycardia devices. *Circulation* 1990, **82**, 1889–99.

Ruskin J. Catheter ablation for SVT. *N. Engl. J. Med.* 1991, **324**, 1660–2.

Ruskin J.N. Primary ventricular fibrillation. *N. Engl. J. Med.* 1987, **317**, 307–9.

# 12 Hypertension

## Summary

Hypertension, defined as abnormal elevation of the blood-pressure, is nearly always the result of increased peripheral vascular resistance. It is an important and potentially treatable cause of cardiovascular disease and death. In about 10% of cases, hypertension is secondary to renal or endocrine disorders, but in the remainder the aetiology is unknown (*essential hypertension*), although evidence points to a complex interaction of hereditary and environmental factors. The hypertensive patient is usually asymptomatic, but examination may reveal a fourth heart sound, reflecting left ventricular (LV) hypertrophy, and signs of hypertensive retinopathy. The major complications are heart-disease (coronary atheroma and left ventricular failure (LVF)), stroke and renal failure. Diagnosis is by sphygmomanometry, but additional investigations are necessary to assess damage to the heart (electrocardiogram (ECG), chest X-ray, echocardiogram) and kidneys (urinalysis and simple renal function tests). Special investigations to identify causes of secondary hypertension are only necessary when clinical suspicion is high, particularly in young patients with no family history of hypertension. Treatment is directed at lowering the blood-pressure to protect against end-organ damage, particularly stroke and ongoing renal disease. General measures, particularly weight reduction and restriction of salt and alcohol intake, are helpful, but the majority of patients require additional drug treatment with either diuretics, beta-blockers, calcium antagonists, angiotensin converting enzyme (ACE) inhibitors or alpha-blockers. Treatment should be tailored to the individual patient and, if a single agent fails to control the blood-pressure, others should be added.

## Definition

It is now well established, from life insurance actuarial analysis, that the risk of morbid complications rises in approximately linear relation to both systolic and diastolic blood-pressure measurements. Indeed, levels of blood-pressure commonly accepted at the upper end of the 'normal' range are usually associated with a significant increase in eventual cardiovascular mortality. Attempts to define normal blood-pressure are further confounded by its diurnal and random variability and the effects of age, sex and race.

## *Diurnal and random variability*

Continuous recording of blood-pressure, with an indwelling arterial cannula, shows a clear diurnal variability — with peak levels occurring during the day (usually in the early morning) and trough levels at night while asleep. Superimposed on this are the effects of anxiety and exertion, both of which cause a variable increase in blood-pressure.

## *Age*

Blood-pressure tends to rise with age and there is a corresponding rise in the prevalence of hypertension. Nevertheless, this does not appear to be a truly physiological phenomenon because it is largely confined to Western cultures and is more marked in urban than rural societies.

## *Sex*

Blood-pressure is usually higher in men than in women, particularly in childhood and early adulthood. Nevertheless, the age-related rise in blood-pressure tends to be steeper in women so that, by middle age, blood-pressure measurements in both sexes are similar.

## *Racial groups*

Studies in the UK and the US indicate that people of African origin have, on average, higher blood-pressures than whites. It is difficult, however, to attribute this entirely to genetic effects because rural populations in Africa usually have low measurements. Other population comparisons confirm that genetic and environmental factors show a complex inter-action; environmental factors of major importance to immigrant popu-lations include psychosocial effects and changes in diet and body-weight (see below).

All this means that any definition of hypertension must be arbitrary. Nevertheless, it is important that levels of 'normality' are defined — in order that decisions can be taken to investigate and treat. Thus, for practical purposes, hypertension in adults may be defined as follows:

*Mild hypertension*: 140/90–160/100 mmHg
*Moderate hypertension*: 160/100–180/115 mmHg
*Severe hypertension*: > 180/115 mmHg

## Mechanisms of hypertension

Blood-pressure is determined by cardiac output and systemic vascular resistance. Although increments in cardiac output may make an early contribution to the pathogenesis of hypertension, in established disease it is nearly always elevated systemic vascular resistance which plays the major role. This may be due to increased arteriolar tone, thickening of the arteriolar wall, or both, but in the majority of patients the underlying mechanisms responsible are unknown. Enhanced secretion of, or sensitivity to, arteriolar vasoconstrictors, particularly angiotensin II, may be important in some hypertensive patients and, although blood levels are not usually elevated, it remains possible that converting-enzyme activity within the arteriolar wall is heightened without detectable changes in blood levels.

Abnormalities of sodium balance have been the basis of many theories of the mechanism of hypertension. One proposal is that reduced renal excretion of sodium leads to salt and water retention, which increases cardiac output, leading to peripheral arteriolar constriction — an auto-regulatory phenomenon which prevents overperfusion. Thus, blood-pressure rises and, as afterload increases, cardiac output falls into the normal range again.

Recently attention has been focused on the handling of sodium at cell membrane level, which is often abnormal in hypertension. Evidence exists for a circulatory inhibitor of the sodium pump (produced in response to subtle expansion of the extracellular fluid volume), which leads to increased intracellular sodium concentration. It has been suggested that this stimulates sodium–calcium exchange in arteriolar smooth muscle, increasing the availability of calcium for vasoconstriction.

At present these remain hypotheses. Hypertension is almost certainly multifactorial in origin and caused by a breakdown of the control mechanisms which regulate cardiac output, blood volume, sodium balance and systemic vascular resistance.

## Aetiology

In the majority of hypertensive patients, no specific aetiological factor can be identified — *essential hypertension*. This must be distinguished from *secondary hypertension*, in which a specific cause can be identified.

### *Essential hypertension*

This accounts for 35–90% of all cases. By definition, the cause is unknown, but evidence points to an interaction between hereditary and environmental factors.

### *Hereditary factors*

The familial incidence of hypertension is due, at least in part, to hereditary factors, although these are often difficult to separate from environmental influences. Thus, concordance for hypertension is greater between monozygotic than dizygotic twins and between natural than adoptive siblings. Nevertheless, the tendency for spouses to have similar blood-pressure reflects the associated importance of the environment in determining the familial incidence of hypertension.

## Environmental factors

The importance of this is emphasized by population studies, in which migrants from rural to industrialized societies often show an increase in blood-pressure to a level characteristic of the indigenous population. Diet plays an important role, particularly when obesity results: several studies have shown a close positive correlation between body fat and blood-pressure. Specific dietary factors have been more difficult to identify, but recent work has shown an important relation with both salt and alcohol consumption. Thus, an increase in sodium intake of 100 mmol/24 hours is associated with an average rise in blood-pressure ranging from 5 mmHg at age 15–19 years to 10 mmHg at age 60–69. Excessive alcohol consumption also has an adverse effect on blood-pressure, systolic blood-pressure being almost 10 mmHg higher in men drinking six to eight drinks daily than in abstainers. Importantly, reductions in salt or alcohol consumption cause parallel reductions in the blood-pressure.

The role of stress and other psychosocial factors is difficult to define. Acute stress produces a physiological rise in blood-pressure, which may be sustained if the stress becomes chronic. Thus, job loss, bereavement, divorce and other life events of this type are all associated with a greater than expected incidence of hypertension.

## Secondary hypertension

In most cases, secondary hypertension is the result of renal disease or hormonal disorders (Table 12.1). Renal causes include both vascular and parenchymal disease, in which activation of the renin–angiotensin system and plasma volume excess, respectively, are seen. Hormonal disorders are responsible for hypertension in primary aldosteronism and Cushing's syndrome (due to excessive mineralocorticoid activity, resulting in sodium retention), and also in phaeochromocytoma (due to catecholamine stimulation). The cause of hypertension in acromegaly is not certain. The most common hormonal cause of hypertension, however, is the oral contraceptive, which almost invariably produces an increase in blood-pressure. Nevertheless, the increase is usually small and reverses promptly on stopping the drug; activation of the renin–angiotensin system is probably responsible. Other iatrogenic causes of hypertension include corticosteroid therapy and treatment with liquorice derivatives.

**Table 12.1**   Causes of secondary hypertension

*Renal parenchymal disease*
Glomerulonephritis
Pyelonephritis
Polycystic disease
Diabetic nephropathy
Connective tissue disease
Hydronephrosis

*Renal artery stenosis*
Atherosclerosis
Fibromuscular hyperplasia
Congenital

*Endocrine disease*
Adrenal cortex — Cushing's syndrome, Conn's syndrome
Adrenal medulla — phaeochromocytoma
Acromegaly
Iatrogenic — contraceptive pill, corticosteroids, sympathomimetic agents

*Miscellaneous*
Coarctation
Pregnancy — pre-eclampsia, eclampsia
Acute porphyria
Increased intracranial pressure

# Pathology

Hypertension is an important risk factor for atherosclerosis, especially in the coronary, cerebral and renal circulations. It may also cause direct vascular damage independently of atherosclerosis, resulting in aortic dissection or haemorrhagic stroke.

## *The heart*

Hypertension is a major risk factor for coronary artery disease and predisposes to myocardial ischaemia, infarction and sudden death. LV hypertrophy occurs, to compensate for the increase in afterload, and, in long-standing disease, irreversible deterioration in systolic and diastolic function may develop, leading to heart failure. The reduction in cardiac output often normalizes the blood-pressure and the condition may become clinically indistinguishable from dilated cardiomyopathy.

## *The brain*

Hypertension is an even more potent risk factor for cerebrovascular disease. The principal lesions are accelerated atherosclerosis in the larger cerebral vessels and mechanical dilatation of the small vessels and arterioles, resulting in microaneurysms. Stroke may result from thrombotic occlusion of atherosclerotic vessels or from intracerebral haemorrhage caused by vascular rupture. Although intracerebral haemorrhage is potentially more devastating in its consequences, the rupture of a micro-aneurysm may be clinically silent, resulting in a typical lacunar infarct. Multiple lacunar infarcts, however, may combine to cause subtle defects of cerebral function, manifested by intellectual deterioration.

Hypertension also predisposes to subarachnoid haemorrhage and transient ischaemic attacks, which precede major stroke in a significant proportion of cases.

## The eye

Fundoscopy provides a unique opportunity to examine the retinal vascular changes in hypertension, which presumably reflect similar changes in small vessels elsewhere in the central nervous system. These are discussed later.

## The kidney

Hypertension is probably the most common cause of chronic renal failure. Nevertheless. because hypertension may also be the result of renal disease, the precise cause-and-effect relationship is often difficult to establish. Hypertension leads to vascular changes in the renal arterioles and glomerular tufts, which produce tubular dysfunction and lower glomerular filtration rate. Proteinuria and haematuria occur and a vicious circle of worsening renal function and increasing hypertension may develop.

## Peripheral vascular disease

Accelerated atherosclerosis in the peripheral vessels predisposes to isch-aemic symptoms — particularly in the legs — and also to aneurysm and dissection of the aorta.

## Clinical manifestations

Uncomplicated hypertension is usually asymptomatic, although indi-vidual patients may complain of occipital headaches (particularly on waking in the morning) or epistaxis. The onset of symptoms usually signals the development of major complications. Angina due to coronary atherosclerosis, LV hypertrophy or a combination of the two is common and, in end-stage disease, LVF with fatigue and dyspnoea may develop. Retinal haemorrhages and exudates produce blurring of vision and field defects, while cerebrovascular disease may lead to transient ischaemic episodes or major stroke.

Examination confirms elevated blood-pressure. The cardiac apex is not usually displaced (before LVF supervenes) but it has a thrusting quality and a double impulse due to a palpable fourth heart sound. Auscultation confirms the fourth sound and may also reveal accentuation of the aortic component of the second sound. A soft mid-systolic murmur at the aortic area is common, due to forceful ejection by the hypertrophied LV. Aortic root dilatation occasionally causes mild aortic regurgitation, with an early diastolic murmur.

Examination of the optic fundus permits direct inspection of the small blood-vessels. Four grades of hypertensive retinopathy are recognized:

*Grade 1*  Narrowing and increased tortuosity of the retinal arteries.

*Grade 2*  Accentuation of the arterial changes and compression of the retinal veins at arteriovenous crossings.

*Grade 3*  Vascular changes associated with haemorrhages and exudates. The haemorrhages are typically flame-shaped and the exudates have a soft 'cotton-wool' appearance.

*Grade 4*  Previous grades with papilloedema. The optic cup is obliterated and the disc is pink with blurred edges.

## Complications

The major complications of hypertension are heart-disease, stroke, retinal damage, renal failure and peripheral vascular disease. These have been discussed previously.

## Diagnosis

Hypertension is diagnosed by sphygmomanometry (see p. 14). Blood-pressure may show considerable variation in an individual and, if found to be elevated, further measurements should be taken after a brief rest and again at a subsequent clinic visit before committing the patient to lifelong treatment. In cases where anxiety-related fluctuations in blood-pressure cause diagnostic difficulties, devices are available for self-measurement of blood-pressure in the more relaxed home environment. Once the diagnosis is established, further investigation is directed at assessing end-organ damage and determining the aetiological diagnosis.

### *Assessment of end-organ damage*

Routine investigations for all hypertensive patients should include an ECG (Fig. 12.1) and a chest X-ray (CXR) for assessment of LV hypertrophy and heart failure, respectively. An echocardiogram permits direct inspection of LV wall thickness and contractile function (Fig. 12.2). Renal status is evaluated by analysis of the urine for blood and protein and measure-

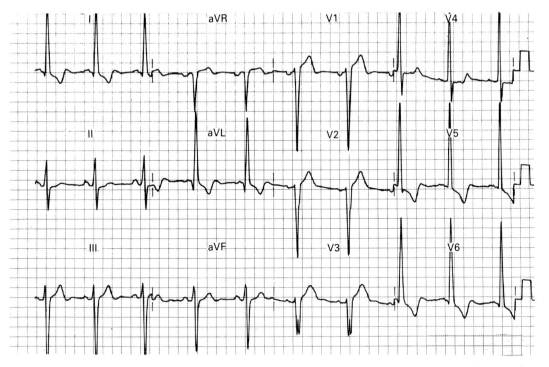

**Fig. 12.1** Hypertension — 12-lead ECG. This recording shows severe left ventricular hypertrophy. The voltage deflexions are exaggerated and there is T-wave inversion in leads I, aVL, V5 and V6 (strain pattern). Note also the broad, notched P waves, indicating associated left atrial enlargement.

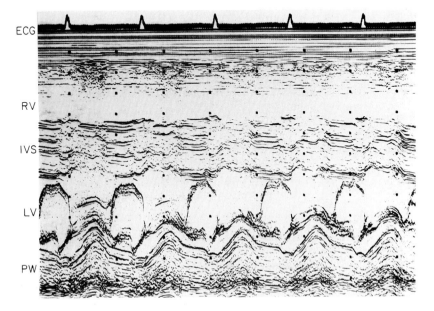

**Fig. 12.2** Hypertension. M-mode echocardiogram. There is severe concentric thickening of the left ventricle involving the interventricular septum (IVS) and posterior wall (PW). The vertical dots are a centimetre scale.

ment of blood urea and creatinine. A blood potassium level is needed as a baseline prior to starting diuretic therapy, and also provides a simple screening test for primary aldosteronism.

## Aetiological diagnosis

Because the large majority of patients have essential hypertension, special investigations to screen for primary renal disease and hormonal disorders are only indicated when the clinical findings suggest that hypertension is secondary. This is more important in hypertensive patients aged under 35 — particularly when there is no family history — because in this group the incidence of secondary hypertension is relatively high.

### Renovascular hypertension

Renal artery stenosis should be suspected in young patients with hypertension (when it is often the result of fibromuscular dysplasia) and in older patients who show an abrupt deterioration in renal function. In the latter age-group, atherosclerosis is the usual cause and may be associated with bruits over the renal arteries. Definitive diagnosis requires renal arteriography but intravenous urography and the radionuclide Hippuran renogram are suggestive if they show delayed opacification of the affected kidney or a delayed rate of rise of radiotracer in the kidney, respectively.

### Renal parenchymal disease

The diagnosis of acute nephritis is suggested by hypertension, oedema and haematuria following a recent throat infection. In chronic renal parenchymal disease, the aetiological diagnosis is often more difficult and it may be unclear whether the renal disease is the cause or the effect of hypertension. Renal biopsy may be helpful because, in a number of cases, specific treatment will be available to halt the progression of disease, e.g. minimal-change nephritis, systemic lupus erythematosus. In end-stage disease, however, when the kidneys are severely reduced in size, establishing the renal diagnosis is less likely to influence treatment, which aims to control uraemia and correct blood-pressure.

### Hormonal disorders

Hypokalaemia is essential for the diagnosis of *primary hyperaldosteronism* (Conn's syndrome) and often causes muscular weakness. Confirmation of hyperaldosteronism first requires correction of hypokalaemia by replacement therapy. Following this, stimuli for renin secretion are given (e.g. intravenous frusemide 40 mg followed by 30 min upright posture), which invariably show an attenuated response. *Cushing's syndrome* is suspected in patients with typical physical findings, including central obesity, moon facies, hirsutism, striae, proximal myopathy and osteoporosis. The diagnosis is confirmed if the dexamethasone suppression test fails to suppress blood cortisol levels and the urinary excretion of 17-hydroxycorticoids. Up to half of all patients with *phaeochromocytoma* have sustained hypertension, although the classical presentation is with fluctuating blood-pressure, in which the hypertensive episodes may be associated with headache, flushing and anxiety. Diagnosis is by demonstration of elevated levels of catecholamines or their metabolites in the blood or urine. In all the adrenal causes of secondary hypertension, computed tomography (CT) will often identify the adrenal hyperplasia or tumour. Nevertheless, failure to image the tumour does not rule out the diagnosis if biochemical tests are conclusive.

## Treatment

Only a small minority of patients have hypertension amenable to surgical correction. This includes those with adrenal disease, renal artery stenosis, unilateral renal parenchymal disease and coarctation. Even so, medical therapy is sometimes preferable, with surgery being reserved for resistant cases. This is particularly true of primary aldosteronism, if a discrete adrenal tumour cannot be identified, and unilateral renal parenchymal disease, in which nephrectomy is the only surgical option.

### *Aims of treatment*

Treatment is aimed at lowering the blood-pressure in order to reduce the incidence of major complications. The efficacy of treatment for preventing stroke is well established. It has also been possible to demonstrate a reduced incidence of renal failure, but effects on coronary artery disease and myocardial infarction are less pronounced. Nevertheless, the overall mortality of treated hypertensives is lower than untreated. In severe hypertension, the mortality reduction during long-term follow-up exceeds 50%.

### *Who to treat*

Despite enthusiastic claims, large-scale studies have failed to show that the treatment of mild hypertension (up to 160/100 mmHg) produces an appreciable benefit in terms of long-term morbidity and mortality. The benefits of treating moderate and severe hypertension, however, are well established. One large study showed that, in patients with diastolic blood-pressure above 115 mmHg (severe hypertension) active treatment reduced the risk of complications from 55% to 18% and more than halved the number of deaths.

There is no evidence that different treatment policies are required in particular racial, sex or age-groups. Although the elderly (over 70 years) are often less able to tolerate antihypertensive drugs, they are most at risk of stroke and benefit from treatment as much, if not more, than younger hypertensives.

## Non-pharmacological measures

Hypertension is not a medical emergency and in many cases can be improved (or even corrected) without drug treatment. Women on the contraceptive pill should, where possible, use an alternative method of contraception. The obese patient should be encouraged to lose weight, because this often produces a significant reduction in blood-pressure. Moderation of alcohol consumption is beneficial, particularly in the heavy drinker. Patients should be advised not to add extra salt to their food. Relief of stress, though difficult to achieve, is beneficial in some patients. A variety of relaxation and meditation techniques have been shown to lower blood-pressure, at least in the short term. Undoubtedly, the most important general measure, however, is the avoidance or correction of other risk factors for arterial disease, particularly smoking and hypercholesterolaemia. In the majority of clinical trials, smoking has emerged as a more important predictor of both myocardial infarction (MI) and stroke than a moderate increase in blood-pressure.

**Table 12.2**   Drugs for the treatment of hypertension

| | |
|---|---|
| *Diuretics* | |
| Bendrofluazide | 2.5 mg daily |
| Cyclopenthiazide | 0.5–1.0 mg daily |
| *Beta-blockers* | |
| Atenolol | 50–200 mg daily |
| Bisoprolol | 5–20 mg daily |
| *Calcium antagonists* | |
| Nifedipine | 10–40 mg twice daily (slow-release preparation) |
| Verapamil | 240 mg daily (slow-release preparation) |
| Amlodipine | 5–10 mg daily |
| *Converting-enzyme inhibitors* | |
| Captopril | 12.5–50 mg twice daily |
| Enalapril | 5–40 mg daily |
| Lisinopril | 2.5–40 mg daily |
| *Alpha-blockers* | |
| Prazosin | 0.5–5 mg three times daily |
| Doxazosin | 1–16 mg daily |

## *Drug therapy* (Table 12.2)

Despite the importance of non-pharmacological methods to control hypertension, many patients will require treatment with antihypertensive drugs and, because this must continue indefinitely, its acceptability in terms of dosage frequency and side-effects must always be a major consideration. Indeed, poor compliance to the treatment regimen is the usual reason for inadequate control of blood-pressure. From the wide range of drugs available, five groups of agents come closest to fulfilling the combined requirement for efficacy and acceptability. These are diuretics, beta-blockers, calcium antagonists, angiotensin-converting enzyme inhibitors and alpha-blockers.

The choice of treatment should be tailored to the individual. In young patients an angiotensin-converting enzyme inhibitor or alpha-blocker is often preferred because side-effects are rarely obtrusive and impotence, in particular, is seldom a problem. In addition, these drugs do not have unfavourable effects on glucose or lipid metabolism and, on theoretical grounds, may protect against development of arterial disease in later life. The elderly are sometimes unwilling to take vasodilators, because of postural hypotension, and often find diuretics more acceptable. Beta-blockers have a useful role in patients with exaggerated tachycardia or an anxiety component to their hypertension, while for many patients calcium antagonists are the best tolerated and most effective drugs. If a single agent provides inadequate blood-pressure control, a second can be added — ideally as a combined preparation for ease of administration and better compliance. Persistent hypertension requires the addition of a third agent and, in the most severe cases, four or more different drugs may be necessary.

## *Diuretics*

Salt and water excretion lowers blood-pressure by reducing plasma volume and cardiac output. Nevertheless, these changes are short-lived and the mechanisms responsible for the long-term antihypertensive efficacy of diuretics are unknown. Although thiazides and loop diuretics are equally effective, thiazides are usually preferred because they produce a less vigorous diuresis. They should be used in combination with potassium-sparing diuretics to prevent hypokalaemia. Impotence may affect up to 15% of patients treated with thiazide diuretics, which are best avoided in younger, sexually active patients. Thiazides cause modest elevations of blood sugar and triglycerides, and there is a theoretical risk of long-term cardiovascular complications in young patients. At present, however, there is no conclusive evidence that the metabolic side-effects of thiazides increase cardiovascular morbidity.

## Beta-blockers

These drugs tend to lower cardiac output by their effect on heart rate and contractility, and they also inhibit sympathetically mediated renin release from the kidney, which reduces angiotensin II synthesis. Nevertheless, it is unlikely that these properties account fully for the antihypertensive efficacy of beta-blockers, the mechanism of which remains uncertain.

Beta-blockers are effective in all degrees of hypertension. They may be used as monotherapy but are particularly useful in combination with thiazides or calcium antagonists, both of which tend to increase renin release — an unwanted effect which is modified by beta-blockers. In addition, beta-blockers prevent reflex tachycardia caused by the vasodilator effects of calcium antagonists and alpha-blockers. The choice of beta-blocker depends principally on patient acceptability, atenolol usually being preferred because it is long-acting and cardioselective and does not cross the blood—brain barrier (see p. 113). The more recently available bisoprolol has similar properties but is longer-acting and more cardioselective and has a neutral effect on blood lipids. Other beta-blockers may cause a small rise in blood cholesterol, though whether this affects the risk of developing arterial disease is not known.

## Calcium antagonists

These drugs relax vascular smooth muscle, producing arteriolar dilatation and reduction in systemic vascular resistance, and are effective in all degrees of hypertension. Nifedipine is best given in combination with a beta-blocker, to prevent reflex tachycardia. Verapamil and diltiazem cause less reflex tachycardia and can be used as single therapy. Although these drugs are relatively short-acting and require to be given three times daily, slow-release preparations are now available for twice-daily dosage, which improves patient compliance. Long-acting calcium antagonists, such as amlodipine, for once-daily administration have recently become available and may have a particularly useful role for the long-term management of hypertension.

## Angiotensin-converting enzyme inhibitors

These drugs produce arteriolar dilatation and reduction in systemic vascular resistance by blocking the synthesis of angiotensin II — a potent vasoconstrictor. They are effective in all degrees of hypertension and are now being used increasingly because side-effects are rarely troublesome and quality of life is often well preserved. Impotence and drowsiness, in particular, seldom occur with angiotensin-converting enzyme inhibitors. These drugs do not have adverse effects on lipid profiles and in many cases cause small reductions in blood cholesterol, though whether this protects against arterial disease during long-term treatment is unknown. A wide variety of different agents are now available, but long-acting drugs for once-daily administration (e.g. enalapril, lisinopril) are usually preferred in the management of hypertension.

## Alpha-blockers

Prazosin, a post-synaptic alpha adrenoceptor-blocker, has been widely used in the past, but doxazosin, a longer-acting drug for once-daily administration, has now largely replaced it in the treatment of hypertension. Doxazosin is effective and well tolerated and, like angiotensin-converting enzyme inhibitors, may cause concomitant small reductions in blood cholesterol levels. Side-effects related to vasodilatation (headache, dizziness) are rarely troublesome and, like ACE inhibitors, the incidence of impotence is low.

## Prognosis

When hypertension is untreated, 50% of patients die of heart-disease, 30% of strokes and 15% of renal failure. The extent of end-organ damage relates principally to the duration of hypertension and its severity: thus, by detecting hypertension at an early stage and treating it effectively, prognosis can be improved. Prognosis is also affected by the age, race and sex of the patient, with young black men being at greatest risk of premature death. The outlook is worse in those patients with associated risk factors for arterial disease, particularly hypercholesterolaemia and smoking.

## Accelerated hypertension

This affects about 1% of all hypertensive patients and occurs in both essential and secondary hypertension. Cigarette smoking is a predisposing factor. Severe elevation of the blood-pressure (often above 200/140 mmHg) may be associated with encephalopathy, characterized by headache, nausea, clouding of consciousness and convulsions. The marked increase in afterload commonly causes LVF and pulmonary oedema. Grade IV retinopathy is invariable. Impairment of renal function usually occurs and if treatment is not instituted rapidly oliguric renal failure develops.

Accelerated hypertension is a medical emergency. Treatment is by reducing the diastolic blood-pressure to between 90 and 110 mmHg. Blood-pressure reduction should be smooth and controlled because there is risk of cerebral infarction if it drops abruptly to very low levels. For this reason, bolus injections of diazoxide or hydralazine are no longer recommended, because the blood-pressure response is unpredictable and difficult to control. Sublingual nifedipine or captopril should be avoided for the same reason. Intravenous infusions of nitroprusside or labetalol are preferred, because incremental dose regimens produce a graded reduction in blood-pressure. These drugs have a short half-life, and potentially dangerous falls in blood-pressure are rapidly reversed by temporarily stopping the infusion. Nitroprusside infusion should start at 25 µg/min, with small increments every 15 min until the desired response is achieved. Labetalol infusion should start at 1 mg/min, with increments every 30 min. Because the drug is a beta-blocker, it should be used cautiously in severe LVF. Following control of the blood-pressure, oral treatment should be prescribed to prevent recurrence of the hypertensive crisis.

## Further reading

Anonymous. Hypertensive emergencies. *Lancet* 1991, **338**, 220–1.
Anonymous. New trials in older hypertensives. *Lancet* 1991, **338**, 1299–1300.
DeQuattro V. The 1980s: a patient-specific therapeutic approach in hypertension. *Am. Heart J.* 1987, **114** (1, part 2), 224–6.
Dunn F.G., Burns J.M. and Hornung R.S. Left ventricular hypertrophy in hypertension. *Am. Heart J.* 1991, **122** (1, part 2), 312–15.
Frohlich E.D. Cardiac hypertrophy in hypertension. *N. Engl. J. Med.* 1987, **317**, 831–3.
Grimm R.H. Treating hypertension and cardiovascular risk: are there trade-offs? *Am. Heart J.* 1990, **119** (3, part 2), 729–32.
Law M.R., Frost C.D. and Wald N.J. By how much does dietary salt reduction lower blood pressure? *Br. Med. J.* 1991, **302**, 811–23.
Messerli F.H. Antihypertensive therapy: going to the heart of the matter. *Circulation* 1990, **81**, 1128–35.
Messerli F.H., Kaesser U.R. and Losem C.J. Effects of antihypertensive therapy on hypertensive heart disease. *Circulation* 1989, **80** (suppl. 6), 145–50.
Middeke M. and Holzgreve H. Review of major intervention studies in hypertension and hyperlipidemia: focus on coronary heart disease. *Am. Heart J.* 1988, **116** (6, part 2), 1708–12.
Ram C.V. Management of hypertensive emergencies: changing therapeutic options. *Am. Heart J.* 1991, **122** (1, part 2), 356–63.
Saunders J.B. Alcohol: an important cause of hypertension. *Br. Med. J.* 1987, **294**, 1045–6.
Semple P.F. and Lever A.F. Glimpses of the mechanisms of hypertension. *Br. Med. J.* 1986, **293**, 901–2.
Swales J.D. First line treatment in hypertension. *Br. Med. J.* 1990, **301**, 1172–3.
Tifft C.P. The hypertensive patient with concomitant cardiovascular disease. *Am. Heart J.* 1988, **116** (1, part 2), 280–7.

# 13  Aortic Aneurysm and Dissection

## Summary

*Aortic aneurysm* is usually abdominal and results from atherosclerosis, although cystic medial necrosis in Marfan's syndrome is a more common cause of ascending aortic aneurysm. Many aneurysms are asymptomatic, though local pressure may cause pain in the lumbar or thoracic spine. Abdominal aneurysms may be palpated as a pulsatile mass in the abdomen but thoracic aneurysms produce no physical signs unless they involve the aortic valve ring, when the early diastolic murmur of aortic regurgitation may be audible. The other principal complication is rupture, unusual in thoracic aneurysms but more common in abdominal aneurysms, particularly those greater than 6 cm in diameter. If the aneurysm is calcified, it is often visible on the plain chest or abdominal X-ray, but ultrasound or computed tomography is required for more precise diagnosis. Blood-pressure control is essential, and surgical resection is indicated for abdominal aneurysms greater than 6 cm or for the correction of complications.

*Aortic dissection* is a medical emergency caused by a tear in the intima of the ascending or arch aorta. The high-pressure arterial blood creates a false lumen through the media, which may either re-enter the true lumen more distally or rupture externally, usually into the pericardial or left pleural spaces. The dissection may partially or completely occlude any of the branch arteries arising from the aorta and, if proximal, may disrupt the aortic valve ring, causing aortic regurgitation. Presentation is with severe chest pain and examination may reveal reduced or absent pulses; coronary occlusion may cause myocardial infarction. Aortic regurgitation is common in proximal dissection, and rupture externally may be associated with signs of tamponade or hypovolaemic shock. Diagnosis requires demonstration of the intimal flap separating true and false aortic lumens. The echocardiogram is helpful (particularly by the transoesophageal approach), but computed tomography is more usually diagnostic. In most cases, however, urgent aortic root angiography is necessary to demonstrate the origin and extent of dissection. For proximal dissections, surgical repair improves prognosis and is the treatment of choice. Distal dissections arising in the aortic arch are best treated medically with beta-blockers to lower blood-pressure.

## Aortic aneurysm

### Aetiology

Aortic aneurysms occur most commonly in the abdominal aorta, where they are usually the result of atherosclerosis. Aneurysms of the descending thoracic aorta are also atherosclerotic in most cases, but in the ascending aorta Marfan's syndrome and other causes of cystic medical necrosis have replaced syphilis as the usual cause.

### Pathology

Risk factors are the same as for atherosclerotic disease elsewhere in the body. Thus, patients at greatest risk are middle-aged or elderly men, particularly when there is a history of cigarette smoking, hypertension or hypercholesterolaemia.

The wall tension in a blood-vessel is determined by the product of intravascular pressure and diameter (law of Laplace). The aorta is the largest artery in the body and its walls, therefore, are under considerable tension. Disease of the aortic wall causes destruction of the elastic fibres in the media, which allows the vessel to dilate. This increases wall tension and a vicious circle becomes established.

Most aortic aneurysms are fusiform, involving the total circumference of a segment of the vessel wall. Occasionally, they are sacular and consist of an outfolding of the vessel wall. Sacular aneurysms are often the result of syphilis or other infections (mycotic aneurysm) and are particularly prone to rupture.

About 76% of aortic aneurysms occur in the abdominal aorta below the renal arteries, where the risk of rupture is greatest and closely related to the size of the aneurysm. When the diameter is less than 6 cm the incidence of rupture within 1 year is 20%, but the incidence approaches 50% for larger aneurysms.

### Clinical manifestations

Aortic aneurysms are usually asymptomatic. When located in the abdominal aorta, low back pain may occur (due to pressure over the lumbar spine), but in many cases aortic rupture is the first manifestation. Examination reveals an expansile pulsating mass in the abdomen, and a bruit is often audible, due to turbulent flow through the aneurysm.

Thoracic aortic aneurysms are more likely to be symptomatic, although rupture is unusual: large aneurysms often cause an aching chest discomfort, which may be associated with pain in the back due to pressure over the thoracic spine. Other symptoms, caused by compression of adjacent structures, include dysphagia, cough and hoarseness. They rarely produce physical signs unless they involve the aortic root, when the early diastolic murmur of aortic regurgitation may be audible. This is particularly common in Marfan's syndrome and other causes of cystic medial necrosis.

## Complications

Rupture is the principal complication, which is a surgical emergency and often rapidly fatal. Abdominal aortic aneurysms are most prone to rupture — usually into the retroperitoneal space. Patients who survive the acute episode present in hypovolaemic shock, with severe pain in the abdomen and the back, often extending into the iliac fossae; emergency surgery salvages about 50% of these patients. Occasionally, rupture is into the duodenum or the inferior vena cava, causing massive gastrointestinal haemorrhage and arteriovenous fistula, respectively.

Unusual complications include thromboembolism, due to thrombosis within the aneurysmal sac, and infection, which produces a syndrome similar to endocarditis. Aneurysm of the ascending aorta is particularly common in Marfan's syndrome and commonly causes aortic regurgitation.

## Diagnosis

Abdominal aortic aneurysms are identified by clinical examination and, if calcified, can usually be seen on the plain abdominal X-ray. The diagnosis is confirmed by ultrasonography, which permits accurate assessment of the size of the aneurysm; computed tomography (CT) provides an

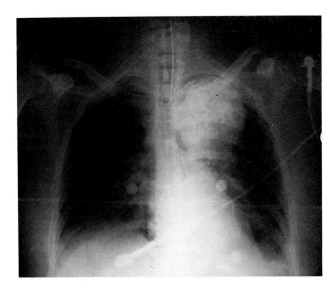

**Fig. 13.1** Thoracic aortic aneurysm. The chest X-ray shows a large calcified mass in the left upper mediastinum. The calcification extends downwards behind the heart in the wall of the aorta, confirming that the mass is an aortic aneurysm.

alternative non-invasive technique for identification of abdominal aortic aneurysms.

Thoracic aortic aneurysms are nearly always visible on the chest X-ray (Fig. 13.1). Echocardiography identifies aortic root aneurysms (see Fig. 16.1), and the transoesophageal technique permits examination of the aortic arch. For most purposes, however, thoracic aortic aneurysms are best examined by CT or aortography.

## Differential diagnosis

Abdominal aortic aneurysms must be differentiated from other masses, particularly those that overlie the aorta and transmit pulsation: non-aneurysmal masses, however, are never expansile. Ultrasound examination is usually sufficient to resolve the differential diagnosis. Thoracic aortic aneurysms require differentiation from other causes of a mediastinal mass.

## Treatment

Specific treatment is usually unnecessary, although blood-pressure control is important. Surgical resection is indicated when symptoms or complications (e.g. aortic regurgitation) cannot be controlled or when rupture threatens (abdominal aneurysms more than 6 cm diameter or those that show rapid radiographic enlargement on serial examinations).

## Prognosis

Patients with atherosclerotic aortic aneurysms nearly always have coronary artery disease and this, together with the size of the aneurysm, has an important influence on prognosis. Thus, 5-year survival is only 20% in patients with symptomatic ischaemic heart-disease, but this rises to 50% in the absence of ischaemic heart-disease. The size is also important, abdominal aneurysms more than 6 cm diameter being at greatest risk of potentially fatal rupture. Aortic root aneurysms in Marfan's syndrome may cause severe aortic regurgitation and ultimately death if surgical replacement of the aortic root is delayed.

### Sinus of Valsalva aneurysm

Sinus of Valsalva aneurysm may be mycotic, occurring as a complication of infective endocarditis. More commonly, however, it is congenital, when it usually affects the right coronary sinus, particularly in men. The fusion between the aortic media and the fibrous ring of the aortic valve

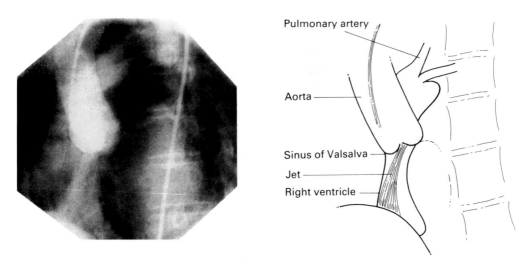

**Fig. 13.2** Aortogram of ruptured sinus of Valsalva aneurysm. A jet of contrast material highlights the communication between the sinus of Valsalva and the right ventricle. The right ventricle and the pulmonary artery are opacified.

is weakened or absent, so that progressive aneurysmal bulging of the affected area occurs. This usually remains asymptomatic until adulthood, when rupture of the aneurysm into a right-sided cardiac chamber (usually the right ventricle) produces an arteriovenous shunt. This volume-loads both sides of the heart, resulting in biventricular failure, and may cause sudden death, although, more commonly, the patient presents with chest pain associated with shortness of breath.

Examination reveals early diastolic collapse of the carotid pulse and a precordial continuous murmur, which is audible throughout the cardiac cycle. The diagnosis is confirmed by ascending thoracic aortography, which demonstrates prompt opacification of the right-sided cardiac chambers due to shunting through the ruptured aneurysm (Fig. 13.2). Treatment is by surgical repair of the defect.

## Aortic dissection

### Aetiology

Like aortic aneurysm, dissection is caused by disease of the aortic media, usually atherosclerosis. Marfan's syndrome and other causes of cystic medial necrosis also predispose to aortic dissection. Patients are often hypertensive, particularly when the dissection arises in the aortic arch.

## Pathology

Dissection nearly always arises in the ascending or arch aorta. The development of a tear in the aortic intima causes the high-pressure aortic blood to create a false lumen for a variable distance through the diseased media. The tear is usually proximal, just above the sinus of Valsalva, but in about 25% of cases it is distal and located within the aortic arch close to the origin of the left subclavian artery. The dissection can partially or completely occlude any of the branch arteries arising from the aorta and, if proximal, may disrupt the aortic valve ring, producing aortic regurgitation. The false lumen may rupture externally (usually into the pericardial sac or left pleural space) or re-enter the true lumen of the aorta more distally.

## Clinical manifestations

Presentation is with the abrupt onset of severe tearing chest pain, which may be experienced in the front or the back of the chest. Pain is maximal at the onset, unlike acute myocardial infarction (MI), in which the pain has a crescendo quality. The patient is cold and sweaty and may be shocked if the aneurysm ruptures externally, causing tamponade or hypovolaemia. Examination commonly reveals an asymmetric pulse deficit due to involvement of the carotid or subclavian arteries arising from the aorta. Pulses may be either absent or reduced so that a difference between the blood-pressures in the arms is detectable. The early diastolic murmur of aortic regurgitation is commonly present in proximal dissection.

## Complications

Branch artery occlusions may cause myocardial infarction and, rarely, stroke, intestinal infarction, renal failure or limb ischaemia; vertebral artery occlusion may result in paraplegia. Because occlusion of the left main coronary artery is usually fatal, MI in survivors of aortic dissection is nearly always located inferiorly and is caused by right coronary occlusion.

When aortic dissection is complicated by external rupture, presentation is with hypovolaemic shock, although rupture into the pericardial sac causes tamponade. In either case, the outcome is usually fatal.

Promixal aortic dissection may disrupt the aortic valve ring, producing aortic regurgitation, the severity of which is variable, but re-suspension or replacement of the aortic valve is often necessary during surgical repair of the dissection.

## Diagnosis

Electrocardiogram (ECG) changes are non-specific, but may show acute MI if the dissection occludes a coronary ostium. The chest X-ray (CXR)

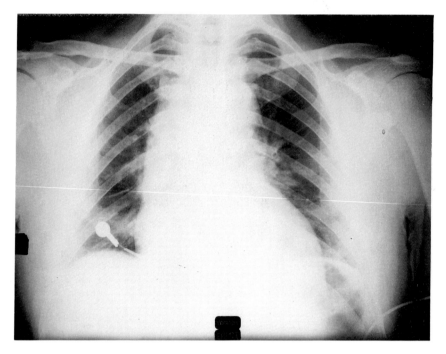

**Fig. 13.3** Aortic dissection. The chest X-ray shows widening of the entire mediastinum. In the patient with chest pain, this is strongly suggestive of aortic dissection.

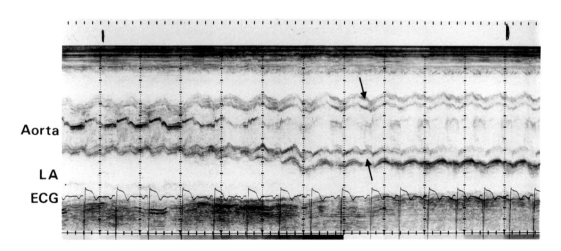

**Fig. 13.4** Aortic dissection — M-mode echocardiogram. This is a scan from the sinuses of Valsalva up the ascending aorta. Just above the sinuses of Valsalva the aorta widens considerably and a false lumen (arrowed) becomes apparent in its wall.

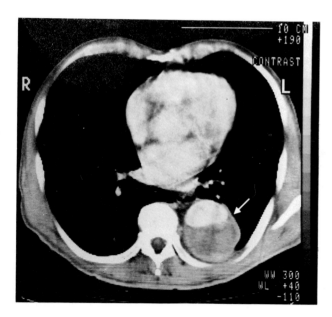

**Fig. 13.5** Aortic dissection — computed tomography. The descending thoracic aorta (arrowed) is grossly dilated. Contrast enhancement of the blood pool reveals two columns within the aorta, separated by an intimal flap. This confirms the diagnosis of dissection.

shows dilatation of the aorta, often with widening of the entire mediastinum (Fig. 13.3). External rupture into the pericardial or pleural spaces causes cardiac enlargement or left pleural effusion, respectively. The echocardiogram often demonstrates the false lumen in proximal dissections (Fig. 13.4) and may also show pericardial haematoma and signs of aortic regurgitation. The transoesophageal technique permits a more complete examination of the ascending aorta and the arch. Nevertheless, computed tomography is probably the most useful non-invasive imaging technique for diagnosis of dissection, reliably demonstrating the true and false aortic lumens separated by an intimal flap (Fig. 13.5). In most cases,

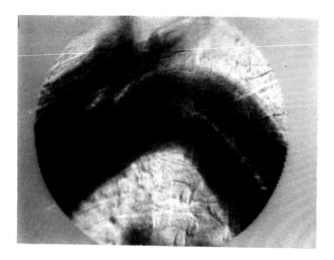

**Fig. 13.6** Aortic dissection. This digital subtraction angiogram of the aortic arch shows abrupt widening of the aorta after the left subclavian branch. The intimal flap (arrowed) is clearly visible, confirming the diagnosis of aortic dissection.

however, urgent aortic angiography is required to define the origin and the extent of the dissection (Fig. 13.6).

## Differential diagnosis

This is from other causes of acute-onset chest pain, particularly MI. The history is helpful (abrupt versus crescendo onset of pain), and serial ECG and enzyme studies indicate acute infarction if the typical evolution of changes occurs. It must be remembered, however, that these differential diagnoses are not necessarily mutually exclusive.

## Treatment

The emergency management requires blood-pressure reduction to reduce the risk of rupture. If rapid control cannot be achieved with oral beta-blockers or calcium antagonists, nitroprusside or labetolol should be infused (see p. 270) to maintain the systolic blood-pressure at no more than 100 mmHg. Transfer to a cardiothoracic centre for aortography must be arranged as soon as possible. If the dissection involves the ascending aorta (whether from a proximal tear or from proximal extension of a distal dissection), the risk of rupture into the pericardial sac and aortic regurgitation is very high. Expeditious surgical repair reduces the risk and is the treatment of choice. In uncomplicated distal dissection, surgery has not been shown to affect prognosis, but strict control of the blood-pressure is essential. Beta-blockers are drugs of choice for maintenance therapy because they reduce the pulse pressure and the systolic pressure.

## Prognosis

Untreated proximal dissection involving the ascending aorta is usually fatal within a month of presentation. Patients with distal dissection fare little better, although lowering the blood-pressure helps prevent rupture and may permit longer survival.

## Further reading

DeSanctis R.W., Doroghazi R.M., Austen W.G. and Buckley M.J. Aortic dissection. *N. Engl. J. Med.* 1987, **317**, 1060–7.
Lindsay J., DeBakey M.E. and Beall A.C. Diseases of the aorta. In Hurst J.W. (ed.), *The Heart* (5th edn). New York, McGraw Hill, 1982, 1432–57.

# 14 Pulmonary Embolism and Pulmonary Heart-disease

## Summary

*Acute pulmonary embolism* is usually a complication of deep venous thrombosis involving the iliofemoral veins. Its severity is determined by the extent of pulmonary vascular obstruction and only when this exceeds 50% (*massive embolism*) does pulmonary resistance rise sufficiently to cause right ventricular failure (RVF). *Minor embolism* is often clinically silent, occasionally causing pleurisy and haemoptysis. Massive embolism presents with abrupt-onset dyspnoea and chest pain, associated with tachypnoea, tachycardia and a loud pulmonary component of the second heart sound (P2); shock and sudden death are not uncommon. Diagnosis is difficult and the electrocardiogram (ECG) and chest X-ray (CXR) are often unhelpful. Arterial gas analysis shows hypoxaemia, hypocapnia and respiratory alkalosis in massive embolism, but definitive diagnosis requires demonstration of ventilation–perfusion mismatch on pulmonary scintigraphy. Treatment is with heparin and oxygen. In severe cases thrombolytic therapy is recommended but failure to respond may require pulmonary angiography and emergency embolectomy.

*Chronic pulmonary embolism* usually remains clinically silent until repeated embolic episodes with progressive obliteration of the vascular bed have caused advanced pulmonary hypertension, evidenced by a left parasternal systolic thrust and a loud P2, often associated with the early diastolic murmur of pulmonary regurgitation. The development of RVF produces elevation of the jugular venous pulse (JVP), usually associated with functional tricuspid regurgitation, hepatomegaly and peripheral oedema. The ECG shows right ventricular (RV) hypertrophy and the CXR an enlarged heart with prominence of the proximal pulmonary arteries and attenuation ('pruning') of the peripheral vessels. Treatment with long-term warfarin is directed at preventing further embolism, but prognosis is poor.

*Primary pulmonary hypertension* is an uncommon disorder, usually affecting young women, in which obliterative pulmonary arteriolar disease of unknown cause results in progressive pulmonary hypertension and RVF. Prognosis is poor and heart–lung transplantation the only effective treatment.

*Pulmonary heart-disease*, also called cor pulmonale, is usually caused by chronic bronchitis and emphysema, in which progressive destruction of the pulmonary vascular bed and hypoxic pulmonary arteriolar constriction lead to pulmonary hypertension and RVF. Initially RVF is intermittent, coinciding with winter exacerbations of bronchitis, but eventually it becomes sustained as pulmonary vascular reserve is exhausted. The patient presents with signs of pulmonary hypertension and RVF. Polycythaemia is common, and respiratory function tests and arterial gas analysis confirm the underlying lung disease. Treatment is directed at preventing progression of pulmonary disease by prophylactic antibiotic therapy and stopping smoking. Diuretics correct peripheral oedema but significant improvement in RV function requires sustained reductions in pulmonary vascular resistance; oxygen therapy is helpful and the role of lung transplantation is under investigation.

## Acute pulmonary embolism

### Aetiology

In the majority of cases, pulmonary embolism (PE) is caused by thrombus, usually deriving from the iliofemoral veins (deep venous thrombosis) and, less commonly, from the right-sided cardiac chambers. Non-thrombotic pulmonary embolism is less common but may be caused by air, amniotic fluid and fat.

### Deep venous thrombosis (DVT)

This is usually a complication of prolonged immobility in bed, particularly following abdominal and hip surgery. Other risk factors are shown in Table 14.1. In about 10% of cases, PE occurs. This is unlikely if thrombosis is confined to the calf veins but becomes more likely with extension to the iliofemoral veins. Symptoms and signs of DVT are variable and non-diagnostic. Indeed, although swelling of the affected leg sometimes occurs, many cases are clinically silent. Doppler ultrasound is

**Table 14.1** Risk factors for deep venous thrombosis

Immobility — particularly following hip and abdominal surgery
Venous stasis in legs — varicose veins, vena cava compression (e.g. gravid uterus), bony fractures of legs
Heart-disease — myocardial infarction, heart failure
Endocrine/metabolic factors — diabetes, obesity, contraceptive pill, post-partum period
Malignant disease — particularly pancreatic and bronchial carcinoma
Miscellaneous — polycythaemia, Behçet's disease

usually diagnostic but in difficult cases venography provides definitive diagnosis.

## Pathology

The severity of PE is largely determined by the extent of pulmonary vascular obstruction; it is classified as *massive* if more than 50% of the major pulmonary arteries are involved, and as *minor* if less extensive. Massive embolism significantly increases pulmonary vascular resistance, causing acute RVF. Pulmonary artery systolic pressure, however, does not usually rise above 40 mmHg because the thin-walled right ventricle is unable to generate sufficient pressure to overcome the vascular obstruction. Occasionally, the increase in pulmonary resistance is out of proportion to the extent of vascular obstruction. It has been proposed, therefore, that pulmonary arteriolar constriction, caused by ill-defined neurohumoral mechanisms, may contribute to the pathophysiology of pulmonary embolism.

Minor pulmonary embolism involving less than 50% of the vascular bed does not compromise right ventricular function because the pulmonary vascular reserve ensures that resistance to flow does not rise significantly. Minor embolism of this type is, therefore, clinically silent unless it causes pulmonary infarction. This affects only about 10% of cases because the lung is protected by the bronchial arterial supply from the thoracic aorta and also obtains oxygen directly from the alveoli.

## Clinical manifestations

These are very variable and usually non-diagnostic. Minor embolism is often asymptomatic but, if it causes pulmonary infarction, pleuritic chest pain with or without haemoptysis may occur.

In massive embolism, patients commonly complain of acute-onset dyspnoea and chest pain, which is usually retrosternal and not necessarily pleuritic in nature. Cough, haemoptysis, diaphoresis and syncope occur less frequently. The most consistent clinical signs are tachypnoea, tachycardia and accentuation of the pulmonary component of the second heart sound; elevation of the JVP, a third heart sound and cyanosis are more variable. In the most severe cases, the patient is shocked, with severe hypotension and other signs of critically impaired cardiac output. Sudden death is not uncommon.

## Complications

Non-fatal PE usually resolves without complications. In patients who develop pulmonary infarction, cavitation and secondary infection of the infarct occasionally occur (Fig. 14.1). In a minority of cases, recurrent

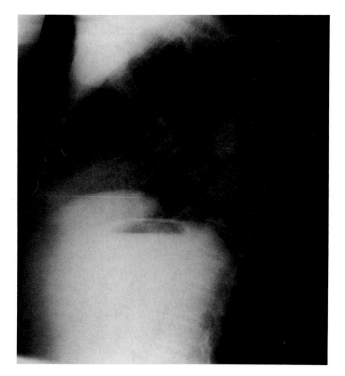

**Fig. 14.1** Pulmonary embolism with cavitating infarct. A week after massive pulmonary embolism, the lateral chest X-ray showed a posteriorly located infarct with a fluid level indicating cavitation.

(often subclinical) thromboembolism results in worsening pulmonary hypertension and right ventricular failure (see below).

## *Diagnosis*

The CXR is often normal, although loss of lung volume (elevated hemidiaphragm) and regional oligaemia are sometimes seen. A pleural reaction is common and may produce a small effusion, although this rarely becomes visible until at least 12–24 hours after the event. When pulmonary infarction occurs, the development of a radiographic density is also a relatively late finding.

The ECG changes are as variable as the clinical features and are rarely diagnostic. Tachycardia may be the only abnormality but, in massive embolism, features of acute right heart strain are sometimes seen. These include P pulmonale, an S wave in lead I and a narrow Q wave in lead III associated with T-wave inversion (S1, Q3, T3). Right bundle branch block and atrial fibrillation may also occur.

Arterial gas analysis is unhelpful in minor embolism but, when more severe, hypoxaemia, associated with hypocapnia and respiratory alkalosis, is a characteristic finding.

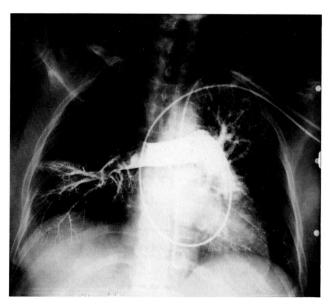

**Fig. 14.2** Massive pulmonary embolism — pulmonary arteriogram. There is extensive pulmonary arterial obstruction, with opacification limited to the left upper lobe and to a few branches in the right lower zone. Note the intraluminal thrombus, which is clearly visible as a filling defect in the right pulmonary artery.

More useful diagnostic information is provided by the radionuclide lung scan. A normal perfusion scan rules out significant pulmonary embolism. However, the demonstration of perfusion defects is suggestive, particularly when simultaneous ventilation scanning confirms ventilation–perfusion mismatch (see Fig. 3.12).

Pulmonary arteriography is the definitive method of diagnosis (Fig. 14.2) but is only indicated in patients suspected of having massive PE, when surgical embolectomy is under consideration. Arteriography is diagnostic if intraluminal filling defects and vessel cut-offs are seen. Other abnormalities, including regional oligaemia, are less specific.

## Differential diagnosis

Minor pulmonary embolism must be differentiated from other causes of pleurisy and haemoptysis, particularly pneumonia. The CXR and the results of blood and sputum culture are usually sufficient to confirm infection, which usually responds promptly to antibiotics. In difficult cases the radionuclide lung scan is helpful because, in pneumonia, ventilation–perfusion defects are matched, unlike PE, when they are mismatched.

Massive PE requires differentiation from myocardial infarction (MI) and other causes of collapse and shock. Typical cardiac pain, associated with the diagnostic evolution of ECG and serum enzyme changes, is usually sufficient to confirm MI. Hypovolaemic and septic shock can be diagnosed from the clinical context in which they occur. Moreover, in neither condition is the JVP elevated.

## Treatment

### Prophylaxis

Treatment to prevent DVT in patients at risk (see Table 14.1) significantly reduces the incidence of PE. Thus, prophylactic heparin is recommended in patients with acute MI and also in patients undergoing surgery. Subcutaneous heparin 5000 units 8-hourly is effective and in surgical patients should start preoperatively. Other techniques to prevent DVT include electrical stimulation and compression or passive movement of the legs, all of which prevent venous stasis during bed-rest and surgery.

### Minor pulmonary embolism

Initial treatment with oxygen and heparin should be given immediately PE is suspected and should not await the results of diagnostic tests. Heparin prevents extension of thrombosis within the lungs and allows endogenous thrombolysis to proceed uninterrupted; it also guards against recurrent thromboembolism. Following an initial intravenous bolus of 10 000 units, treatment should continue with up to 40 000 units daily in order to keep the partial thromboplastin time at least twice normal. After 7 days, warfarin should be substituted and continued for 3–6 months. The dose is titrated against the prothrombin time, which should be maintained at least twice to three times normal.

### Massive pulmonary embolism

Initial treatment again is with heparin and oxygen. Low-output heart failure requires haemodynamic support with inotropic agents (see p. 88). If recovery is delayed, thrombolytic therapy with streptokinase is recommended to hasten resolution of the embolus. Although streptokinase is often given through a catheter positioned in the pulmonary artery, delivery by a peripheral vein is probably equally effective. A loading dose of 600 000 units is followed by an infusion of 100 000 units/hour. In the shocked patient who fails to respond rapidly to these measures, pulmonary arteriography with a view to embolectomy must be considered, though the mortality is high.

## Prognosis

In minor PE, spontaneous resolution usually occurs and, provided that no further emboli occur, the prognosis is good, albeit dependent on the underlying disorder. In massive PE, sudden death is common. In those patients who survive the acute episode, however, complete resolution of the embolus can be expected, following which prognosis is usually good, depending again on the underlying disorder.

## Non-thrombotic pulmonary embolism

### Air embolism

Major air embolism into the venous circulation is rare. Relatively large volumes (in excess of 50–100 ml) delivered rapidly are required to cause significant haemodynamic disturbance. Air usually gains access through indwelling venous sheaths which do not have haemostatic valves, although, occasionally, faulty intravenous infusion equipment is responsible. In the most severe cases, shock or cardiac arrest occurs; nevertheless, vigorous resuscitation may permit absorption of the air into the bloodstream, following which recovery is possible.

### Fat embolism

This is seen following extensive accidental or surgical bony injury. Marrow fat gains access to the venous circulation and embolizes to the lungs. Presentation is usually after a latent period of 12–36 hours and is due not only to pulmonary vascular obstruction by globules of fat but also to local toxic vasculitis caused by free fatty acid release. Mental confusion and severe cardiopulmonary embarrassment occur and mortality is high.

### Amniotic fluid embolism

This may complicate both normal and Caesarean deliveries. Significant quantities of amniotic fluid leaking into the venous circulation cause massive pulmonary embolism, which is often abruptly fatal. In those patients who survive the acute episode, the subsequent course is complicated by disseminated intravascular coagulation because of the thromboplastic properties of amniotic fluid. Mortality is high.

## Chronic pulmonary embolism

Repeated, often subclinical, episodes of pulmonary thromboembolism may lead to progressive obliteration of the pulmonary vascular tree. This is a chronic process, associated with a slowly rising pulmonary vascular resistance, which provides time for the development of compensatory right ventricular hypertrophy. Pulmonary hypertension is always severe, and right ventricular failure eventually supervenes (see p. 84).

The ECG usually shows evidence of RV hypertrophy with right axis deviation and prominent R waves in leads V1 to V3, which may be

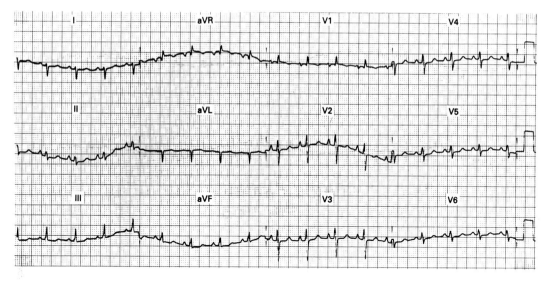

**Fig. 14.3** Chronic pulmonary embolism. The ECG shows P pulmonale, right axis deviation and a dominant R wave in lead V1, associated with T-wave inversion. These are typical features of pulmonary hypertension.

associated with T-wave inversion (Fig. 14.3). The CXR shows cardiac enlargement and considerable dilatation of the proximal pulmonary arteries, although the peripheral lung fields often appear oligaemic (peripheral 'pruning', Fig. 14.4). Nevertheless, these changes are non-specific and occur in other conditions associated with pulmonary hypertension.

By the time the patient presents, the pulmonary vascular disease is usually irreversible and treatment must be directed at preventing further embolic events. Lifelong anticoagulation with warfarin is essential and, in some cases, surgical procedures are undertaken to prevent further embolism from the iliofemoral veins. Ligation or plication of the inferior vena cava has been widely used but the beneficial effects are usually only temporary because, as large venous collaterals open up, thromboembolism continues. More recently, intraluminal filters (introduced into the inferior vena cava by the percutaneous transvenous route) have been used; these filter the blood and remove small emboli without impeding flow. Whether this improves prognosis is uncertain, however, and few patients survive more than 5 years from the time of diagnosis.

## Primary pulmonary hypertension

Primary pulmonary hypertension is an uncommon condition, usually affecting young women. It is characterized pathologically by muscular hypertrophy and intimal hyperplasia of the small pulmonary arteries — the cause of which is, by definition, unknown. Pulmonary hypertension is

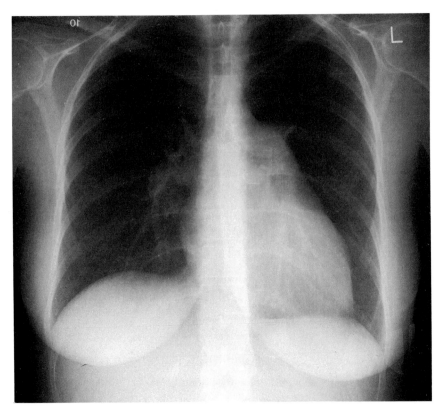

**Fig. 14.4**   Chronic pulmonary embolism. The chest X-ray shows enlargement of the proximal pulmonary arteries and oligaemic lung fields.

unremitting and progressive, resulting in severe hypertrophy of the RV, which eventually dilates and fails. Exertional dyspnoea and fatigue are the predominant symptoms, although up to 50% of patients also complain of exertional chest discomfort. Physical signs are those of severe pulmonary hypertension and include a left parasternal systolic thrust (due to RV hypertrophy) and accentuation of the pulmonary component of the second heart sound, sometimes associated with the early diastolic murmur of pulmonary regurgitation. The ECG and CXR show changes consistent with right ventricular hypertrophy, pulmonary hypertension and pulmonary vascular obstruction, similar to those seen in chronic pulmonary embolism and other causes of pulmonary hypertension (see above). It is essential, therefore, that other potentially treatable conditions, particularly chronic PE, are excluded before the diagnosis of primary pulmonary hypertension is made.

Treatment is usually with vasodilators (e.g. calcium antagonists, beta-2 agonists), most of which have been shown to lower pulmonary artery pressure when given acutely. However, there is no evidence that drugs of this type are of long-term benefit. Indeed, the only treatment of potential long-term value is heart–lung transplantation and, at present, this is only indicated in severely incapacitated patients with end-stage disease.

The prognosis is poor, most patients dying within 10 years of diagnosis. In many cases death is sudden, presumably due to ventricular arrhythmias; the remainder die of progressive right ventricular failure (RVF).

## Pulmonary heart-disease

Pulmonary heart-disease — also called cor pulmonale — is diagnosed when right ventricular hypertrophy and dilatation result from disease of the lungs or pulmonary circulation. Because the basic problem resides in the lungs (or less commonly in the mechanisms of respiratory control), prevention of progressive right heart failure can be achieved only by correction of the pulmonary disorder.

### *Aetiology* (Table 14.2)

Chronic obstructive pulmonary disease caused by bronchitis and emphysema is responsible for the large majority of cases of pulmonary heart-disease. Destruction of the pulmonary vascular bed as a result of alveolar damage and interstitial fibrosis increases the pulmonary vascular resistance. Air trapping and hypoxia exacerbate the process by capillary compression and stimulation of bronchial arteriolar constriction, respectively. These factors combine to produce pulmonary hypertension, which overloads the RV, leading eventually to heart failure.

**Table 14.2**   Causes of pulmonary heart-disease

| | |
|---|---|
| **1** | *Obstructive airways disease* |
| | Bronchitis |
| | Emphysema |
| | Asthma |
| **2** | *Parenchymal lung disease* |
| | Sarcoidosis |
| | Pneumoconiosis |
| | Bronchiectasis |
| **3** | *Neuromuscular and chest wall diseases* |
| | Poliomyelitis |
| | Kyphoscoliosis |
| **4** | *Impaired respiratory drive* |
| | Pickwickian syndrome |
| **5** | *Pulmonary vascular disease* |
| | Primary pulmonary hypertension |
| | Chronic pulmonary embolism |

Pulmonary parenchymal disease due to fibrotic, infective or granulomatous disorders (e.g. pneumoconiosis, bronchiectasis, sarcoidosis) is not often so severe as to cause significant pulmonary hypertension. Obliterative pulmonary vascular disease (e.g. chronic pulmonary embolism), on the other hand, almost invariably leads to pulmonary hypertension and right heart failure.

In certain neuromuscular and chest wall disorders, hypoxaemia, due to inadequate pulmonary ventilation, stimulates pulmonary arteriolar constriction. Increments in pulmonary vascular resistance may be sufficient to cause right heart failure. Impaired respiratory drive — sometimes seen in severe obesity (Pickwickian syndrome) — causes pulmonary heart-disease by a similar mechanism.

## *Pathology*

Pulmonary heart-disease is always the result of chronic (sustained or episodic) pulmonary hypertension. The increase in pulmonary vascular resistance which characterizes pulmonary hypertension is caused either by destructive or obliterative disease of the vascular bed or by pulmonary arteriolar constriction, or both.

The vascular reserve of the pulmonary circulation is considerable. Thus, a threefold increase in cardiac output during exercise causes only a small increase in pulmonary artery pressure; even after pneumonectomy, increments in pulmonary artery pressure during exercise remain small. Therefore, pulmonary disease must be extensive before anatomical reductions in vascular reserve are sufficient to cause pulmonary hypertension. The effects of alveolar hypoxia — a potent stimulus for pulmonary arteriolar constriction — exacerbate anatomical reductions in pulmonary vascular reserve. Indeed, in patients with neuromuscular disorders or diminished respiratory drive, alveolar hypoxia is the primary mechanism.

The interaction between anatomical reductions in pulmonary vascular reserve and hypoxia is important. In patients with chronic bronchitis and emphysema, for example, pulmonary hypertension is usually episodic, coinciding with infective exacerbations of the lung disease. The exacerbations produce alveolar hypoxia, which triggers pulmonary vasoconstriction, unmasking the underlying reduction in pulmonary vascular reserve. Similarly, in other parenchymal lung disorders, superimposed infection is often the trigger for episodes of pulmonary hypertension and right heart failure. Only when the pulmonary vascular reserve is completely exhausted by the destructive effects of the underlying disease do pulmonary hypertension and right heart failure become sustained. The pattern is often different, however, in obliterative pulmonary vascular disease caused by chronic pulmonary embolism. In this, there is an unremitting increase in pulmonary artery pressure, associated with worsening right ventricular hypertrophy as the pulmonary vascular bed becomes progressively obliterated.

An additional factor in the development of pulmonary hypertension is polycythaemia, which occurs in response to chronic hypoxia. The increase in red cell mass increases blood viscosity and pulmonary resistance; nevertheless, only when the haematocrit exceeds 60% does the disadvantage of increased viscosity exceed the benefit of increased oxygen-carrying capacity.

Pulmonary heart-disease exerts its major effects on the RV, which hypertrophies in response to the chronic increase in afterload, leading eventually to ventricular dilatation and contractile failure. Nevertheless, abnormalities of left ventricular (LV) function may also exist, although the cause is not always clear. Occult ischaemia — due to the effects of hypoxaemia and coronary artery disease — may be important in certain cases, while in others hypertrophy and bulging of the interventricular septum interfere with LV filling, particularly when RV hypertrophy and dilatation are severe.

## Clinical manifestations

The typical patient is a middle-aged or elderly man with a long history of winter bronchitis caused by cigarette smoking. Clinical manifestations are those of the underlying respiratory disorder, associated with pulmonary hypertension and right heart failure (RHF). Common complaints are dyspnoea, fatigue, abdominal discomfort (caused by hepatic congestion) and peripheral oedema. The patient is often centrally cyanosed — particularly during exacerbations of obstructive pulmonary disease — and may be jaundiced or clubbed. Carbon dioxide retention produces a bounding pulse (due to peripheral vasodilatation) and, when severe, tremor and clouding of consciousness may occur.

Signs of pulmonary hypertension are usually prominent. These include a left parasternal systolic thrust, due to RV hypertrophy, and a loud pulmonary component of the second heart sound, sometimes associated with the early diastolic murmur of pulmonary regurgitation. Nevertheless, hyperinflation of the lungs may make palpation of the RV impulse difficult and may also muffle the heart sounds. The development of frank RVF produces elevation of the JVP, hepatomegaly and peripheral oedema. Functional tricuspid regurgitation is almost invariable in advanced cases.

## Complications

Complications of pulmonary heart-disease are the same as occur in other cases of right heart failure. They include cardiac arrhythmias, particularly

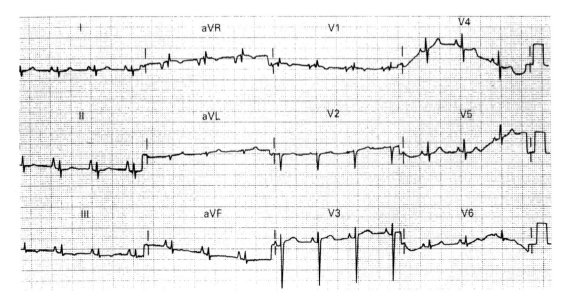

**Fig. 14.5** Pulmonary heart-disease — 12-lead ECG. Note P pulmonale, right axis deviation and the dominant R wave in lead V1, associated with T-wave inversion. The ECG is in all respects similar to that of chronic pulmonary embolism (see Fig. 14.3) and other causes of pulmonary hypertension.

atrial fibrillation (AF) and deep venous and intracardiac thrombosis, which predispose to PE. In end-stage disease, progressive renal and hepatic failure usually occur.

## Diagnosis

Polycythaemia is commonly present but the haematocrit rarely rises above 65%. In obstructive pulmonary disease arterial gas analysis shows hypoxaemia and hypercapnia, with partially compensated respiratory acidosis. Respiratory function tests confirm an obstructive defect, although in other causes of pulmonary heart-disease a restrictive defect may be more prominent. The ECG shows signs suggestive of right ventricular hypertrophy, including dominant R waves in leads V1 and V2 (see Fig. 2.12), P pulmonale and right axis deviation, sometimes associated with right bundle branch block (Fig. 14.5). The CXR shows an enlarged heart and, on the lateral film, obliteration of the retrosternal space indicates dilatation of the RV. The proximal pulmonary arteries are prominent and, in advanced pulmonary hypertension, attenuation ('pruning') of the peripheral vessels may be present. The echocardiogram confirms dilatation of the right-sided cardiac chambers.

## Differential diagnosis

Pulmonary heart-disease must be differentiated from other causes of right heart failure, including left ventricular failure (LVF), mitral valve disease, cardiomyopathy, pulmonary and tricuspid valve disease and constrictive pericarditis. In these conditions, however, signs of pulmonary hypertension, if present, are rarely as marked as those that characterize pulmonary heart-disease. Indeed, only in mitral stenosis is the severity of pulmonary hypertension sometimes comparable. The echocardiogram, however, is diagnostic of mitral stenosis; it also identifies right-sided valvular disease and LV impairment in patients with congestive heart failure and cardiomyopathy.

## Treatment

Treatment is directed towards the underlying pulmonary disease as well as RVF.

### Pulmonary disease

In patients with pulmonary heart-disease caused by chronic bronchitis and emphysema, presentation is usually with an acute exacerbation which precipitates RVF. Treatment with antibiotics, bronchodilators, inhaled oxygen and physiotherapy is directed at resolving the exacerbation and lowering pulmonary artery pressure in order to correct RVF. Prophylaxis is by prompt antibiotic therapy at the first sign of a chest infection and encouragement to stop cigarette smoking.

Measures directed at controlling progressive disease in other causes of pulmonary hypertension include antibiotics and physiotherapy in bronchiectasis, steroid therapy in asthma and advanced pulmonary sarcoidosis, anticoagulant therapy in chronic pulmonary embolism and weight reduction in severe obesity.

### Right ventricular failure

Diuretic therapy is usually effective for controlling peripheral oedema and visceral congestion. Moreover, by reducing right ventricular volume, diuretics may correct functional tricuspid regurgitation and increase cardiac output. Generally speaking, however, significant improvements in RV function can be achieved only by inotropic stimulation or reductions in afterload. Inotropic therapy (e.g. intravenous dobutamine) is certainly of value in acute exacerbations of RVF associated with severe low-output states. In chronic RVF, however, there are no orally active inotropic agents of value for long-term outpatient management, although digitalis plays an important role in patients with AF.

Afterload reduction in pulmonary heart-disease requires effective pulmonary arteriolar dilatation. Drugs such as hydralazine and calcium antagonists reduce pulmonary vascular resistance and improve cardiac output acutely. In some patients, significant symptomatic improvement occurs but, in the majority, sustained benefit during long-term therapy is difficult to demonstrate. Continuous oxygen therapy is of greater value for afterload reduction in pulmonary heart-disease. For domiciliary management, oxygen is conveniently delivered by nasal catheters at a flow rate of 2 litres/min. If an arterial oxygen tension of at least 8 kPa (60 mmHg) can be achieved and sustained for 15 hours/day, pulmonary vascular resistance will usually fall. The improvement is often sustained and has been associated with a significant mortality reduction in patients with advanced pulmonary heart-disease.

Oxygen therapy also provides the most effective means of reducing haematocrit. The associated reduction in blood viscosity lowers pulmonary vascular resistance and improves RV function. In patients for whom continuous oxygen therapy is inappropriate (advanced age, continued cigarette smoking), polycythaemia can be treated by regular venesection, which is only necessary, however, for haematocrit values above 65% because, at this level, the effect on pulmonary vascular resistance and the risk of intravascular thrombosis become excessive.

The role of lung transplantation for correcting pulmonary hypertension in end-stage pulmonary heart-disease is now receiving attention, but at present the long-term result is not satisfactory.

## Prognosis

In pulmonary heart-disease, prognosis is poor once RVF develops. Following the first episode of RVF in patients with chronic bronchitis, survival beyond 5 years is unusual.

## Further reading

Anonymous. Surgery for pulmonary emboli? *Lancet* 1989, **i**, 198.

Goldhaber S.Z., Meyerovitz M.F., Markis J.E. *et al.* Thrombolytic therapy of acute pulmonary embolism: current status and future potential. *J. Am. Coll. Cardiol.* 1987, **10** (suppl. B), 96–104.

Hall R.J.C. and Haworth S.G. Disorders of the pulmonary circulation. In Julian D.G., Camm A.J., Fox K.M., Hall R.J.C. and Poole-Wilson P.A. (eds), *Diseases of the Heart*. London, Baillière Tindall, 1989, pp. 1293–328.

Moser K.M., Auger W.R. and Fedullo P.F. Chronic major vessel thromboembolic pulmonary hypertension. *Circulation* 1990, **81**, 1735–43.

Peacock A. Pulmonary hypertension due to chronic hypoxia. *Br. Med. J.* 1990, **300**, 763.

Rich S. and Brundage B.H. Pulmonary hypertension: a cellular basis for understanding the pathophysiology and treatment. *J. Am. Coll. Cardiol.* 1989, **14**, 545–50.

Uren N.G. and Oakley C.M. The treatment of primary pulmonary hypertension. *Br. Heart J.* 1991, **66**, 119–21.

# 15 Congenital Heart-disease

## Summary

Congenital heart-disease affects 0.8% of live-born babies, 70% of whom die by the age of 5. Genetic factors can be identified in less than 1% of cases, and in the remainder environmental factors are assumed to play an important role. Echo–Doppler techniques now permit non-invasive diagnosis of nearly all congenital cardiac defects.

*Anomalies of septation*   *Ventricular septal defect* is the most common anomaly at birth although 40% close spontaneously. Blood shunts from left to right across the defect into the low-resistance pulmonary circulation causing a pansystolic murmur and palpable thrill. It may present in infancy with heart failure or later in life if complicated by obliterative pulmonary vascular disease and Eisenmenger's syndrome — pulmonary hypertension and right-to-left shunting with central cyanosis and clubbing. Very small defects remain asymptomatic and are compatible with a normal lifespan. Surgery should be offered if the pulmonary–systemic flow ratio is more than 2:1 but, in established Eisenmenger's syndrome, heart–lung transplantation is the only option. *Atrial septal defect* is usually caused by the 'secundum' defect of the oval fossa. The left-to-right shunt causes fixed splitting of S2 and a pulmonary flow murmur. Presentation is usually in adulthood with either atrial fibrillation and right ventricular failure or Eisenmenger's syndrome, depending on whether or not obliterative pulmonary vascular disease develops. Surgery is recommended if the pulmonary–systemic flow ratio is more than 2:1. In *patent ductus arteriosus*, the aortopulmonary shunt causes a continuous murmur. Large shunts may cause heart failure in infancy or lead to Eisenmenger's syndrome in later life, but in many cases it remains asymptomatic.

*Anomalies of the atrioventricular junction*   These include *Ebstein's anomaly* (downward displacement of the tricuspid valve with tricuspid regurgitation and right atrial enlargement), *tricuspid atresia* (absent right atrioventricular connection such that pulmonary flow becomes dependent on shunting through associated septal defects), *hypoplastic left heart syndrome* (complete absence of left atrioventricular connection) and various *abnormalities of atrial situs*.

*Anomalies of the ventriculoarterial junction* *Aortic stenosis*, caused by a bicuspid valve, may present with heart failure in infancy, but more commonly stenosis remains insignificant until middle age, when calcification of the valve occurs. Treatment is surgical. *Pulmonary stenosis* is a common anomaly and, if severe, can be treated by balloon valvuloplasty. In *Fallot's tetralogy*, subvalvular pulmonary outflow obstruction is associated with ventricular septal defect, overriding of the aorta and right ventricular (RV) hypertrophy. If outflow obstruction is severe, right-to-left shunting ensures cyanosis at birth, but in other cases progressive obstruction usually leads to cyanosis in childhood. Palliative surgery is directed at improving pulmonary flow, pending total correction in later life. *Transposition of the great arteries*, in which the aorta arises from the morphological RV and the pulmonary artery from the morphological left ventricle (LV), results in parallel systemic and pulmonary circulations. Survival depends on associated septal defects allowing mixing of arterial and venous blood and, if these are not present, the creation of an atrial septal defect by the emergency Rashkind procedure is potentially life-saving. *Coarctation of the aorta* is a fibrotic narrowing just beyond the left subclavian branch, close to the ductus arteriosus. It may cause heart failure in infancy but more commonly remains asymptomatic, as compensatory LV hypertrophy and collaterals around the coarctation combine to preserve haemodynamic stability. Examination reveals radiofemoral pulse delay and hypertension in the arms. Presentation is commonly before the age of 40 with left ventricular failure (LVF) or sudden death, caused by stroke, aortic dissection or arrhythmias.

## Introduction

Cardiac defects are the most common of all major congenital abnormalities (Table 15.1). About eight in every thousand babies born alive have con-

**Table 15.1** Prevalence of congenital heart-disease

| Live-born babies | Adults |
| --- | --- |
| Ventricular septal defect | Atrial septal defect (secundum) |
| Patent ductus arteriosus | Aortic stenosis |
| Pulmonary stenosis | Pulmonary stenosis |
| Atrial septal defect (secundum) | Patent ductus arteriosus |
| Tetralogy of Fallot | Coarctation |
| Aortic stenosis | Tetralogy of Fallot |
| Coarctation of the aorta | Congenital complete heart block |
| Atrial septal defect (primum) | Situs inversus |
| Complete transposition | Corrected transposition |
| Univentricular heart | Ebstein's anomaly |

**Table 15.2**  Aetiology of congenital heart-disease

---

**Genetic factors**

*Chromosomal abnormalities*
| | |
|---|---|
| Trisomy 21 (Down's syndrome) | — ASD, VSD, Fallot's tetralogy |
| XO (Turner's syndrome) | — VSD, PDA, pulmonary stenosis |
| XXXY | — PDA, ASD |

*Single-gene disorders*
| | |
|---|---|
| Autosomal dominant | — ASD (secundum), hypertrophic cardiomyopathy, mitral valve prolapse |
| Autosomal recessive | — ASD (primum) |

*Congenital syndromes*
Autosomal dominant
| | |
|---|---|
| Marfan | — Aortic and mitral regurgitation |
| Leopard | — Pulmonary stenosis, hypertrophic cardiomyopathy |
| Holt–Oram | — ASD, VSD |
| Romano–Ward | — Prolonged QT interval |

Autosomal recessive
| | |
|---|---|
| Osteogenesis imperfecta | — Aortic regurgitation |
| Pseudoxanthoma elasticum | — Mitral regurgitation |
| Lawrence–Moon–Biedl | — VSD |

**Environmental factors**

*Viral infection*
| | |
|---|---|
| Rubella | — PDA, pulmonary stenosis, ASD |

*Drugs*
| | |
|---|---|
| Alcohol | — ASD, PDA |
| Trimethadione | — Complete transposition, Fallot's tetralogy |
| Lithium | — Ebstein's anomaly, ASD |
| Amphetamines | — VSD, PDA, complete transposition |

---

ASD — atrial septal defect; PDA — patent ductus arteriosus; VSD — ventricular septal defect.

genital heart-disease — a figure that excludes non-stenotic bicuspid aortic valve and mitral valve prolapse. Untreated, the mortality is high, and, by the age of 5, 70% of affected children are dead. Those who survive have less severe cardiac lesions but few live beyond the age of 40.

## Aetiology

The aetiology of congenital heart-disease is complex and poorly understood (Table 15.2). Genetic factors can be identified in less than 1% of cases, cardiac disorders occurring in a number of congenital syndromes and also exhibiting a variable association with recognizable chromosomal abnormalities, ranging from over 90% in trisomy to between 18% and 35% in Turner's syndrome. Single-gene disorders account for the familial incidence of certain isolated cardiac defects but, in most cases, the siblings or children of patients with congenital heart-disease have only a slightly increased risk of being affected. Moreover, concordance for con-

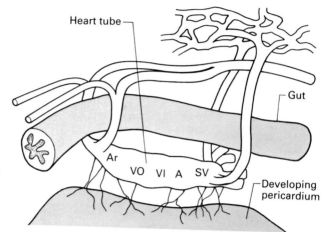

**Fig. 15.1** The embryonic heart tube. SV — sinus venosus; A — atrium; VI — ventricular inlet; VO — ventricular outlet; Ar — arterial segment (adapted from Anderson R.H. and Becker A.E. *Cardiac Anatomy*. London, Gower Medical Publishing, 1980).

genital cardiac defects is unusual in monozygotic twins. Thus, environmental factors are likely to play an important role. Environmental factors known to influence development of the heart during early pregnancy include maternal rubella and certain drugs.

## *Embryology of the heart*

Two endothelial tubes run in the belly of the developing embryo and fuse in the neck region to form the single heart tube. Venous inflow and arterial outflow are at the caudal and cephalic ends of the heart tube, respectively. Serial constrictions in the heart tube divide it into five segments: sinus venosus, atrium, ventricular inlet component, ventricular outlet component and arterial segment (Fig. 15.1). During the fourth week of gestation, complex looping of the heart tube provides the basis of adult cardiac structure, with the ventricle lying in front of and beneath the atrium, and the outflow component of the ventricle lying beside the inflow component, closely related to the atrium. The four-chamber arrangement requires separation and septation of the atrial and ventricular components and division of the arterial segment into aorta and pulmonary artery. This occurs during the fifth and sixth weeks of gestation and is the process most prone to aberrant development. By the end of the eighth week, cardiovascular development is complete and no further change takes place until birth.

## *Circulatory changes at birth*

In the fetus, gas exchange takes place at the placenta, which receives desaturated blood from the umbilical arteries and returns saturated blood to the fetal vena cava via the umbilical vein and the ductus venosus (Fig. 15.2). Vascular resistance in the fetal pulmonary circulation is consider-

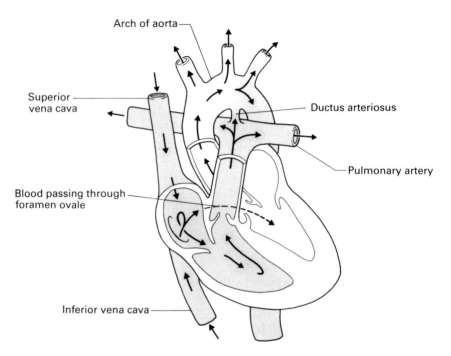

Arch of aorta

Superior
vena cava

Ductus arteriosus

Pulmonary artery

Blood passing through
foramen ovale

Inferior vena cava

**Fig. 15.2**   The fetal circulation (adapted from Beck F., Moffat D.B. and Davies D.P., *Human Embryology*. Oxford, Blackwell Scientific Publications, 1985).

ably higher than in the systemic and placental circulations. Thus, much of the saturated vena-caval blood which returns to the right side of the fetal heart bypasses the lung, by shunting directly into the low-resistance systemic circulation. Shunting occurs through the valve-like oval fossa in the atrial septum or through the ductus arteriosus, which joins the main pulmonary trunk to the aorta. Fetal survival is not threatened by cardiac defects so long as one or other side of the heart can drive saturated blood from the great veins into the systemic circulation.

At birth the lungs take over the role of gas exchange. Clamping of the umbilical cord deprives the systemic circulation of the low-resistance placental circuit. Systemic resistance rises and shunting through the oval fossa and the ductus arteriosus falls abruptly. Substantial increments in pulmonary flow therefore occur, facilitated by the reduction in pulmonary resistance that coincides with inflation of the lungs. The delivery of saturated blood into the proximal aorta and the effects of local prostaglandins stimulate constriction of the ductus arteriosus. In mature babies, closure is usually complete within 12 hours of birth, but prematurity may delay closure.

## Clinical manifestations

### Heart failure

Heart failure in the neonatal period is a medical emergency and may be caused by almost any major cardiac defect. In the preterm baby, heart failure is usually the result of a persistent ductus arteriosus; in the mature baby the major causes of heart failure are large left-to-right shunts, obstructive left-sided lesions, myocardial disease and arrhythmias. Generally speaking, left-to-right shunts do not present until after the first week of life, when shunting peaks as pulmonary vascular resistance declines to its lowest level.

The clinical manifestations of heart failure in the infant result from pulmonary and systemic congestion and reductions in cardiac output, in the same way as in the adult. The infant is pale and breathless with a cool skin, dyspnoea and rapid tachycardia (160–190 beats/min). The blood-pressure is often low and a gallop rhythm is audible. The liver is usually palpable but peripheral oedema is rare. Poor feeding and failure to thrive are invariable.

Treatment is with rest in an oxygen tent, with careful temperature and humidity control. Diuretics and, occasionally, inotropic agents may be necessary, but definitive surgical treatment, if feasible, should not be delayed.

### Cyanosis

Central cyanosis occurs in severe pulmonary oedema and also when there is significant mixing of venous and arterial blood, caused either by a right-to-left shunt or by other lesions which produce inadequate separation of the right and left sides of the heart (e.g. single ventricle and solitary arterial trunk). Complete transposition of the great arteries, in which there are two separate and parallel circulations, causes cyanosis at birth.

### Squatting

Children with cyanotic heart-disease, particularly Fallot's tetralogy, commonly squat following exertion. This tends to improve arterial oxygen saturation by increasing systemic vascular resistance, which reduces right-to-left shunting through septal defects. Squatting also increases venous return to the right side of the heart, improving pulmonary flow.

### Clubbing and polycythaemia

Cyanotic congenital heart-disease is nearly always associated with the development of digital clubbing and polycythaemia, though neither is present at birth. The cause of clubbing is unknown, but polycythaemia is a physiological response to arterial desaturation, directed at maintaining systemic oxygen delivery. In severe polycythaemia (more than 20 g/100 ml), venesection is often recommended, particularly in patients with heart failure or venous thrombosis. Venesection reduces blood viscosity and improves peripheral flow.

## Pulmonary hypertension

Left-to-right intracardiac shunts (e.g. septal defects and persistent ductus arteriosus) inevitably increase pulmonary flow. In certain patients — depending largely on the size of the shunt — this causes obliterative changes in the pulmonary arterioles, characterized by intimal proliferation, hyalinization and fibrosis. Once established, these changes are not reversible. Obliterative disease produces progressive increments in pulmonary vascular resistance. Pulmonary artery pressure rises, leading to reductions in left-to-right intracardiac shunting. Eventually, the pressures in the pulmonary and systemic circulations equilibrate and shunting becomes negligible or even reverses.

The time course of obliterative pulmonary vascular disease in patients with left-to-right intracardiac shunts is very variable, but it usually occurs

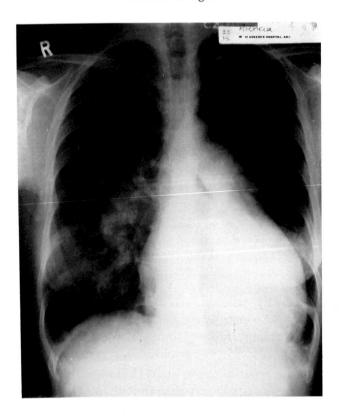

**Fig. 15.3**  Eisenmenger's syndrome — chest X-ray. Note the massive dilatation of the proximal pulmonary arteries and the relative paucity of vessels in the peripheral lung fields (pruning).

in infancy. It may be delayed until adulthood, however, or may never occur at all, particularly when the shunt is very small.

The syndrome of severe pulmonary hypertension and cyanosis in patients with septal defects or patent ductus arteriosus is called Eisenmenger's syndrome. Clinical manifestations reflect the specific cardiac lesion and, in addition, the patient is cyanosed (due to reduced pulmonary flow and venous/arterial mixing through the defect), with polycythaemia and clubbing. Signs of pulmonary hypertension are always prominent, and include a left parasternal systolic thrust, due to RV hypertrophy, and a loud pulmonary component of the second heart sound, often associated with the early diastolic murmur of pulmonary regurgitation. The development of right ventricular failure produces elevation of the jugular venous pulse (JVP), with hepatomegaly and peripheral oedema. Functional tricuspid regurgitation is almost invariable. The electrocardiogram (ECG) shows RV hypertrophy. The chest X-ray (CXR) shows an enlarged heart, with prominence of the proximal pulmonary arteries and attenuation ('pruning') of the peripheral vessels (Fig. 15.3).

Because the obliterative pulmonary vascular changes are irreversible, surgical correction of the congenital cardiac defect does not relieve pulmonary hypertension and right ventricular failure (RVF) (cf. mitral stenosis, p. 186). Thus, diuretics and oxygen provide the only means of treatment, short of total heart–lung transplantation, and death by the age of 40 usually occurs.

### Failure to thrive

Babies with congenital heart-disease often fail to thrive normally. In older children, growth and physical development may be impaired, particularly in cyanotic heart-disease, unlike mental development, which is usually normal. The mechanisms responsible for growth impairment are likely to be complex but include anorexia, chronic heart failure, hypoxaemia and recurrent chest infections.

### Other clinical manifestations

Angina is unusual in congenital heart-disease but may occur in severe aortic stenosis or pulmonary hypertension, due to left or right ventricular hypertrophy, respectively. Coronary artery anomalies — such as anomalous origin from the pulmonary artery — may also cause angina.

Syncope and sudden death in congenital heart-disease are usually caused by cardiac arrhythmias in conditions such as severe aortic stenosis, Eisenmenger's syndrome and hypertrophic cardiomyopathy. Congenital atrioventricular (AV) heart block (see p. 219) rarely causes symptoms, but heart block complicating cardiac surgical procedures is more ominous and always requires pacemaker therapy to prevent Stokes–Adams attacks and sudden death.

## Intracardiac shunts

### Atrial septal defect (ASD)

#### Pathology

Communications between the atria may be caused by sinus venosus defects high in the septum or 'primum' defects low in the septum, which are often associated with anomalous pulmonary venous drainage and mitral valve abnormalities, respectively. Nevertheless, the most common ASD is the 'secundum' defect of the oval fossa. Blood shunts preferentially from left to right into the low-resistance pulmonary circulation, and the ratio of pulmonary to systemic flow (the shunt ratio) often exceeds 2:1. Increased pulmonary flow predisposes to obliterative pulmonary vascular disease.

#### Clinical manifestations

ASD often remains asymptomatic, at least until middle age, when presentation is usually with atrial fibrillation and symptoms of mild heart failure, particularly dyspnoea and fatigue. In some cases the chronic increase in pulmonary flow leads to obliterative pulmonary vascular disease and Eisenmenger's syndrome. The cardinal physical signs are fixed splitting of the second heart sound (see Fig. 1.9) and a mid-systolic murmur at the pulmonary area, due to increased flow through the valve. When the left-to-right shunt is large, a mid-diastolic tricuspid flow murmur may also be present. The primum type of defect is often associated with an apical pansystolic murmur and other signs of mitral regurgitation.

#### Complications

Atrial fibrillation (AF) commonly complicates ASD. The major complication, however, is severe pulmonary hypertension leading to RVF which affects some patients with large shunts. Infective endocarditis is rare except in the primum type of defect, when infection of the mitral valve may occur. Nevertheless, antibiotic prophylaxis is recommended prior to dental surgery and other invasive non-sterile procedures.

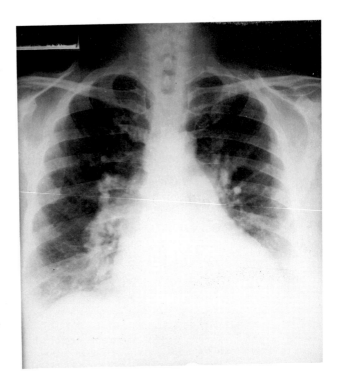

**Fig. 15.4** Atrial septal defect — chest X-ray. Note the cardiac enlargement, the dilatation of the proximal pulmonary arteries and the plethoric lung fields.

## Diagnosis

The ECG shows left axis deviation in primum ASD but, in the more common secundum defect, the axis is usually to the right. An rSR' pattern is often seen in lead V1, due to partial or complete right bundle branch block. The CXR shows cardiac enlargement, with dilatation of the proximal pulmonary arteries and plethoric lung fields, reflecting increased pulmonary flow (Fig. 15.4), which disappears as obliterative pulmonary vascular disease develops. Echocardiography shows dilatation of the right-sided cardiac chambers, but the defect cannot always be imaged directly, although echo-contrast techniques may be helpful (Fig. 15.5). Doppler studies are more helpful, and colour flow imaging permits visualization of the left-to-right shunt across the atrial septum.

Cardiac catheterization confirms the diagnosis. Serial measurements of oxygen saturation in the vena cava, right-sided cardiac chambers and pulmonary artery show an abrupt 'step-up' at right atrial level, due to shunting of oxygenated blood through the defect (see Table 3.1). The catheter can be directed across the defect into the left atrium. Measurements of pulmonary and systemic flow, using the Fick principle, permit quantification of the shunt ratio. When a high oxygen saturation is found in the superior vena cava or when the catheter enters a pulmonary vein directly from the high right atrium, a sinus venosus defect with anomalous

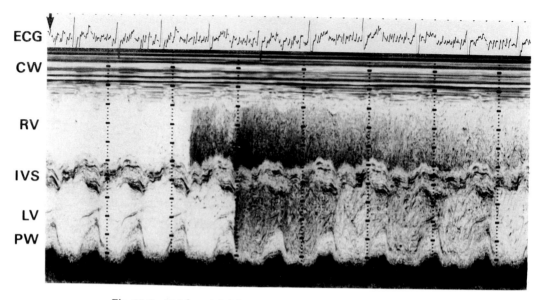

**Fig. 15.5**   Atrial septal defect — contrast echocardiography. Hand-agitated saline solution has been injected into a peripheral vein at the time indicated by the arrow. Bubble contrast appears first in the right side of the heart. Opacification of the left side of the heart is also seen due to passage of bubbles through an atrial septal defect. Note the relative dilatation of the right ventricle compared with the left ventricle.

pulmonary venous drainage is the likely diagnosis. The demonstration of mitral regurgitation during LV angiography, on the other hand, suggests a primum defect.

**Differential diagnosis**

The flow murmurs that characterize ASD must be differentiated from those that occur in organic pulmonary and tricuspid stenosis. In neither of these conditions, however, is there fixed splitting of the second heart sound. Echocardiography confirms the valvular abnormalities.

## Treatment

The risk of pulmonary hypertension and Eisenmenger's syndrome demands surgical correction if the shunt ratio is more than 2:1. In secundum and sinus venosus defects, the procedure has a very low mortality (less than 0.1%), but correction of primum defects is more complex because of the associated mitral valve abnormalities. In established Eisenmenger's syndrome, pulmonary hypertension is irreversible and closure of the defect is unhelpful. At this stage, heart–lung transplantation is the only surgical option.

## Prognosis

Obliterative pulmonary vascular disease in infancy is incompatible with survival beyond middle age. In other cases, life expectancy may be normal if the shunt is small, but larger shunts (more than 2:1) usually lead to RVF and death by the age of 60, unless the defect is closed.

# Ventricular septal defect (VSD)

## Pathology

VSD is the most common congenital cardiac anomaly. Defects usually occur in the perimembranous septum but may also occur lower, in the muscular septum. Blood shunts preferentially from left to right unless there is obstruction to pulmonary flow (e.g. Fallot's tetralogy). About 40% of defects close spontaneously in early childhood but, in those that remain patent, the chronic increase in pulmonary flow predisposes to obliterative pulmonary vascular disease and Eisenmenger's syndrome.

## Clinical manifestations

If the shunt is large, it may cause heart failure in infancy. This is usually delayed until pulmonary vascular resistance has fallen to its nadir after the first week of life and shunting is at its peak. Smaller shunts may remain asymptomatic until adulthood, when fatigue and shortness of breath are common. These symptoms are accentuated by the development of obliterative pulmonary vascular disease. Examination reveals cardiac enlargement, with a prominent LV impulse. A systolic thrill at the lower left sternal edge can often be felt in association with a pansystolic murmur at the same location. Signs of pulmonary hypertension develop in patients with obliterative pulmonary vascular disease.

## Complications

Recirculation of blood through the pulmonary bed volume-loads the LV and predisposes to LV failure, depending on the size of the shunt. The chronic increase in pulmonary flow may lead to Eisenmenger's syndrome in infancy or, less commonly, in adulthood. There is a significant (approximately 4%) risk of endocarditis in patients with VSD. The risk is unaffected by surgical closure of the defect but abolished by spontaneous closure. Antibiotic prophylaxis against endocarditis is essential in all patients.

## Diagnosis

The ECG and CXR may be normal if the defect is small. Larger defects produce LV hypertrophy and cardiomegaly with pulmonary plethora caused by increased pulmonary flow. The echocardiogram is diagnostic if the defect can be imaged, and Doppler studies identify the abnormal flow across the septum. Cardiac catheterization confirms the diagnosis. There is a step-up in oxygen saturation at RV level (see Table 3.1), and LV angiography produces prompt opacification of the RV through the defect.

## Treatment

VSD requires urgent repair if it causes heart failure in infancy. In asymptomatic cases, conservative management is usually appropriate but, if signs of pulmonary hypertension develop during follow-up, cardiac catheterization is required with a view to closure. In established Eisenmenger's syndrome, closure of the defect is unhelpful and total heart–lung transplantation is the only option.

## Prognosis

When spontaneous closure of a VSD occurs in infancy, life expectancy is normal. Persistent small defects (maladie de Roger) are consistent with a normal lifespan, but larger defects may produce heart failure and death in infancy or lead to Eisenmenger's syndrome with death by middle age.

# Extracardiac shunts

## Patent ductus arteriosus (PDA)

### Pathology

In the fetus, the ductus arteriosus joins the main pulmonary trunk to the aorta. Persistent patency after birth is common in premature infants because normal mechanisms for its closure (see p. 300) are not developed. Persistent patency in the full-term baby may be caused by relative hypoxaemia (high altitude, pulmonary disease, cyanotic heart-disease), which delays normal closure. In other cases, persistent patency of the ductus arteriosus is properly regarded as a congenital defect. It occurs more commonly in females and is sometimes a complication of first-trimester rubella. Blood shunts from left to right across the defect into the low-resistance pulmonary circulation, increasing pulmonary flow and volume-loading the left side of the heart. Large shunts may cause heart failure in infancy or lead to obliterative pulmonary vascular disease and Eisenmenger's syndrome.

## Clinical manifestations

In the premature infant, patency of the ductus arteriosus commonly causes heart failure, which exacerbates the respiratory distress of hyaline membrane disease. Apnoeic episodes and respirator dependency are common. Heart failure may also occur in the full-term infant but in many cases the condition remains asymptomatic. Examination reveals a collapsing carotid pulse due to diastolic shunting through the ductus, and a continuous 'machinery' murmur is audible at the upper left sternal edge, caused by turbulent flow through the ductus, which occurs throughout the cardiac cycle. The murmur is loudest at end-systole/early diastole when flow is greatest.

## Complications

When the shunt is large, PDA may cause heart failure in infancy or obliterative pulmonary vascular disease and Eisenmenger's syndrome. Even with a small shunt there is a risk of infective endocarditis.

## Diagnosis

The CXR is often normal but may show cardiac enlargement and pulmonary plethora if the shunt is large, and, in adults, calcification of the ductus arteriosus may be visible (Fig. 15.6). The echocardiogram shows dilatation of the left-sided cardiac chambers, and Doppler studies identify the abnormal flow across the ductus. At cardiac catheterization, serial blood sampling (see Table 3.1) shows a step-up in oxygen saturation at pulmonary artery level; the catheter can often be passed across the ductus into the descending thoracic aorta.

### Differential diagnosis

The collapsing pulse and early diastolic accentuation of the murmur may cause confusion with aortic regurgitation. Echocardiography and Doppler studies are helpful and cardiac catheterization confirms the diagnosis.

## Treatment

PDA always requires closure, regardless of the size of the shunt. It is a low-risk procedure and guards against the development of complications, particularly endocarditis. In the premature infant, prostaglandin inhibitors

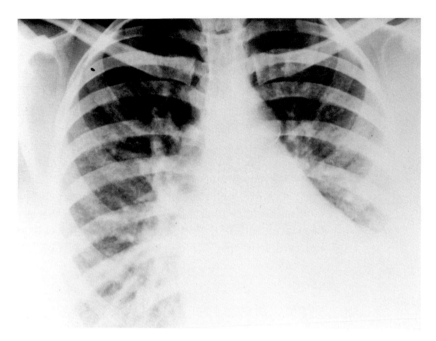

**Fig. 15.6** Patent ductus arteriosus — chest X-ray. A thin line of calcification is seen just below the aortic knuckle. This is the 'comma' sign and represents a calcified ductus arteriosus. Cardiomegaly and pulmonary plethora indicate that the shunt is large.

(e.g. indomethacin) may be effective, but in the full-term infant surgical closure is required. In the absence of symptoms, however, this may be delayed until school age, when the risk is very low. Recently, catheterization techniques have been developed which permit closure of the defect by an intraluminal obstructor device, thereby avoiding the small risk of surgery.

## Prognosis

If the shunt is large, it leads to premature death, caused either by heart failure in infancy or obliterative pulmonary vascular disease. A small shunt is consistent with a normal lifespan.

## Anomalies of the atrioventricular junction

### Ebstein's anomaly

#### Pathology

Displacement of the septal attachment of the tricuspid valve towards the cardiac apex causes a variable increase in the size of the right atrium at the expense of the right ventricle. Tricuspid regurgitation is almost invariable and exacerbates the tendency to RV failure. In over 50% of cases, there is an ASD and, because right atrial pressure is elevated, shunting may be from right to left. This produces cyanosis, particularly in the new-born, when pulmonary vascular resistance is at its height. As pulmonary resistance falls, however, shunting decreases and cyanosis often disappears.

## Clinical manifestations

Ebstein's anomaly may present with heart failure and cyanosis at birth. In many cases, however, symptoms develop insidiously over several years, as RV function deteriorates: the patient complains of fatigue and dyspnoea, and examination reveals signs of tricuspid regurgitation.

## Complications

Life-threatening cardiac arrhythmias are common and right ventricular failure almost invariable.

## Diagnosis

The ECG characteristically shows right bundle branch block and signs of right atrial enlargement (P pulmonale). The echocardiogram is diagnostic, showing right atrial enlargement and displacement of the septal attachment of the tricuspid valve towards the cardiac apex (Fig. 15.7).

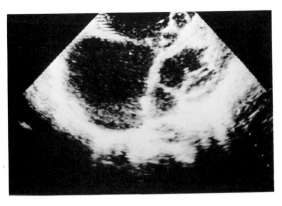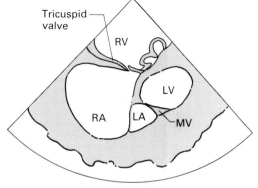

**Fig. 15.7** Ebstein's anomaly. This two-dimensional echocardiogram (apical four-chamber view) shows displacement of the septal attachment of the tricuspid valve towards the cardiac apex, associated with massive dilatation of the right atrium. These findings are diagnostic of Ebstein's anomaly.

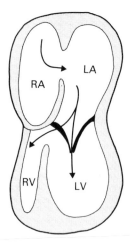

Fig. 15.8   Tricuspid atresia.

## Prognosis

Sudden death may occur in patients with ventricular arrhythmias. The development of RVF rarely permits survival beyond middle age.

### Tricuspid atresia

Tricuspid atresia is characterized by complete absence of the right atrio-ventricular connection (Fig. 15.8). An atrial septal defect is invariable and right atrial outflow is into the left atrium across the defect. A VSD is also invariable and pulmonary flow depends on the degree of shunting into the diminutive right ventricle. Infants with tricuspid atresia have severe heart failure and are always cyanosed because of obligatory mixing of systemic and pulmonary venous blood in the left atrium; pulmonary flow is reduced, intensifying cyanosis.

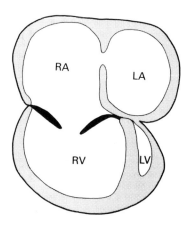

Fig. 15.9   Hypoplastic left heart syndrome.

The ECG shows right atrial enlargement and LV hypertrophy (an unusual combination of features) with left axis deviation (see Chapter 2). The CXR shows diminished pulmonary vascular markings and a small main pulmonary artery. Echocardiography confirms a small right ventricle, a large left ventricle and absence of the tricuspid valve.

Emergency surgery in infancy may be life-saving. An aortopulmonary shunt increases pulmonary flow and provides useful palliation; definitive repair, however, is by the Fontan procedure, performed when the child is older. A valved conduit is placed between the right atrium and the pulmonary artery and the atrial septal defect is closed. This establishes flow of desaturated systemic venous blood from the right atrium into the pulmonary circulation and permits survival to adulthood.

## Hypoplastic left heart syndrome

Hypoplastic left heart syndrome is characterized by complete absence of the left atrioventricular connection (Fig. 15.9). Saturated pulmonary venous blood enters the left atrium and passes across a patent foramen ovale into the right atrium, where it mixes with systemic venous blood. The RV drives flow through the pulmonary circulation and also the systemic circulation by a patent ductus arteriosus. The echocardiogram is diagnostic, showing absence of the mitral valve and a diminutive left ventricle and aortic root. The affected baby is cyanosed and usually dies when the ductus arteriosus constricts shortly after birth. There is no effective treatment.

## Atrial situs and dextrocardia

There are always two recognizable atrial chambers, which show four possible arrangements (Fig. 15.10). The normal right–left arrangement (solitus) may be mirror-imaged (inversus). Alternatively, two morphologically right or two morphologically left atria may be present (isomerism). In general, the atrial situs may be inferred from the visceral situs. Thus, if the CXR shows a left-sided stomach bubble, the atrial situs is likely to be solitus. If the visceral arrangement is mirror-imaged, on the other hand, the atrial situs is likely to be inversus.

The AV connection may be concordant or discordant, depending on whether the atria are connected to their morphologically appropriate ventricles (Fig. 15.10). Thus, if the atrial situs is inversus and the atrioventricular connections remain concordant, there exists the anatomical basis for dextrocardia (right-sided heart), which is compatible with a normal circulation. However, when dextrocardia occurs with situs solitus (or atrial isomerism), the atrioventricular connections cannot be concordant and survival depends on the coexistence of other anomalies.

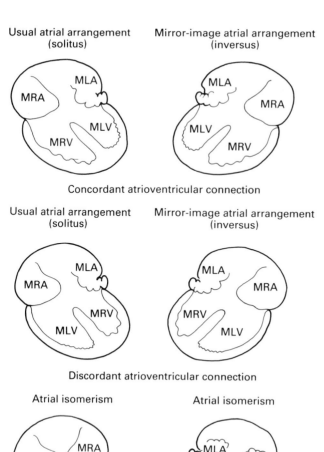

Usual atrial arrangement (solitus)

Mirror-image atrial arrangement (inversus)

Concordant atrioventricular connection

Usual atrial arrangement (solitus)

Mirror-image atrial arrangement (inversus)

Discordant atrioventricular connection

Atrial isomerism

Atrial isomerism

Discordant atrioventricular connection

**Fig. 15.10** Atrial situs and the atrioventricular connections. (Reproduced with permission from Anderson R.H. and Ho S.Y. The diagnosis and naming of congenitally malformed hearts. In Macartney F.J. (ed.) *Congenital Heart Disease*. Lancaster, MTP Press Ltd., 1986.) MLA = morphological left atrium, MRA = morphological right atrium, MLV = morphological left ventricle, MRV = morphological right ventricle.

Dextrocardia is readily apparent in the CXR and the ECG shows a bizarre frontal-plane axis (Fig. 15.11).

## Anomalies of the ventriculoarterial junction

### Aortic stenosis

Congenital aortic stenosis (AS) is caused by commissural fusion, which results most commonly in a bicuspid valve (Fig. 15.12). Rarely, the valve is unicuspid with a central orifice. Associated abnormalities may include patent ductus arteriosus and coarctation of the aorta. Bicuspid aortic valve may present in infancy with severe AS but, more commonly, in

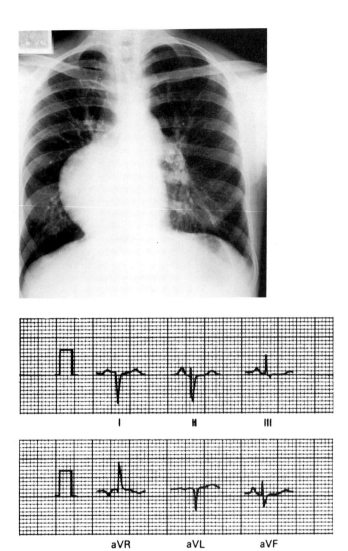

**Fig. 15.11** Dextrocardia — chest X-ray and ECG. The left-sided gastric air bubble indicates situs solitus. The cardiac apex, however, is situated on the right side of the chest and the QRS vector is therefore negative in leads I and aVL but positive in aVR. The positive P waves in I, II and III distinguish this from accidental reversal of the left and right arm leads.

adulthood, following calcification of the valve cusps (see p. 195). Indications for surgery are essentially the same as for adult AS. However, the procedure of choice in children is now balloon valvotomy (see p. 199). Surgical valvotomy, in which the valve commissures are separated under direct vision, has an operative mortality of about 2%.

Discrete subvalvular obstruction caused by a muscular band or diaphragm accounts for up to 10% of cases of congenital AS. The clinical manifestations are almost identical to valvular stenosis, except that there

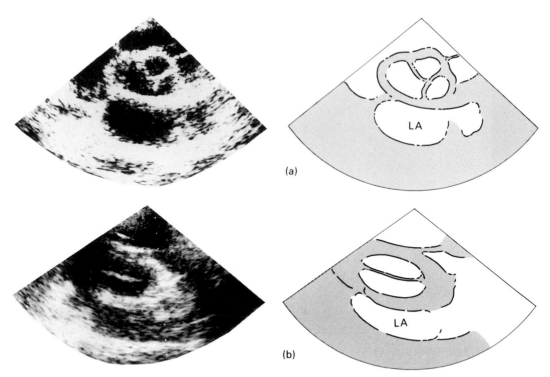

**Fig. 15.12** Bicuspid aortic valve — two-dimensional echocardiogram. (a) This is a normal aortic valve showing clearly the 'Mercedes Benz' configuration of the three commissures. (b) This is a bicuspid aortic valve in which the two valve commissures form a single line across the aorta.

is no ejection click. The echocardiogram confirms that the valve leaflets are normal and may also demonstrate the muscular band or diaphragm. Surgical correction carries no greater risk than other forms of aortic valve surgery.

Supravalvular aortic stenosis occurs at the superior margin of the sinuses of Valsalva, above the coronary arteries. The condition is commonly associated with idiopathic hypercalcaemia, mental retardation and a characteristic 'elfin-like' facies. The cardiac manifestations are almost identical to valvular AS, although an ejection click is uncommon. Surgical correction is possible but the results are often less satisfactory than those obtained following valvular or subvalvular surgery.

## Pulmonary stenosis

### Pathology

This is caused by fusion of the valve commissures and it is one of the most common congenital anomalies. The obstruction to RV outflow produces a pressure gradient across the valve, with variable RV hypertrophy.

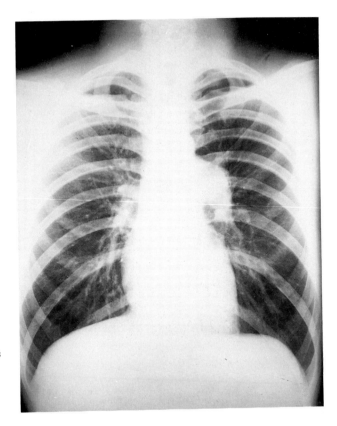

**Fig. 15.13** Congenital pulmonary stenosis — chest X-ray. Post-stenotic dilatation of the main pulmonary artery is clearly visible. In more severe cases cardiac enlargement and diminished pulmonary vascularity may also be present.

## Clinical manifestations

Mild to moderate pulmonary stenosis (PS) (peak systolic pressure gradient 75 mmHg) is only rarely symptomatic. More severe cases may present in infancy with cyanosis and heart failure but, more commonly, present in later life with exertional dyspnoea progressing to frank RVF. On examination, the JVP may be elevated and the RV impulse is palpable in the left parasternal area. Auscultation at the pulmonary area reveals an ejection click, followed by a mid-systolic murmur. The pulmonary component of the second heart sound is delayed and in severe PS is soft or inaudible.

## Diagnosis

The ECG may be normal but, in severe cases, shows right axis deviation and RV hypertrophy. The CXR shows post-stenotic dilatation of the main pulmonary artery (Fig. 15.13), and pulmonary vascularity may be reduced in severe PS. The echocardiogram confirms the diagnosis, if adequate views of the pulmonary valve can be obtained. Doppler studies permit non-invasive measurement of the pressure gradient. In severe cases cardiac catheterization is required before proceeding to correction of the defect.

## Treatment

In symptomatic patients, and all patients with a peak systolic gradient greater than 75 mmHg, balloon dilatation of the pulmonary valve is the procedure of choice. This carries a low risk and protects against right ventricular failure.

## Prognosis

Mild to moderate PS is consistent with a normal lifespan but, in severe cases, the development of right ventricular failure ensures a worse prognosis unless the defect is corrected.

## Tetralogy of Fallot

### Pathology

The tetralogy consists of subvalvular pulmonary outflow obstruction, ventricular septal defect, overriding of the aorta and right ventricular hypertrophy. Associated anomalies, including atrial septal defect and patent ductus arteriosus, are present in about 40% of cases. Depending largely on the severity of right ventricular outflow obstruction, blood shunts from right to left across the VSD. In severe outflow obstruction, the shunt is large and cyanosis severe, but, in mild outflow obstruction, pulmonary flow may be close to normal and shunting negligible — acyanotic Fallot's. Nevertheless, the outflow obstruction is often progressive and cyanosis usually develops early during childhood.

### Clinical manifestations

Tetralogy of Fallot presents with cyanosis at birth or during the first year of life, as pulmonary outflow obstruction increases. Indeed, it is the most common cardiac cause of cyanosis after the first year of life. When pulmonary outflow obstruction is severe, the right-to-left shunt is considerable and volume-overloads the left ventricle, which fails in infancy. Unprovoked attacks of intense cyanosis may occur, leading to syncope, convulsions and death. In less severe cases, important symptoms do not occur until later, when the child is troubled by exertional dyspnoea and may squat to relieve symptoms (see p. 301). Examination reveals central cyanosis and clubbing, associated with physical underdevelopment; a

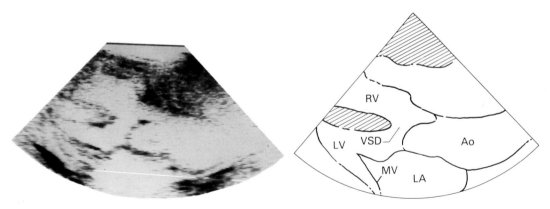

**Fig. 15.14**  Tetralogy of Fallot — two-dimensional echocardiogram (long-axis view). The VSD (arrowed) with the dilated overriding aorta is clearly visible.

mid-systolic ejection murmur is present in the pulmonary area, but the pulmonary component of the second heart sound is absent. Bronchial collaterals make an important contribution to pulmonary flow and may produce a soft continuous murmur, audible over the back of the chest.

## Complications

It may be complicated by severe LVF in infancy if severe pulmonary outflow obstruction causes excessive right to left shunting. In children and adults, however, right ventricular failure (RVF) is more common, due to chronic pulmonary outflow obstruction. Other complications include cyanotic attacks (infants), cardiac arrhythmias and endocarditis.

## Diagnosis

The ECG shows variable RV hypertrophy, depending on the degree of outflow obstruction. The CXR typically shows a boot-shaped heart, with deep concavity of the left heart border, due to a diminutive pulmonary artery and dilated left ventricle. Pulmonary vascularity is reduced. The echocardiogram is diagnostic if the VSD and the overriding aorta are imaged (Fig. 15.14). Doppler studies are helpful but cardiac catheterization may be necessary to confirm the diagnosis.

### Differential diagnosis

Fallot's tetralogy can usually be distinguished from other cardiac causes of central cyanosis by the echocardiographic and Doppler findings. In the adult, Eisenmenger's syndrome is the major differential diagnosis, both conditions being associated with central cyanosis, clubbing and heart murmurs. However, the pulmonary component of the second heart sound, which is loud in Eisenmenger's syndrome, is absent in tetralogy of Fallot.

## Treatment

Treatment is by total correction of the abnormality, involving closure of the VSD and relief of pulmonary outflow obstruction. In infants, however, palliative procedures are usually performed, pending total correction in later life. These procedures are directed at improving pulmonary flow by creating anastomoses between the ascending aorta and the pulmonary artery (Waterston shunt) or the subclavian artery and the pulmonary artery (Blalock shunt).

## Prognosis

It may be fatal in infancy if RV outflow obstruction is severe, but, in less severe cases, survival to adulthood may occur, although few patients live beyond middle age without surgical correction. In babies, cyanotic attacks are the major cause of death, but in children and adults RVF, arrhythmias and endocarditis are more important.

## Transposition of the great arteries

If the ventriculoarterial junctions are discordant, the aorta arises from the morphological RV and the pulmonary artery from the morphological LV. This provides the anatomical basis for parallel systemic and pulmonary circulations, when survival depends upon mixing of blood through a septal defect or a patent ductus arteriosus. In the absence of associated anomalies, however, the baby presents soon after birth (following physiological closure of the ductus arteriosus) with severe cyanosis and heart failure. Diagnosis is by echocardiography. In the critically ill baby, the Rashkind procedure is potentially life-saving: a balloon catheter is introduced into the right atrium by the femoral vein and directed across the foramen ovale into the left atrium. The balloon is inflated and the catheter is drawn back abruptly into the right atrium, which tears the atrial septum, allowing the systemic and pulmonary venous blood to mix. The procedure is palliative pending surgical correction, in which the venous return to the two ventricles is switched by insertion of an atrial baffle (Mustard's operation). This directs the pulmonary and systemic venous return to the morphological RV and LV, respectively.

Very occasionally, ventriculoarterial discordance (transposition) is compatible with a normal circulation, requiring simultaneous AV discordance ('corrected' transposition). Although corrected transposition is compatible with a normal lifespan, troublesome and potentially life-threatening arrhythmias are common.

## Coarctation of the aorta

### Pathology

Coarctation is not strictly an anomaly of the ventriculoarterial junction because it rises more distally in the aorta, in association with the ductus arteriosus. It is a localized fibrotic narrowing just beyond the origin of the left subclavian artery. Coarctation is more common in males, and may be associated with bicuspid aortic valve, Berry aneurysm or gonadal dysgenesis (Turner's syndrome).

Coarctation does not cause significant obstruction to aortic flow until the ductus arteriosus constricts following birth, which may precipitate acute LVF if obstruction to flow is complete. More commonly, however, the obstruction is partial and heart failure is avoided by compensatory LV hypertrophy, providing time for development of an extensive collateral supply around the coarctation.

### Clinical manifestations

Coarctation is usually asymptomatic if heart failure in infancy does not occur. Characteristic physical findings include delayed and diminished femoral pulses compared with the radial pulses (radiofemoral delay). The blood-pressure in the arms is elevated, but in the legs it is normal or low. LV hypertrophy produces a prominent apical impulse and a fourth heart sound; a systolic murmur is always present, due to turbulent flow through the coarctation and collateral vessels. The murmur is often louder over the back of the chest and may be continuous if the collateral circulation is extensive. In adults with coarctation, the shoulders and arms are often noticeably better developed that the lower extremities.

### Complications

Hypertension in the upper half of the body is almost invariable and predisposes to LVF, stroke and aortic dissection. Ruptured Berry aneurysm, endocarditis and arrhythmias also occur.

### Diagnosis

The ECG is usually normal in infancy but features of LV hypertrophy develop thereafter. The CXR may show pre- and post-ductal aortic dilatation, giving a 3-shaped contour to the left upper mediastinum. More

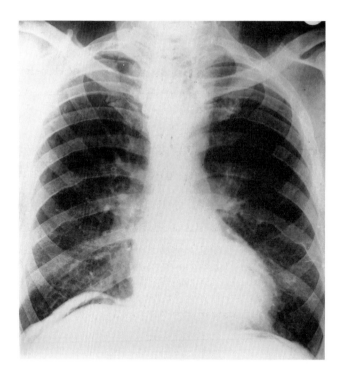

**Fig. 15.15** Coarctation of the aorta — chest X-ray. Notching of the inferior margins of the ribs is clearly visible. The gas under the diaphragm is the result of recent abdominal surgery.

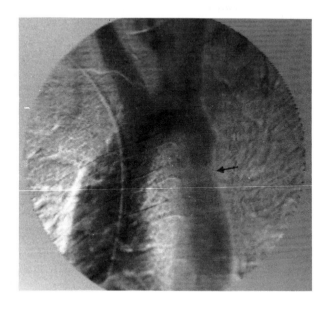

**Fig. 15.16** Coarctation of the aorta — aortogram. This digital subtraction aortogram shows a discrete coarctation (arrowed) in the thoracic aorta just beyond the left subclavian branch.

characteristic is rib-notching, but this rarely develops before the age of 10 (Fig. 15.15). The notches occur on the underside of the ribs and are the result of erosion by dilated intercostal collateral arteries. Aortic angiography confirms the diagnosis (Fig. 15.16).

**Differential diagnosis**

Diminished or absent femoral pulses may also be caused by advanced atherosclerosis. However, this usually affects an older age-group and produces ischaemia with intermittent claudication or frank gangrene, neither of which are seen in patients with coarctation.

## Treatment

Treatment is surgical and is usually by resection of the coarctation, with end-to-end anastomosis of the aorta. If the coarctation is long, however, a Dacron graft may be required for the aortic anastomosis. Elective surgery in childhood corrects hypertension and removes the risk of LVF and stroke; if delayed, hypertension may become irreversible.

## Prognosis

Complications of coarctation rarely permit survival beyond the age of 40 unless surgically corrected.

## Further reading

Anonymous. Coarctation repair: the first forty years. *Lancet* 1991, **338**, 546–7.

Borow K.M. and Karp R. Atrial septal defect: lessons from the past, directions for the future. *N. Engl. J. Med.* 1990, **323**, 1698–700.

Bull C. Interventional catheterisation in infants and children. *Br. Heart J.* 1986, **56**, 197–200.

Ferencz C. On the birth prevalence of congenital heart disease. *J. Am. Coll. Cardiol.* 1990, **16**, 1701–2.

Kugler J.D. and Danford D.A. Pacemakers in children: an update. *Am. Heart J.* 1989, **117**, 665–79.

Mullins C.E. Pediatric and congenital therapeutic cardiac catheterization. *Circulation* 1989, **79**, 1153–9.

Rao P.S. Indications for balloon pulmonary valvuloplasty. *Am. Heart J.* 1988, **116**, 1661–2.

Riemenschneider T.A. Management of hypoplastic left heart syndrome: a challenge to those who care for children with heart disease. *Am. Heart J.* 1986, **112**, 864–6.

Somerville J. Congenital heart disease in adults and adolescents. *Br. Heart J.* 1986, **56**, 395–7.

# 16 Pregnancy, Systemic Disorders and the Heart

## Summary

*Pregnancy* is associated with increased plasma volume, vasodilatation, hyperdynamic circulation and variable compression of the heart by the uterine fundus. These changes often produce flow murmurs, added heart sounds, peripheral oedema and minor electrocardiogram (ECG) and chest X-ray abnormalities, any of which may give rise to a spurious impression of heart-disease. When organic heart-disease does occur, it is mitral stenosis and cardiomyopathy that are most hazardous, because of the risk of life-threatening pulmonary oedema in the third trimester. Echocardiography is the safest and most reliable diagnostic technique.

*Endocrine disorders* Diabetes and thyroid disease are the most important endocrine disorders affecting the heart. Diabetes is a major risk factor for atherosclerosis and is commonly associated with premature coronary and peripheral vascular disease. Specific heart muscle disease, indistinguishable from dilated cardiomyopathy, may also occur. The effects of thyrotoxicosis on the heart, including tachycardia and arrhythmias (particularly atrial fibrillation), largely resemble those of sympathetic overstimulation and respond to beta-blockers. Hypothyroidism causes bradycardia and pericardial effusion and, in long-standing disease, may result in cardiac dilatation and congestive failure.

*Connective tissue disorders* These are associated with vasculitis, which may affect almost any part of the heart. Pericarditis is the most common cardiac manifestation of rheumatoid arthritis and systemic lupus erythematosus, while aortic root disease leading to aortic regurgitation is the characteristic lesion in ankylosing spondylitis and Marfan's syndrome.

*Infiltrative disorders*, such as amyloidosis and haemochromatosis, are important causes of specific heart muscle disease, but in sarcoidosis granulomatous destruction of conducting tissue, with varying degrees of atrioventicular (AV) block, is a more frequent mode of presentation.

*Infective disease* is usually either viral, causing pericarditis or myocarditis, or bacterial, causing endocarditis. However, tubercle remains an important cause of pericarditis in many parts of the world, and the specific heart muscle and conducting tissue disease that complicates chronic trypanosomiasis is commonly seen in Central and South America.

*Neoplastic disease* affecting the heart is usually metastatic from lung or breast and, when clinically evident, presents with pericardial effusion and tamponade. Of the primary cardiac tumours, the histologically benign left atrial myxoma is the most common. Typically, it is pedunculated and attached to the interatrial septum, causing variable obstruction to mitral flow during diastole. Symptoms and signs are similar to mitral stenosis, but the echocardiogram permits reliable differential diagnosis. Primary malignant tumours are rare and are nearly all sarcomas; death early in the clinical course is invariable.

## Pregnancy

### Circulatory changes

During pregnancy, plasma volume and cardiac output increase to meet the requirements of the uterus. By the third trimester, plasma volume may be increased by 40–50%. Plasma volume expansion is associated with a fall in colloid osmotic pressure, which predisposes to oedema, even in the absence of pre-eclampsia. Oedema is usually mild and tends to affect the lower limbs, due to compression of the pelvic veins by the uterus. Elevated venous pressure is also an important factor in the development of varicose veins and haemorrhoids, which are common in pregnancy. Following delivery, there is a sharp drop in plasma volume, due to blood loss associated with shedding of the placenta. Thereafter, plasma volume and cardiac output decline more gradually, returning to pre-pregnancy levels after about 6 weeks.

### Clinical manifestations

The skin is warm and often flushed, due to peripheral vasodilatation. The heart rate is increased and the pulse has a collapsing quality. During the third trimester, the pregnant uterus may cause upward displacement of the diaphragm. This compresses the heart so that the apex beat becomes palpable in the fourth intercostal space in the anterior axillary line. Auscultation during this period commonly reveals an 'innocent' ejection murmur at the base of the heart and a third heart sound — both manifestations of the hyperdynamic circulation.

The ECG and chest X-ray (CXR) are usually normal but, late in pregnancy, may show changes, reflecting cardiac compression. These include a degree of left axis deviation and apparent radiological cardiac enlargement. Atrial and ventricular premature beats are frequently found.

## *Heart-disease in pregnancy*

Flow murmurs, added heart sounds, peripheral oedema and minor ECG and CXR abnormalities often give rise to a spurious impression of heart-disease in the pregnant woman. In such cases, the echocardiogram provides a safe and useful means of ruling out valvular and myocardial disorders.

Coronary artery disease is unusual in premenopausal women but valvular and myocardial disease are seen more often. Presentation is typically during the third trimester, or at the time of delivery, when increments in plasma volume and cardiac output are at their peak. Mitral stenosis, in particular, is poorly tolerated and there is a considerable risk of acute pulmonary oedema. It is best treated by valvotomy before the onset of labour but, if valvular calcification or regurgitation contraindicate this procedure, medical management is preferable. Aortic and right-sided valvular disorders are better tolerated during pregnancy and definitive surgical treatment can usually be delayed until after delivery. In women with valvular disease, antibiotic prophylaxis against endocarditis (intravenous gentamicin and amoxycillin) is unnecessary for normal vaginal deliveries but is recommended for instrumented deliveries and for all women with prosthetic valves or a history of previous endocarditis. Generally speaking, if valve replacement is required in pregnancy (or in women who may become pregnant at a future date), a porcine xenograft should be chosen (see p. 184) since this avoids the need for anticoagulation, which poses special problems during pregnancy.

Women with cardiomyopathy usually tolerate pregnancy well, although in severe cases there is always a risk of pulmonary oedema during the third trimester or at delivery. Dilated cardiomyopathy presenting 3 months before or after labour has been named peripartum cardiomyopathy. This appears to be a specific entity related to pregnancy and is particularly common in women of West African origin. Nevertheless, it remains unclear whether peripartum cardiomyopathy represents the direct effects of pregnancy on a previously normal heart or merely a deterioration in a pre-existing cardiomyopathy. Peripartum cardiomyopathy can present with life-threatening pulmonary oedema in the peripartum period, demanding urgent Caesarean section and, although variable (sometimes complete) clinical recovery usually occurs following delivery, the risk of recurrent decompensation in future pregnancies is considerable.

## Endocrine disease

## *Thyroid disease*

Cardiovascular manifestations of thyrotoxicosis include palpitation, dyspnoea, tachycardia, systolic hypertension and the third heart sound.

Arrhythmias are common, particularly atrial fibrillation, which may be the only sign of thyrotoxicosis in the elderly patient. Tachycardia and arrhythmias exacerbate angina in patients with coronary artery disease and may lead to heart failure. It is noteworthy that the effects of thyrotoxicosis on the cardiovascular system largely resemble those of sympathetic overstimulation, and beta-blockers provide the most effective treatment, pending definitive measures to reduce secretion of thyroid hormone.

Hypothyroidism has a direct effect on myocardial structure and function, which leads ultimately to cardiac dilatation and congestive failure. Bradycardia, hypotension and pericardial effusion are common findings. The ECG shows low-voltage QRS complexes, which often persist despite removal of pericardial fluid. The hypercholesterolaemia that accompanies hypothyroidism may predispose to coronary artery disease. Following thyroid replacement therapy, reversal of cardiovascular abnormalities nearly always occurs. Nevertheless, treatment must be given cautiously — particularly in the elderly and those known to have underlying organic heart-disease — because abrupt myocardial stimulation by thyroid hormone may precipitate acute ischaemia or cardiac arrhythmias. Thus, initial therapy is with very low doses of thyroid hormone, which are gradually increased over a period of weeks.

## *Diabetes*

Cardiovascular disease in diabetic patients is common, due to the heightened risk of atherosclerosis. This affects the coronary and peripheral arteries and predisposes to angina, myocardial infarction (MI), stroke and limb ischaemia. The distribution of disease differs from that of non-diabetic patients in that the small distal arteries in the coronary circulation and the legs tend to be involved, often to the same extent as the proximal arteries. This increases the technical difficulties of vascular bypass surgery and angioplasty procedures.

The sensory supply of the heart runs with the autonomic innervation, and silent ischaemia (see p. 107) is therefore common in patients with diabetic neuropathy. Painless MI is common for the same reason but, in other respects, MI is usually more severe than in the non-diabetic patient and the incidence of all complications (including arrhythmias, heart failure and death) is higher. Catecholamine release exacerbates the diabetic state and adequate metabolic control in the coronary care unit demands regular administration of short-acting insulin, even in patients usually controlled with oral hypoglycaemic agents.

Diabetes may cause specific heart muscle disease, which is clinically indistinguishable from dilated cardiomyopathy and unrelated to coronary artery disease. The precise cause is uncertain, but some studies of myocardial histology have provided evidence of microvascular obliterative disease. Treatment is the same as for dilated cardiomyopathy (see p. 146).

## Acromegaly

Cardiac enlargement is almost invariable in acromegaly and is due principally to the effects of growth hormone on the myocardium, but hypertension, which affects up to 50% of patients, contributes to this. Premature coronary artery disease is common in acromegaly, not only because of hypertension but also because of abnormal lipid and carbohydrate metabolism.

## Adrenal disease

In Cushing's disease, hypertension and abnormalities of lipid and carbohydrate metabolism commonly lead to accelerated atherosclerosis. MI is a common cause of death in untreated cases. Primary hyperaldosteronism (Conn's syndrome) is associated with hypertension and hypokalaemia, which predispose to myocardial disease, coronary artery disease and arrhythmias. The only important cardiovascular manifestation of Addison's disease is hypotension, which may cause postural dizziness or syncope. Hyperkalaemia is rarely so severe as to disturb cardiac rhythm.

Catecholamine-secreting tumours of the adrenal medulla (phaeochromocytoma) are an important cause of secondary hypertension. The tumours are usually benign but may occur bilaterally or in extra-adrenal locations. Hypertension caused by phaeochromocytoma is characteristically labile, due to episodic release of catecholamines. Arrhythmias are not uncommon and in severe cases diffuse myocardial dysfunction leads to heart failure and death. Myocardial disease is due in part to the effects of hypertension, but has also been attributed to the direct action of catecholamines, which cause focal myocardial necrosis.

## Carcinoid syndrome

Carcinoid tumours in the appendix and other parts of the small bowel secrete kinin peptides and serotonin, which are largely inactivated in the liver. Following metastasis to the liver, however, the systemic circulation is no longer protected from these toxic substances, which are responsible for the characteristic clinical manifestations of carcinoid syndrome. These include diarrhoea, bronchospasm, flushing attacks and telangiectasia. Cardiac manifestations are the result of toxic damage to the tricuspid and pulmonary valves; variable stenosis or regurgitation often develops (see Fig. 9.12). Left-sided valvular disease is rare but is occasionally seen in patients with pulmonary metastases.

## Nutritional disease

### Obesity

The excess mortality in severe obesity is largely related to cardiovascular disease. Hypertension is common (see p. 259) and associated metabolic abnormalities include diabetes and hyperlipidaemia, which are both major risk factors for atherosclerosis and predispose to MI and stroke. Obesity is also associated with increased plasma volume and myocardial mass. In advanced disease, plasma volume overload and myocardial hypertrophy lead to congestive heart failure. In certain cases, chronic hypoventilation (Pickwickian syndrome) produces pulmonary hypertension and cor pulmonale (see p. 290).

### Malnutrition

Although anorexia nervosa is associated with reduced myocardial mass and hypotension, there is no demonstrable impairment of left ventricular contractile function. However, in advanced protein–calorie malnutrition (marasmus, kwashiorkor), cardiac atrophy and interstitial oedema commonly lead to left ventricular (LV) dysfunction and there is a major risk of acute pulmonary oedema during rehydration of these patients.

Beriberi, caused by thiamine deficiency, is the only hypovitaminosis associated with heart-disease; it occurs in parts of the world where polished rice is the staple carbohydrate source. Reductions in systemic vascular resistance (due probably to autonomic neuropathy) produce a chronically elevated cardiac output, which may lead to high-output failure (see p. 78). Physical signs are those of a hyperkinetic circulation and include the third heart sound and an ejection systolic murmur.

## Connective tissue disease

### Rheumatoid arthritis

Fibrinous pericarditis commonly occurs in rheumatoid disease and is a well-recognized cause of pericardial effusion and tamponade. In patients with widespread subcutaneous rheumatoid nodules, myocardial and valvular nodules also occur. These are granulomatous lesions but they rarely affect myocardial or valvular function. Coronary arteritis can often be demonstrated in post-mortem studies but this rarely causes myocardial ischaemia or infarction.

### Systemic lupus erythematosus

The diffuse vasculitis characterizing this condition nearly always involves the heart; however, cardiac disease is rarely prominent. Pericarditis is the most common lesion and may produce effusion and tamponade. Myo-carditis is subclinical in most cases and, although congestive heart failure occurs, it is usually the result of hypertension secondary to renal disease. Inflammatory endocarditis, originally described by Libman and Sacks, may affect any of the heart valves and consists of extrusions of degenerative tissue on the valve surfaces, which, though large (up to 4 mm), rarely cause significant valvular dysfunction.

## Polyarteritis nodosa

Vasculitis affecting the pericardial and coronary vessels may lead to pericarditis and MI, though the latter is rare. Myocardial disease and congestive failure are usually the result of hypertension secondary to renal disease.

## Ankylosing spondylitis

Though diffuse carditis with pericardial, myocardial and endocardial involvement may occur in ankylosing spondylitis, aortic regurgitation is the most characteristic cardiac manifestation. This is partly the result of valve scarring, but dilatation of the aorta due to destruction of elastic tissue is the major cause.

## Marfan's syndrome

This is a generalized connective tissue disorder, with an autosomal dominant mode of inheritance; about 15% of cases occur sporadically. Phenotypic expression is variable, but typical manifestations include long limbs, mobile joints, dislocation of the lens and chest deformities.

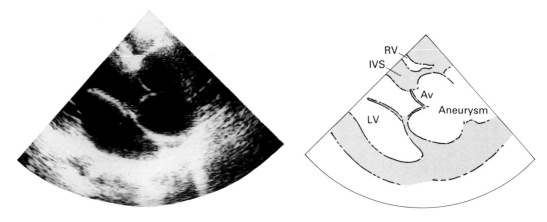

**Fig. 16.1**  Marfan's syndrome — two-dimensional echocardiogram (long-axis view). There is a large aneurysm of the aortic root involving the sinuses of Valsalva.

Cardiovascular complications are the major cause of death in Marfan's syndrome. Mitral valve prolapse is the most common, but more important is cystic medial necrosis of the aorta, leading to aortic root dilatation and aortic regurgitation (Fig. 16.1). Death is usually the result of left ventricular failure (LVF), aortic dissection or aneurysmal rupture.

## Scleroderma

Cardiac involvement is common but usually silent, affecting up to 50% of cases. Myocardial fibrosis may present as dilated (or occasionally restrictive) heart muscle disease, while pericarditis sometimes results in significant effusion and tamponade. Lung disease in scleroderma causes pulmonary hypertension and may lead to severe right-sided heart failure.

## Infiltrative disease

### Amyloidosis

In this condition extracellular deposits of the fibrous protein amyloid occur in various sites of the body. Almost any organ may be involved. When amyloidosis is secondary to chronic infection (e.g. tuberculosis) or inflammation (e.g. rheumatoid arthritis), cardiac involvement is unusual. In primary amyloidosis, however, heart failure is the most common cause of death. Myocardial deposits of amyloid may cause contractile dysfunction, leading to cardiac dilatation and congestive failure. More commonly, however, the defect is one of diastolic relaxation and the syndrome resembles restrictive cardiomyopathy (see p. 152). Cardiac enlargement may not be prominent but echocardiography demonstrates variable ventricular hypertrophy and, in the most severe cases, characteristic myocardial stippling is seen. Nevertheless, definitive diagnosis is only possible by endomyocardial biopsy. There is no treatment that influences the progression of cardiac amyloidosis.

### Haemochromatosis

This is a genetic disorder characterized by excessive intestinal absorption of iron, leading to parenchymal deposition of iron in multiple organs, particularly the liver, pancreas, pituitary and heart. Clinical manifestations are rare before the age of 20 and an identical syndrome may result from iron overload secondary to liver disease and multiple blood transfusions. Myocardial deposition of iron leads to fibrosis and contractile dysfunction, resulting in cardiac dilatation and congestive failure; definitive diagnosis of cardiac involvement requires endomyocardial biopsy. Regular phlebotomy provides the best means of treating iron overload, but chelating agents, such as desferrioxamine, may also be used. Nevertheless, once congestive heart failure is established, it is always progressive.

## Sarcoidosis

This is a multisystem granulomatous disorder of unknown aetiology. Pulmonary sarcoidosis may lead to progressive fibrosis and cor pulmonale, which is the most common cardiac manifestation. Although primary cardiac involvement can be demonstrated in up to 25% of post-mortem cases, clinical sarcoid heart-disease occurs in less than 5%. Granulomatous destruction of the conducting tissues may cause AV block, which is the most frequent clinical manifestation of cardiac sarcoidosis. Atrial and ventricular arrhythmias also occur. In patients with extensive granulomatous disease of the ventricular myocardium, congestive heart failure may develop. Sudden death due to heart block or arrhythmias is not uncommon in patients with cardiac sarcoidosis.

## Neurological disease

### Muscular dystrophy

Sinus tachycardia and ECG abnormalities are common in Duchenne's muscular dystrophy, although the mechanisms are uncertain. Myocardial contractile dysfunction occasionally leads to heart failure, but severe cardiac dilatation is unusual.

### Dystrophia myotonica

Clinical manifestations of cardiac involvement occur in over 50% of cases. Most common are conduction disturbances, including all degrees of AV block and bundle branch block. Sinus bradycardia and atrial and ventricular arrhythmias also occur.

### Friedreich's ataxia

Up to 50% of patients have symptomatic myocardial disease and nearly all patients have ECG abnormalities. Hypertrophic cardiomyopathy is the most common cardiac disorder and is often responsible for death.

### Guillain–Barré syndrome

Despite mechanical ventilation, Guillain–Barré syndrome remains fatal in up to 20% of cases; a proportion of these deaths are sudden, and may

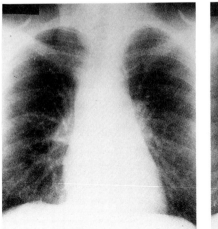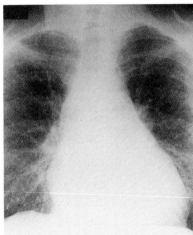

**Fig. 16.2** Tuberculous pericardial effusion. The chest X-ray on the left shows hilar lymphadenopathy. Cervical lymph node biopsy 3 weeks later confirmed tuberculosis. Meanwhile, a repeat chest X-ray had shown considerable cardiac enlargement due to pericardial effusion.

be attributed to cardiac arrhythmias. Both brady- and tachyarrhythmias occur, and ECG monitoring is recommended, particularly in severe cases.

## Infective disease

Infective endocarditis, viral myocarditis and pericarditis have been previously discussed (see Chapters 7 to 9) and will not be considered further in this section.

### Tuberculosis (TB)

In many parts of the world TB remains a common cause of pericarditis tamponade and constriction, although it is seen less often in developed countries (Fig. 16.2). Myocardial involvement is very rare but may lead to AV block, ventricular aneurysm, arrhythmias or heart failure.

### Syphilis

Cardiovascular syphilis is now rarely seen, due to effective treatment in the early stages of the disease. Spirochaetal invasion of the aortic media occurs soon after the initial infection and is usually localized in the ascending aorta. Medial necrosis, fibrosis and calcification lead to aortic dilatation after a latent period of up to 25 years. Aneurysm formation in the ascending aorta is the most common manifestation and when this involves the aortic valve ring it leads to aortic regurgitation. Ostial stenoses of the coronary arteries also occur. Aneurysmal compression or erosion of adjacent mediastinal or bony structures may produce a variety of symptoms and signs, including pain, dysphagia, stridor and hoarseness. Aortic regurgitation commonly leads to LVF, while coronary ostial stenoses are a cause of angina and, less frequently, MI. Death is usually the result of LVF or aneurysmal rupture.

## Diphtheria

This is now rarely seen due to effective immunization in infancy. The diphtheria bacillus infects the pharynx and secretes an exotoxin which, in 20% of cases, causes acute myocarditis, which is the most common cause of death. By the end of the first week of the illness, the heart is dilated, with severe contractile dysfunction, and all grades of heart block may occur. Pulmonary congestion and low-output failure commonly develop. Treatment is with antitoxin and penicillin; if the patient survives, recovery of normal myocardial function can be expected in most, but not all, cases.

## Trypanosomiasis (Chagas' disease)

This disease, caused by the protozoon parasite *Trypanosoma cruzi*, is endemic in Central and South America, where it is responsible for about 30% of all deaths. It is transmitted by the reduviid bug. Occasionally, an acute illness develops at the time of the initial infection but in the majority of cases there is a latent period of up to 25 years before chronic Chagas' disease develops. This is characterized by biventricular dilatation and contractile failure, with involvement of the conducting tissues. Symptoms and signs are those of congestive heart failure. The ECG usually shows bundle branch block and, in many patients, complete AV block develops. Ventricular arrhythmias are common.

## Acquired immunodeficiency syndrome (AIDS)

Cardiac involvement in AIDS is common but rarely clinically prominent, usually being obscured by the systemic manifestations of the syndrome. Myocarditis is a consequence of opportunistic infection and a variety of organisms have been implicated, including *Pneumocystis carinii*, *Mycobacterium tuberculosis* and *Candida albicans*. In most cases it is asymptomatic and diagnosed only at post-mortem, but occasionally it causes severe congestive heart failure and cardiac arrhythmias. Endocarditis is nearly always the non-bacterial thrombotic variety (marantic endocarditis), which is known to be associated with long-term wasting illnesses and malignancies. Embolic complications have occasionally

Systole

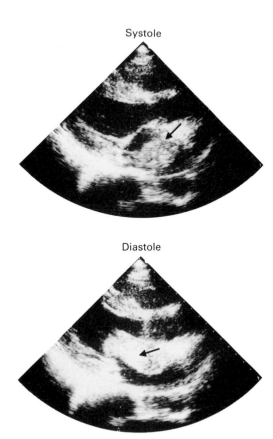

Diastole

**Fig. 16.3** Left atrial myxoma — two-dimensional echocardiogram (long-axis view). Note that during diastole the tumour (arrowed) prolapses through the valve, obstructing left ventricular filling.

been reported. Pericarditis is usually associated with concomitant myocardial disease and is caused by infiltration with Kaposi's sarcoma or opportunistic infection.

## Cardiac tumours

### Primary tumours

Primary cardiac tumours are rare, the histologically benign myxoma accounting for at least half of all cases. Myxomas usually arise in the left atrium but are also found in the other cardiac chambers. Typically the tumour is pedunculated and attached to the interatrial septum, prolapsing into the mitral valve orifice during diastole (Fig. 16.3). This impedes diastolic filling of the LV and produces symptoms similar to those of mitral stenosis (MS). Nevertheless, the dyspnoea is often episodic and provoked by changes in posture, which encourage gravitational prolapse of the tumour into the mitral valve. On examination, there is a low-pitched noise in mid-diastole (tumour plop), probably caused by the

*Benign*
Myxoma
Lipoma
Rhabdomyoma
Fibroma
Hamartoma

*Malignant*
Angiosarcoma
Rhabdomyosarcoma
Fibrosarcoma

myxoma striking the LV wall. This may be mistaken for the mid-diastolic murmur of MS. Other symptoms and signs variably present include fever, weight loss and clubbing. The erythrocyte sedimentation rate (ESR) may be raised and systemic thromboembolism is common. Sudden death may occur if the tumour causes unrelieved obstruction of the mitral valve. In the past, left atrial myxoma was usually misdiagnosed as MS, but the echocardiogram now permits visualization of the tumour and rules out mitral valve disease. Treatment is by surgical excision of the tumour.

Other benign tumours of the heart (Table 16.1) usually present with heart failure due to intracavity obstruction to flow, and may also cause myocardial contractile dysfunction (particularly if very large) and conduction disturbance. Rhabdomyomas are most commonly seen in infants and, if large, may be a cause of still birth. About half of all cases occur in association with tuberous sclerosis. Fibromas and hamartomas occur principally in children but lipomas occur in all age-groups. Malignant tumours of the heart are nearly all sarcomas and include angiosarcomas, rhabdomyosarcomas and fibrosarcomas. They usually present in adults and, because they proliferate rapidly, death occurs early in the clinical course (Fig. 16.4).

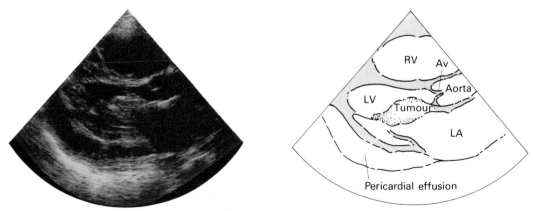

**Fig. 16.4**  Fibrosarcoma — two-dimensional echocardiogram (long-axis view). The large tumour applied to the anterior leaflet of the mitral valve is seen. Pericardial seeding has led to pericardial effusion.

## *Metastatic tumours*

Metastases account for the majority of cardiac tumours and usually originate from the breast or lung. The pericardium is most commonly affected but any other part of the heart may also be involved. Most cases are clinically silent, but pericardial effusion and tamponade is the most common clinical presentation. Invasion of the conducting tissue may produce heart block, and occasionally extensive myocardial involvement or valvular obstruction leads to heart failure.

## Further reading

Buckley B.H. and Hutchins G.M. Atrial myxoma: a fifty year review. *Am. Heart J.* 1979, **97**, 639–43.

Doherty N.E. and Siegel R.J. Cardiovascular manifestations of systemic lupus erythematosus. *Am. Heart J.* 1985, **110**, 1257–65.

Fleming H.A. Sarcoid heart disease. *Br. Med. J.* 1986, **292**, 1095–6.

Fyke F.E., Seward J.B., Edwards W.D. *et al.* Primary cardiac tumors: experience with 30 consecutive patients since the introduction of two-dimensional echocardiography. *J. Am. Coll. Cardiol.* 1985, **5**, 1965–73.

Goldman A.P. and Kotler M.N. Heart disease in scleroderma. *Am. Heart J.* 1985, **110**, 1043–6.

Gottdiener J.S., Hawley R.J., Maron B.J., Bertorini T.F. and Engle W.K. Characteristics of the cardiac hypertrophy in Friedreich's ataxia. *Am. Heart J.* 1982, **103**, 525–31.

Hayward R.P., Emanuel R.W. and Nabarro J.B.N. Acromegalic heart disease: influence of treatment of the acromegaly of the heart. *Q. J. Med.* 1987, **237**, 41–58.

Hiromasa S., Ikeda T. and Kubota K. Myotonic dystrophy: ambulatory electrocardiogram, electrophysiologic study, and echocardiographic evaluation. *Am. Heart J.* 1987, **113**, 1482–8.

Homans D. Peripartum cardiomyopathy. *N. Engl. J. Med.* 1985, **312**, 1432–7.

Hunsacker R.H., Fulkerson P.K., Barry F.J., Lewis R.O., Leier C.V. and Unverferth D.V. Cardiac function in Duchenne's muscular dystrophy. *Am. J. Med.* 1982, **73**, 235–8.

Jacob A.J. and Boon N.A. HIV cardiomyopathy: a dark cloud with a silver lining? *Br. Heart J.* 1991, **66**, 1–2.

Kaul S., Fishbein M.C. and Siegel R.J. Cardiac manifestations of acquired immune deficiency syndrome: a 1991 update. *Am. Heart J.* 1991, **122**, 535–44.

Kirk J. and Cosh J. The pericarditis of rheumatoid arthritis. *Q. J. Med.* 1969, **38**, 397–402.

Oakley C.M. Pregnancy in heart disease. In Jackson, G. (ed.), *Difficult Cardiology: Practical Management and Decision Making*. London, Martin Dunitz, 1990, pp. 1–20.

Oliveira J.S. A natural model of intrinsic heart nervous system denervation: Chagas' cardiopathy. *Am. Heart J.* 1985, **110**, 1092–8.

Roberts W.C. and Honig H.S. The spectrum of cardiovascular disease in the Marfan syndrome: a clinico-morphologic study of 18 necropsy patients and comparison to 151 previously reported patients. *Am. Heart J.* 1982, **104**, 115–35.

Schrader M.L., Hochman J.S. and Bulkley B.H. The heart in polyarteritis nodosa: a clinicopathologic study. *Am. Heart J* 1985, **109**, 1353–9.

Stevens M.B. Lupus carditis. *N. Engl. J. Med.* 1988, **319**, 861–2.

Sullivan J.M. and Ramanathan K.B. Management of medical problems in pregnancy: severe cardiac disease. *N. Engl. J. Med.* 1985, **313**, 304–9.

Symons C. Thyroid heart disease. *Br. Heart J.* 1979, **41**, 257–62.

Zarich S.W. and Nesto R.W. Diabetic cardiomyopathy. *Am. Heart J.* 1989, **118**, 1000–12.

# 17 Surgery and Heart-disease

## Summary

*Preoperative factors*  Heart failure increases surgical risk considerably and should always be controlled in the preoperative period. Coronary disease also increases risk, particularly for patients with myocardial infarction in the previous 6 months, in whom elective surgical procedures are contraindicated because of the 16% risk of recurrent perioperative infarction. Valvular disease requires antibiotic prophylaxis against endocarditis only if the risk of bacteraemia is high (bowel or dental surgery). Anticoagulation with subcutaneous heparin is recommended for all patients prior to surgery to protect against pulmonary embolism.

*Perioperative factors*  Anaesthetic agents can cause severe hypotension, through direct effects on the myocardium and the autonomic nervous system, leading to coronary hypoperfusion and low-output failure. Risk is particularly high during induction, when careful monitoring of blood-pressure is essential. The arrhythmogenic properties of anaesthetic agents may also be troublesome and demand continuous electrocardiogram (ECG) monitoring. Myocardial injury may complicate severe hypotension and coronary hypoperfusion, but the risk is particularly high during cardiopulmonary bypass, when the incidence of perioperative infarction is related to the duration of the procedure and the adequacy of myocardial protection.

*Postoperative factors*  Fluid imbalance is the major cause of cardiovascular instability in the postoperative period. Requirements can be monitored with a central venous catheter but, in patients with left ventricular disease, a pulmonary artery (Swan–Ganz) catheter provides more useful information about fluid balance, by providing an indirect measure of left ventricular filling pressure.

## Preoperative factors

### Heart failure

The patient with heart failure is a considerably higher operative risk than the patient with a normal heart, regardless of the cause of heart failure and the nature of the surgical procedure. In major non-cardiac surgery, perioperative mortality rises from 4% in mild heart failure to 67% in severe heart failure. A similar pattern of risk exists in patients undergoing cardiac procedures. Mitral valve replacement, for example, carries a 3% mortality for moderately symptomatic patients but a 17% mortality for the severely symptomatic patient who is dyspnoeic at rest. Thus, heart failure should always be controlled before submitting the patient to elective surgical procedures.

## Coronary artery disease

Patients with coronary artery disease are at risk of perioperative myocardial infarction, which is an important cause of surgical death. The risk is particularly high in patients undergoing peripheral vascular surgery, who often have severe coronary artery disease. Thus, patients with troublesome angina, particularly when there is a recent history of unstable symptoms or myocardial infarction, should undergo coronary angiography preoperatively with a view to coronary bypass grafting before peripheral revascularization. This policy of 'prophylactic' coronary bypass grafting has been shown to reduce the risk of vascular surgery significantly.

The risk of perioperative myocardial infarction is also increased in those patients who have suffered a previous myocardial infarction. Indeed, patients undergoing surgery during the first 6 months after myocardial infarction have a 16% risk of recurrent infarction during the perioperative period. For this reason, recent myocardial infarction should be regarded as a contraindication to elective surgical procedures.

## Valvular disease

Where possible elective surgery should be avoided in the patient with severe valvular heart disease until after valve replacement. In those patients with less severe lesions undergoing surgery, antibiotic prophylaxis against endocarditis is not necessary unless there is an important risk of bacteraemia, e.g. bowel surgery, dental surgery.

## Arrhythmias

Careful control of cardiac arrhythmias is essential before patients are submitted to surgery.

## Anticoagulant therapy

Oral anticoagulant therapy (warfarin) should be discontinued at least 3 days before elective surgical procedures, because of the risk of bleeding. Subcutaneous heparin (5000 units 8-hourly) can be substituted and continued into the early postoperative period. Indeed, heparin is recommended for all surgical procedures to protect against pulmonary embolism, particularly in patients undergoing pelvic or hip surgery. In the event of bleeding complications, heparin (unlike warfarin) can be rapidly reversed with protamine.

## Perioperative factors

### Heart failure

The cardiovascular properties of anaesthetic agents, mediated through direct effects on the heart and the autonomic nervous system, can have a profound influence on the circulation during surgery. Induction of anaesthesia with thiopentone, for example, can cause myocardial depression and vasodilatation, leading to severe hypotension. This is particularly undesirable in patients with coronary artery disease, in whom reductions in blood-pressure may threaten the perfusion of regionally ischaemic myocardium and lead to myocardial infarction. Thus, careful monitoring of blood-pressure is essential during this critical part of the anaesthetic procedure. Many other anaesthetic agents depress the myocardium and can exacerbate heart failure, although the degree to which this occurs in practice is modified by the extent of simultaneous stimulation of the sympathetic nervous system. Halothane produces little sympathetic stimulation and can cause severe hypotension and myocardial contractile failure in susceptible subjects.

### Arrhythmias

Anaesthetic agents also have important arrhythmogenic properties, which are heightened by hypoxaemia, electrolyte disorders and acid–base imbalance, all of which may occur during prolonged surgical procedures. Intubation at the start of the anaesthetic procedure elicits a profound vagal response, which may cause heart block or asystole.

### Myocardial injury

The risk of myocardial infarction during surgery has already been discussed. Myocardial injury may also occur as a complication of heart surgery. The risk is greatest for open-heart procedures, when the heart is isolated from the circulation during cardiopulmonary bypass. The incidence of myocardial injury is related to both the duration of the procedure and the adequacy of myocardial protection. Myocardial protection is provided by cooling the heart and, in some cases, by selective perfusion of the coronary arteries with oxygenated blood. In a few cases, however, myocardial injury develops, which is not always reversible in the postoperative period. Factors unrelated to the bypass procedure can also contribute to myocardial injury during open-heart surgery. These include embolization of air or platelet fragments into the coronary circulation and inadvertent damage to the coronary arteries.

## Postoperative factors

### *Fluid balance*

Early after major surgical procedures, the patient is particularly sensitive to the consequences of fluid imbalance. Under normal circumstances, fluctuations in plasma volume are compensated for by reflex adjustments of venous capacity, such that cardiac filling remains constant within a narrow range. However, these homoeostatic responses may be attenuated during the postoperative period, due to the effects of anaesthetic and analgesic agents on venous tone. Thus, a relatively minor plasma volume deficit can produce severe reductions in ventricular filling and cardiac output, whilst excessive fluid replacement readily causes pulmonary oedema.

Maintenance of haemodynamic stability after major surgery is made easier by measuring ventricular filling pressures. In most patients, fluid requirements can be titrated against right atrial pressure, measured with a central venous catheter. The right atrial pressure should be maintained in the normal range, between 5 and 8 mmHg (equivalent to a left atrial pressure of 9–13 mmHg). In the patient with heart failure, however, the relation between the ventricular filling pressures is variable and it is more difficult to predict left atrial pressure from measurements of central venous pressure. Under these circumstances a Swan–Ganz catheter may be inserted for titration of fluid replacement against measurements of pulmonary artery wedge pressure, which provides an indirect measure of left atrial pressure (see p. 70). Patients with left ventricular (LV) disease recovering from major surgery often depend upon a high left atrial pressure to maintain adequate cardiac output. A pulmonary artery wedge pressure of 15–20 mmHg is optimal because this takes maximal advantage of the Starling effect, without producing pulmonary oedema. If cardiac output remains inadequate, despite adjustment of plasma volume, treatment with vasodilators or inotropes is indicated to improve LV performance.

The patient recovering from open-heart surgery can present special problems if recovery of myocardial contractile function is delayed. The 'stunned' heart does not always respond to inotropic stimulation, and intra-aortic balloon pump therapy may be necessary. This is a useful temporizing measure pending recovery of normal contractile function.

# Further reading

Anonymous. Perioperative myocardial ischaemia and non-cardiac surgery. *Lancet* 1991, **337**, 1516–17.

Collins R., Scrimgeour A., Yusuf S. and Peto R. Reduction in fatal pulmonary embolism and venous thrombosis by perioperative administration of subcutaneous heparin: overview of results of randomized trials in general, orthopedic and urologic surgery. *N. Engl. J. Med.* 1988, **318**, 1162–73.

Deron S.J. and Kotler M.N. Noncardiac surgery in the cardiac patient. *Am. Heart J. 1988*, **116**, 831–8.

Eagle K.A. and Boucher C.A. Cardiac risk of noncardiac surgery. *N. Engl. J. Med.* 1989, **321**, 1330–2.

# Index

Principal entries are set in **bold** type